Pharmaceutical Crystals (Volume II)

Pharmaceutical Crystals (Volume II)

Editors

Etsuo Yonemochi
Hidehiro Uekusa

MDPI • Basel • Beijing • Wuhan • Barcelona • Belgrade • Manchester • Tokyo • Cluj • Tianjin

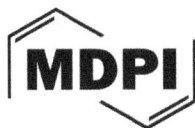

Editors
Etsuo Yonemochi
Hoshi University
Japan

Hidehiro Uekusa
Tokyo Institute of Technology
Japan

Editorial Office
MDPI
St. Alban-Anlage 66
4052 Basel, Switzerland

This is a reprint of articles from the Special Issue published online in the open access journal *Crystals* (ISSN 2073-4352) (available at: https://www.mdpi.com/journal/crystals/special_issues/pharmaceutical_crystals_VolumeII).

For citation purposes, cite each article independently as indicated on the article page online and as indicated below:

LastName, A.A.; LastName, B.B.; LastName, C.C. Article Title. *Journal Name* **Year**, *Volume Number*, Page Range.

ISBN 978-3-0365-5473-0 (Hbk)
ISBN 978-3-0365-5474-7 (PDF)

Cover image courtesy of Hidehiro Uekusa

© 2023 by the authors. Articles in this book are Open Access and distributed under the Creative Commons Attribution (CC BY) license, which allows users to download, copy and build upon published articles, as long as the author and publisher are properly credited, which ensures maximum dissemination and a wider impact of our publications.
The book as a whole is distributed by MDPI under the terms and conditions of the Creative Commons license CC BY-NC-ND.

Contents

About the Editors vii

Preface to "Pharmaceutical Crystals (Volume II)" ix

Hironaga Oyama, Takashi Miyamoto, Akiko Sekine, Ilma Nugrahani and Hidehiro Uekusa
Solid-State Dehydration Mechanism of Diclofenac Sodium Salt Hydrates
Reprinted from: *Crystals* **2021**, *11*, 412, doi:10.3390/cryst11040412 1

Majid Ismail Tamboli, Yushi Okamoto, Yohei Utsumi, Takayuki Furuishi, Siran Wang, Daiki Umeda, Okky Dwichandra Putra, Kaori Fukuzawa, Hidehiro Uekusa and Etsuo Yonemochi
Crystal Structures of Antiarrhythmic Drug Disopyramide and Its Salt with Phthalic Acid
Reprinted from: *Crystals* **2021**, *11*, 379, doi:10.3390/cryst11040379 17

Majid Ismail Tamboli, Yohei Utusmi, Takayuki Furuishi, Kaori Fukuzawa and Etsuo Yonemochi
Crystal Structure of Novel Terephthalate Salt of Antiarrhythmic Drug Disopyramide
Reprinted from: *Crystals* **2021**, *11*, 368, doi:10.3390/cryst11040368 37

Mariya A. Kryukova, Alexander V. Sapegin, Alexander S. Novikov, Mikhail Krasavin and Daniil M. Ivanov
New Crystal Forms for Biologically Active Compounds. Part 2: Anastrozole as N-Substituted 1,2,4-Triazole in Halogen Bonding and Lp-π Interactions with 1,4-Diiodotetrafluorobenzene
Reprinted from: *Crystals* **2020**, *10*, 371, doi:10.3390/cryst10050371 49

Hong Pang, Yu-Bin Sun, Jun-Wen Zhou, Meng-Juan Xie, Hao Lin, Yan Yong, Liang-Zhu Chen and Bing-Hu Fang
Pharmaceutical Salts of Enrofloxacin with Organic Acids
Reprinted from: *Crystals* **2020**, *10*, 646, doi:10.3390/cryst10080646 63

Soon Young Shin, Young Han Lee, Yoongho Lim, Ha Jin Lee, Ji Hye Lee, Miri Yoo, Seunghyun Ahn and Dongsoo Koh
Single Crystal X-Ray Structure for the Disordered Two Independent Molecules of Novel Isoflavone: Synthesis, Hirshfeld Surface Analysis, Inhibition and Docking Studies on IKKβ of 3-(2,3-dihydrobenzo [b][1,4]dioxin-6-yl)-6,7-dimethoxy-4H-chromen-4-one
Reprinted from: *Crystals* **2020**, *10*, 911, doi:10.3390/cryst10100911 81

Franc Perdih, Nina Žigart and Zdenko Časar
Crystal Structure and Solid-State Conformational Analysis of Active Pharmaceutical Ingredient Venetoclax
Reprinted from: *Crystals* **2021**, *11*, 261, doi:10.3390/cryst11030261 97

Leo Štefan, Dubravka Matković-Čalogović, Darko Filić and Miljenko Dumić
Synthesis, Crystal Structure and Solid State Transformation of 1,2-Bis[(1-methyl-1H-imidazole-2-yl)thio]ethane
Reprinted from: *Crystals* **2020**, *10*, 667, doi:10.3390/cryst10080667 113

Ke-Jie Xiong and Feng-Pei Du
Design, Synthesis, Crystal Structure, and Fungicidal Activity of Two Fenclorim Derivatives
Reprinted from: *Crystals* **2020**, *10*, 587, doi:10.3390/cryst10070587 125

Bwalya A. Witika, Marique Aucamp, Larry L. Mweetwa and Pedzisai A. Makoni
Application of Fundamental Techniques for Physicochemical Characterizations to Understand Post-Formulation Performance of Pharmaceutical Nanocrystalline Materials
Reprinted from: *Crystals* **2021**, *11*, 310, doi:10.3390/cryst11030310 137

About the Editors

Etsuo Yonemochi

Etsuo Yonemochi, Pharmacist and Professor of Department of Physical Chemistry at Hoshi University, was born in 1961. He graduated Faculty of Pharmaceutical Sciences, Chiba University (1985), and received Ph. D. (1991). In 1987, he joined the Faculty of Pharmaceutical Sciences, Chiba University as a Research Associate, then he spent two years at the School of Pharmacy, University of London as a research fellow. He moved to Toho University as an Associate Professor in 1996 and moved to Hoshi University in 2013. His main fields of interests are Characterization of pharmaceutical products and Application of in silico simulation and various analytical method to pharmaceutical formulation. He is a Chairman of the Japanese Pharmacopoeia Analytical Methods Committee, a President of Japan Society of Pharmaceutical Machinery and Engineering, and Board of directors of the Pharmaceutical Society of Japan and the Academy of Pharmaceutical Science and Technology Japan. His hobby is putting his horses into racing.

Hidehiro Uekusa

Hidehiro Uekusa, Associate Professor of Department of Chemistry at Tokyo Institute of Technology, was born in 1964 in Tokyo. He received B. of Science (1987), M. of Science (1989), and D. of Science (1992) degrees from Keio University. In 1992, he joined the Department of Chemistry at Tokyo Institute of Technology as a Research Associate (1992–1999), then was appointed to Associate Professor in 1999. His primary field is chemical crystallography. His current interests include 1) pharmaceutical crystals and its phase transition, 2) analysis of crystalline state reactions, and 3) crystal structure analysis from powder diffraction data. He was a senior co-editor of X-ray Structure Analysis Online journal, and also co-editor of Acta Crystallographica Section C, and editor of journal of Crystallographic Society of Japan. He is a council member of the Crystallographic Society of Japan and a board member of the Organic Crystals Division of the Chemical Society of Japan. He enjoys teatime with his students.

Preface to "Pharmaceutical Crystals (Volume II)"

We are delighted to deliver the second book of the series of "Pharmaceutical Crystals (Volume II)", a Special Issue of *Crystals*.

The crystalline state is the most used and essential form of solid active pharmaceutical ingredients (APIs) in manufacturing, processing, storing, and administering. The center of the characterization of pharmaceutical crystals is crystal structure analysis, which reveals the molecular structure and the alignment of the molecules of important pharmaceutical compounds. This structural information is the key to understanding intermolecular interactions, and a wide range of physicochemical and biological properties of the APIs (e.g., solubility, stability, tablet ability, color, hygroscopicity, etc.).

The second book of the Special Issue series on "Pharmaceutical Crystals" aimed to publish novel molecular and crystal structures of pharmaceutical compounds, especially new crystal structures of APIs, including polymorphs and solvate crystals, and multi-component crystals of APIs, such as co-crystals and salts.

Thus, this Special Issue demonstrates the importance of crystal structure information in many sectors of pharmaceutical science. Ten articles present the latest research findings, including in areas of morphology, spectroscopic, theoretical calculation, and thermal analysis with the crystallographic study. This wide variety of studies is the essence of this Special Issue, presenting current trends in the structure-property study of pharmaceutical crystals.

This Special Issue focuses on physicochemical properties and crystal structure, correlating various physical properties to crystal structure.

Multi-component crystals (MCCs), a generic term for crystals, such as co-crystals, salt crystals, and hydrates, have been the focus of recent research on pharmaceutical crystals. Half of the articles in this Special Issue deal with MCCs. MCCs are essential for improving other crystals' properties with challenging physical properties since they can contain the same drug substance but have different physicochemical properties due to their unique crystal structure.

Tamboli et al. [1, 2] newly synthesized 1:1 salt crystals (MCC) of the anti-arrhythmic drug, Disopyramide, with phthalates and studied their crystal structures in detail. Strong charge-assisted hydrogen bonding interactions are observed between ionized molecules in the crystal. The conformations of the API molecules in the "mother crystal" and in the MCC are different. The differences in physicochemical properties between these two crystals were further characterized by differential calorimetric analysis, thermal gravimetric analysis, powder X-ray diffraction and infrared spectroscopy. It is important to analyze and evaluate crystals using various methods, along with crystal structure analysis.

Research to improve the solubility of drug crystals by MCC formation is one of the most exciting topics because crystals with low solubility result in low bioavailability of the API. For example, Enrofloxacin is an antibacterial drug of fluoroquinolones, and its low solubility is a problem. Pang et al. [3] synthesized three new organic salt crystals of Enrofloxacin (with tartaric acid, nicotinic acid, and suberinic acid). They performed crystal structure analysis to compare the structures and study the molecular interactions' characteristics. Solubility measurements revealed that these new salt crystals exhibit excellent water solubility. Combined crystal characterization (field emission scanning electron microscopy, powder X-ray diffraction, Fourier transform infrared spectroscopy, and differential scanning calorimetry) was also performed in this research, and new data were reported.

A wide variety of intermolecular interactions are observed in MCC, and, in recent years, halogen bonding has been attracting attention in addition to traditional hydrogen bonding, which is understood as an electrostatic attraction interaction between a positive region on a halogen atom and a negative part on another molecule, which has strength and directionality similar to hydrogen bonds. Kryukova et al. [4] targeted anastrozole, a well-known aromatase inhibitor, and successfully made MCCs by halogen bonding. This research used advanced analysis using quantum chemical calculations and QTAIM analysis to study the intermolecular interactions quantitatively.

Hydrate crystals are important MCCs. By studying the relative positions and interactions between API molecules and water molecules in crystals and comparing them to the structure of anhydrous crystals, we can gain insight into the stability of hydrate crystals. In addition, by making hydrate crystals with various hydration numbers and examining the conditions of dehydration, one can establish a landscape encompassing various crystals of the API molecule and gain insight into the stability of the crystals. Štefan et al. [5] synthesized chemical derivatives of the thyreostatic drug methimazole and successfully made tetrahydrate, dihydrate, and anhydrous crystals, which were analyzed for crystal structures. These crystal structures are being evaluated with spectroscopy, microscopy, and thermal analysis.

The sodium salts of pharmaceutical molecules often form hydrate crystals. Hydrate crystals are considered potentially unstable because they dehydrate depending on environmental conditions such as temperature and humidity. To utilize sodium salt hydrates as pharmaceuticals, it is important to clarify the changes in crystal structure by dehydration/hydration via crystallographic analysis. Oyama et al. [6] studied the structural change of diclofenac sodium salt 4.75 hydrate, a non-steroidal anti-inflammatory drug, to 3.5 hydrates and then to anhydrate crystals upon dehydration. They elucidated the complex mechanism of dehydration and hydration involving the coordination of water to sodium ions.

Determination of the three-dimensional structure of molecules is important in docking research of drug molecules for developing novel anticancer drugs. Shin et al. [7] synthesized an isoflavone compound and revealed its crystal structure by single crystal X-ray structure analysis. Interestingly, they found two independent molecules in the crystal, each with its disorder, and compared their molecular structures. Information on crystal structures leads to research on intermolecular interactions and then to intermolecular docking studies. This study suggests that this isoflavone compound has the potential to bind to the active site of IKKβ, which may be explored as an anticancer drug targeting IKKβ inhibition.

On the other hand, crystallographic analysis of protein complexes in which disease-related protein molecules and API molecules are docked has been performed. Would the structure of the API molecule change with or without docking? For example, Venetoclax is an API molecule used as a selective inhibitor of B-cell lymphoma-2 that can be administered orally. Until now, only the molecule's structure docked with a protein molecule was known, but Perdih et al. [8] reported the first crystal structure of API alone. By comparing the conformations of two independent molecules with the molecular structure of the bound state, they revealed that the supramolecular structure is achieved through various intermolecular interactions.

The elucidation of molecular and crystal structures is also important for developing new pharmaceuticals. Crystal structure analysis is an essential tool to confirm the chemical synthesis of compounds, and it can also provide information on intermolecular interactions in solids, such as hydrogen bonding. Furthermore, the three-dimensional structure of a compound can be used for research on the expression of its activity as a drug. Xiong et al. [9] designed and synthesized two fenclorim derivatives and revealed their molecular structures by crystallographic analysis. These compounds showed superior in vitro activity compared to known pharmaceuticals, suggesting their potential as new pyrimidine fungicides.

As a parallel topic to the detailed discussion on crystal structures, we present an important, review of crystals in the last article.

Nanocrystalline materials (NCMs) are crystalline materials composed of nanoparticles with dimensions less than 1000 nm. Their application in drug crystals and co-crystals is an example of NCMs with attractive physicochemical properties. They have attracted significant attention as an important material class with great potential in drug delivery. This review article by Witika et al.[10] summarizes recent advances in therapeutic options using drug NCMs. It also provides a detailed description of the basic characterization methods of drug NCMs and their applications, as well as their impact on the performance of NCMs after formulation.

In conclusion, this Special Issue presents a wide range of recent studies about pharmaceutical crystals and provides valuable information for future studies in the related field. The guest editors hope the readers enjoy this fruitful Special Issue of "Pharmaceutical Crystals (Volume II)".

References:

1. Tamboli, M.I.; Okamoto, Y.; Utsumi, Y.; Furuishi, T.; Wang, S.; Umeda, D.; Putra, O.D.; Fukuzawa, K.; Uekusa, H.; Yonemochi, E. Crystal Structures of Antiarrhythmic Drug Disopyramide and Its Salt with Phthalic Acid. *Crystals* **2021**, *11*, 379. https://doi.org/10.3390/cryst11040379

2. Tamboli, M.I.; Utusmi, Y.; Furuishi, T.; Fukuzawa, K.; Yonemochi, E. Crystal Structure of Novel Terephthalate Salt of Antiarrhythmic Drug Disopyramide. *Crystals* **2021**, *11*, 368. https://doi.org/10.3390/cryst11040368

3. Pang, H.; Sun, Y.-B.; Zhou, J.-W.; Xie, M.-J.; Lin, H.; Yong, Y.; Chen, L.-Z.; Fang, B.-H. Pharmaceutical Salts of Enrofloxacin with Organic Acids. *Crystals* **2020**, *10*, 646. https://doi.org/10.3390/cryst10080646

4. Kryukova, M.A.; Sapegin, A.V.; Novikov, A.S.; Krasavin, M.; Ivanov, D.M. New Crystal Forms for Biologically Active Compounds. Part 2: Anastrozole as N-Substituted 1,2,4-Triazole in Halogen Bonding and Lp-π Interactions with 1,4-Diiodotetrafluorobenzene. *Crystals* **2020**, *10*, 371. https://doi.org/10.3390/cryst10050371

5. Štefan, L.; Matković-Čalogović, D.; Filić, D.; Dumić, M. Synthesis, Crystal Structure and Solid State Transformation of 1,2-Bis[(1-methyl-1H-imidazole-2-yl)thio]ethane. *Crystals* **2020**, *10*, 667. https://doi.org/10.3390/cryst10080667

6. Oyama, H.; Miyamoto, T.; Sekine, A.; Nugrahani, I.; Uekusa, H. Solid-State Dehydration Mechanism of Diclofenac Sodium Salt Hydrates. *Crystals* **2021**, *11*, 412. https://doi.org/10.3390/cryst11040412

7. Shin, S.Y.; Lee, Y.H.; Lim, Y.; Lee, H.J.; Lee, J.H.; Yoo, M.; Ahn, S.; Koh, D. Single Crystal X-Ray Structure for the Disordered Two Independent Molecules of Novel Isoflavone: Synthesis, Hirshfeld Surface Analysis, Inhibition and Docking Studies on IKKβ of 3-(2,3-dihydrobenzo[b][1,4]dioxin-6-yl)-6,7-dimethoxy-4H-chromen-4-one. *Crystals* **2020**, *10*, 911. https://doi.org/10.3390/cryst10100911

8. Perdih, F.; Žigart, N.; Časar, Z. Crystal Structure and Solid-State Conformational Analysis of Active Pharmaceutical Ingredient Venetoclax. *Crystals* **2021**, *11*, 261. https://doi.org/10.3390/cryst11030261

9. Xiong, K.-J.; Du, F.-P. Design, Synthesis, Crystal Structure, and Fungicidal Activity of Two Fenclorim Derivatives. *Crystals* **2020**, *10*, 587. https://doi.org/10.3390/cryst10070587

10. Witika, B.A.; Aucamp, M.; Mweetwa, L.L.; Makoni, P.A. Application of Fundamental Techniques for Physicochemical Characterizations to Understand Post-Formulation Performance of Pharmaceutical Nanocrystalline Materials. *Crystals* **2021**, *11*, 310. https://doi.org/10.3390/cryst11030310

Etsuo Yonemochi and Hidehiro Uekusa
Editors

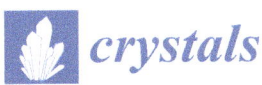

Article

Solid-State Dehydration Mechanism of Diclofenac Sodium Salt Hydrates

Hironaga Oyama [1], Takashi Miyamoto [1], Akiko Sekine [1], Ilma Nugrahani [2] and Hidehiro Uekusa [1,*]

[1] Department of Chemistry, School of Science, Tokyo Institute of Technology, 2-12-1 Ookayama, Meguro-ku, Tokyo 152-8550, Japan; oyama.h.ab@m.titech.ac.jp (H.O.); tmiyamoto388@gmail.com (T.M.); asekine@chem.titech.ac.jp (A.S.)
[2] Department of Pharmacochemistry, School of Pharmacy, Bandung Institute of Technology, Bandung 40132, Indonesia; ilma_nugrahani@fa.itb.ac.id
* Correspondence: uekusa@chem.titech.ac.jp

Citation: Oyama, H.; Miyamoto, T.; Sekine, A.; Nugrahani, I.; Uekusa, H. Solid-State Dehydration Mechanism of Diclofenac Sodium Salt Hydrates. Crystals 2021, 11, 412. https://doi.org/10.3390/cryst11040412

Academic Editor: Sławomir Grabowski

Received: 25 February 2021
Accepted: 7 April 2021
Published: 12 April 2021

Publisher's Note: MDPI stays neutral with regard to jurisdictional claims in published maps and institutional affiliations.

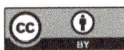

Copyright: © 2021 by the authors. Licensee MDPI, Basel, Switzerland. This article is an open access article distributed under the terms and conditions of the Creative Commons Attribution (CC BY) license (https://creativecommons.org/licenses/by/4.0/).

Abstract: Salt formation is a useful technique for improving the solubility of active pharmaceutical ingredients (APIs). For instance, a nonsteroidal anti-inflammatory drug, diclofenac (DIC), is used in a sodium salt form, and it has been reported to form several hydrate forms. However, the crystal structure of the anhydrous form of diclofenac sodium (DIC-Na) and the structural relationship among the anhydrate and hydrated forms have not yet been revealed. In this study, DIC-Na anhydrate was analyzed using single-crystal X-ray diffraction (XRD). To determine the solid-state dehydration/hydration mechanism of DIC-Na hydrates based on both the present and previously reported crystal structures (4.75-hydrate and 3.5-hydrate), additional experiments including simultaneous powder XRD and differential scanning calorimetry, thermogravimetry, dynamic vapor sorption measurements, and a comparison of the crystal structures were performed. The dehydration of the 4.75-hydrate form was found to occur in two steps. During the first step, only water molecules that were not coordinated to Na$^+$ ions were lost, which led to the formation of the 3.5-hydrate while retaining alternating layered structures. The subsequent dehydration step into the anhydrous phase accompanied a substantial structural reconstruction. This study elucidated the complete landscape of the dehydration/hydration transformation of DIC-Na for the first time through a crystal structure investigation. These findings contribute to understanding the mechanism underlying these dehydration/hydration phenomena and the physicochemical properties of pharmaceutical crystals.

Keywords: crystal structure analysis; diclofenac; diclofenac sodium; hydration–dehydration mechanism; hydrate; anhydrate

1. Introduction

In drug development, improving the poor water solubility of many active pharmaceutical ingredients (APIs) is an attractive area of research. In addition to the formulation of low-crystallinity solids such as solid dispersions [1,2] and cyclodextrin inclusion compounds [3], other methods can increase solubility through the formation of a stable multi-component crystalline state such as salt formation [4], co-crystallization [5], and salt co-crystallization [6–8], in which the crystal structure differs from the mother API crystal, providing an opportunity to change the solubility. Among these strategies, salt formation is a common method for enhancing the solubility of some APIs with acidic or basic functional groups (carboxy, conjugated hydroxy, amino, etc.) [9,10]. In particular, sodium salt formation is a well-known technique for increasing the solubility of poorly soluble acidic APIs in drug development, and sodium ions account for approximately 60% of the counter cations of acidic API salts [11].

Sodium API salts often form hydrate crystals in which the water coordination geometry around Na$^+$ is more flexible than the structure of the transition metal ion hydrate owing to the s-block atomic nature of Na [12]. This "pseudo-coordination bond" property of Na$^+$–O(water) interactions contributes the specific hydration–dehydration behaviors of sodium API salts [13–19].

Hydrate crystals often undergo dehydration according to variations in the ambient temperature or humidity and transform into an anhydrous phase with different physicochemical properties [20,21]. Approximately one in three pharmaceutical compounds form hydrate crystals [22], and analyzing the X-ray crystal structure is essential [23] because the physicochemical properties of crystalline materials, such as their solubility [24], hygroscopicity [25,26], and tableting properties [27] depend on their crystal structure [28]. Sometimes, alternations in the crystal structure induced by a dehydration/hydration result in a color change [29,30]. For pharmaceutical hydrates, such property changes may affect their bioavailability and safety as pharmaceutical products. Therefore, the structural investigation of polymorphic transitions and the establishment of dehydration mechanisms of drug hydrates are both important processes in drug development [31].

The nonsteroidal anti-inflammatory drug diclofenac (DIC, 2-[2-((2,6-dichlorophenyl) amino)phenyl]acetic acid; Figure 1) is a widely used analgesic, and owing to its high permeability but low solubility, it is categorized as a Biopharmaceutics Classification System (BCS) Class II [32]. Since DIC has an acidic carboxyl group, it can be formulated as a salt with sodium or potassium to improve its solubility. Diclofenac sodium (DIC-Na) has been reported to form several hydrate crystals (Table S1, the Supplementary Materials). Until now, however, the crystal structure of the anhydrous form of DIC-Na and the structural relationship among this anhydrate and DIC-Na hydrates have not yet been elucidated. The crystal structures of DIC-Na pentahydrate, 4.75-hydrate (4.75H), and tetrahydrate were investigated independently, and the reported lattice parameters were almost identical [33–35], implying either that they are isostructural hydrates or that hydrate water molecules are misplaced. The trihydrate has also been recognized in the literature, but its crystal structure is still unknown, and the number of water molecules it contains is not clear [36]. In addition, a hemi-heptahydrate (3.5H) form was reported very recently [37]. Multi-component crystals of DIC-Na with organic agents such as phenanthroline [38] and L-proline [39] have also been reported. In particular, the DIC solubility achieved by forming the DIC-Na L-proline salt cocrystal was significantly higher than that of DIC-Na [39]. In the DIC-Na L-proline study, a new hydrate form was observed, but the structure was not revealed. Furthermore, in order to complete the overall picture of the DIC-Na hydrate structures, analyzing the crystal structure of the anhydrous form of DIC-Na is essential, which would also establish the complicated hydration–dehydration mechanism of DIC-Na hydrates. The elucidation of such mechanisms is important in the pharmaceutical sciences.

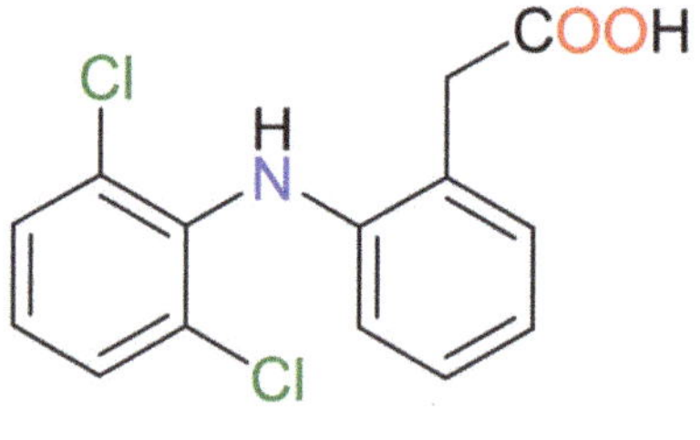

Figure 1. Molecular structure of diclofenac (DIC).

In this study, a novel crystalline phase, anhydrate (AH), was revealed by single-crystal X-ray diffraction (SCXRD) analysis, and the 4.75H and 3.5H crystal structures were re-analyzed for an accurate structural comparison under the same measurement conditions, such as temperature. Simultaneous powder X-ray diffraction (PXRD) and differential scanning calorimetry (DSC) measurements were used to visualize the multi-step dehydration process of DIC-Na 4.75H. Based on the crystal structures, the dehydration mechanism of DIC-Na 4.75H is discussed.

2. Materials and Methods

2.1. Materials

DIC-Na (anhydrous) was purchased from Tokyo Chemical Industry Co., Ltd. (Tokyo, Japan). Solvents (tetrahydrofuran, acetonitrile, and methanol) were obtained from Tokyo Chemical Industry Co., Ltd., Nacalai Tesque, Inc. (Kyoto, Japan), and Sigma-Aldrich Japan (Tokyo, Japan), respectively.

2.2. Preparation of Solid Samples

2.2.1. Diclofenac Sodium 4.75-Hydrate

Dissolving anhydrous DIC-Na (ca. 40 mg) in distilled water (5 mL) and then slowly evaporating the solution yielded plate-like DIC-Na 4.75-hydrate crystals.

2.2.2. Diclofenac Sodium Hemiheptahydrate

Anhydrous DIC-Na (ca. 50 mg) was dissolved in tetrahydrofuran (5 mL), followed by the slow evaporation of the solution, which yielded plate-like 3.5H crystals.

2.2.3. Diclofenac Sodium Anhydrate

After dissolving anhydrous DIC-Na (ca. 50 mg) in a mixed acetonitrile–methanol (4:1 by volume, 5 mL) solvent, the solution was subsequently evaporated, resulting in needle-like anhydrous crystals.

2.3. Powder X-ray Diffraction (PXRD)

PXRD was performed using SmartLab (Rigaku, Japan) in the manner of transmission geometry. The data were collected from $2\theta = 3°$ to $40°$ at an ambient temperature at step and scan speeds of $0.01°$ and $3°\,min^{-1}$, respectively, using a Cu Kα source (45 kV, 200 mA). The conditions for simultaneous PXRD and DSC measurements are discussed in Section 2.6.

2.4. Single-Crystal X-ray Diffraction (SCXRD)

Single crystals of DIC-Na hydrates and anhydrate were prepared by the method described in Section 2.2, and the SCXRD data were collected using R-AXIS RAPID (Rigaku Tokyo, Japan) with Mo Kα radiation ($\lambda = 0.71075$ Å). Data reduction and correction were performed using RAPID-AUTO (Rigaku) with ABSCOR (T. Higashi Rigaku, Tokyo, Japan). The space group was determined using PLATON [40]. The structure was solved using a dual-space algorithm of SHELXT [41] and then refined on F^2 using SHELXL-2017/1 [42]. All non-hydrogen atoms were refined anisotropically. Hydrogen atoms attached to oxygen (water) and nitrogen atoms were found in the differential Fourier map. The water hydrogen atoms were refined using standard distance restraints and constrained isotropic thermal parameters. The hydrogen atoms attached to nitrogen were refined with lax distance restraints of 0.88 Å and thermal parameters set to 1.2 times those of the parent atom. Other hydrogen atoms were located in the geometrically calculated position and refined using the riding model. The 3D structures of the molecules were drawn using Mercury 4.3.1 [43].

2.5. Thermogravimetric (TG) Analysis

Thermogravimetric (TG) and differential thermal analysis (DTA) measurements were performed using a Thermo plus EVO (Rigaku, Tokyo, Japan). A sample of powdery 4.75H (7.856 mg) in an unsealed aluminum pan was heated at 5 °C min^{-1} up to 150 °C under flowing N_2 gas (100 mL min^{-1}).

2.6. Differential Scanning Calorimetry (DSC)

PXRD and DSC measurements were performed simultaneously using an XRD-DSC (Rigaku, Japan) equipped with a D/tex Ultra detector and Cu Kα source (40 kV, 40 mA). A powdery sample of DIC-Na 4.75H was heated at +1 °C min^{-1} up to 120 °C in an unsealed Al pan with flowing N_2 gas (100 mL min^{-1}). The preliminary DSC measurement was performed up to 300 °C to confirm the absence of phase transformation over 150 °C (Figure S1, the Supplementary Materials).

2.7. Dynamic Vapor Sorption (DVS)

The critical relative humidity (RH) where the hydration of the anhydrous DIC-Na AH occurs was determined by dynamic vapor sorption (DVS) using a Dynamic Vapor Sorption Advantage instrument (Surface Measurement Systems Ltd., Wembley, UK) at 25 °C. The RH was increased from 0% to 90% and then decreased to 0% with a step width of 5%.

3. Results

3.1. Crystal Structure of DIC-Na Hydrates

The crystal structures of DIC-Na 4.75H, 3.5H, and AH were successfully analyzed by SCXRD, and the crystallographic data are shown in Table 1. The phase agreement between the solid powder samples obtained by the method described in Section 2.2 and the analyzed single crystals was confirmed by their PXRD patterns.

Table 1. Crystallographic data of diclofenac sodium (DIC-Na) hydrates and anhydrate.

	4.75H	3.5H	AH
Chemical formula	$C_{14}H_{10}Cl_2NNaO_2$ 4.75(H_2O)	$C_{14}H_{10}Cl_2NNaO_2$ 3.5(H_2O)	$C_{14}H_{10}Cl_2NNaO_2$
Formula weight	403.69	381.17	318.12
Temperature/K	173	173	173
Crystal system	Monoclinic	Triclinic	Orthorhombic
Space group	$P2_1$	$P\bar{1}$	$Pbca$
a/Å	9.5552(3)	9.3628(3)	26.3664(5)
b/Å	39.5393(8)	9.4844(3)	6.44256(12)
c/Å	9.8346(2)	19.0742(6)	32.8255(6)
α/°	90	90.1187(11)	90
β/°	90.7122(8)	99.5439(12)	90
γ/°	90	90.5134(11)	90
Volume/Å^3	3715.28(16)	1670.28(9)	5575.97(18)
Z, Z'	8, 4	4, 2	16, 2
Density/g cm^{-3}	1.443	1.516	1.516
$R\,[F^2 > 2\sigma(F^2)]$	0.0379	0.0347	0.0646
CCDC number	2065085	2065083	2065086

The lattice parameters of DIC-Na 4.75H shown in Table 2 are identical to those reported by Llinàs et al. (Table S1) [34]. The asymmetric unit contained four DIC anions and 19 water molecules (Figure 2). Na$^+$ ions were surrounded by a large amount of water, and Na$^+$ was coordinated to either six or five water molecules (6-coordination or 5-coordination, respectively), while DIC anions formed no coordination bonds with Na$^+$ ions. Five of the 19 water molecules did not coordinate with Na$^+$ ions and existed as crystalline water molecules in the crystal.

Similarly, the lattice parameters of DIC-Na 3.5H in Table 1 are the same as those reported by Nieto et al. (Table S1) [37]. DIC-Na 3.5H crystallized in the triclinic $P\bar{1}$ space group, and its asymmetric unit, consisted of two DIC anions, two Na$^+$ cations, and seven water molecules (Figure 3). All water in the crystal was bound to Na$^+$. One Na$^+$ ion was coordinated to either five water oxygens and a carboxylate oxygen or to four water oxygens and two carboxylate oxygens of DIC, resulting in a 6-coordination configuration in both cases (Figure 4). Although the unit cell of 3.5H was relatively similar to that of 4.75H, its crystallographic symmetry was reduced from monoclinic to triclinic.

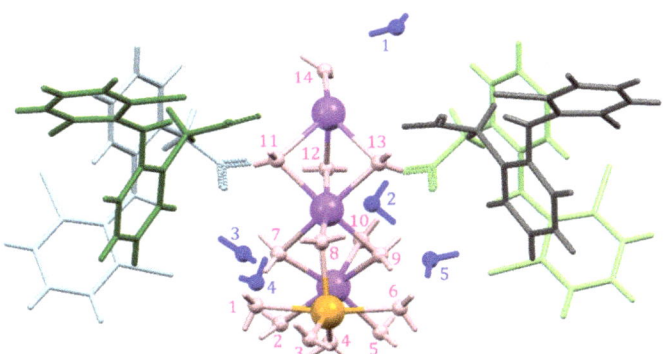

Figure 2. Asymmetric unit of DIC-Na 4.75H, with fourteen bonded (pink) and five non-bonded (blue) water molecules and 6-coordinated (purple) and 5-coordinated (orange) Na$^+$ ions.

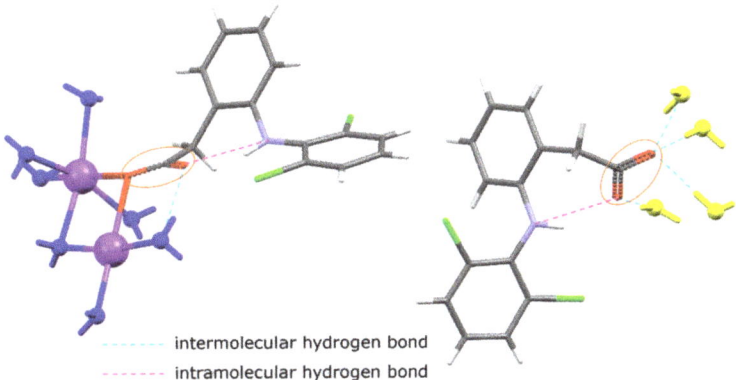

Figure 3. Asymmetric unit of DIC-Na 3.5H (yellow water molecules are not included). One (**left**) DIC is connected to Na$^+$ ions, but the other (**right**) forms hydrogen bonds with water and does not bond with Na$^+$ ions.

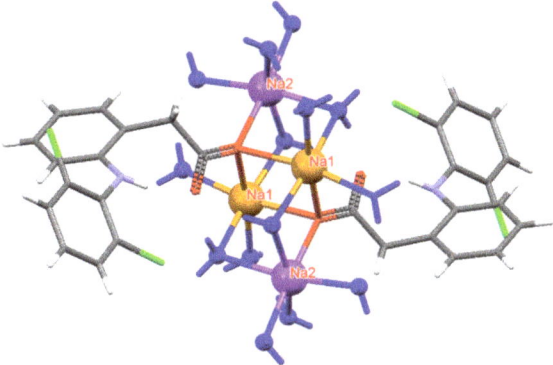

Figure 4. Coordination environment around Na$^+$ ions in DIC-Na 3.5H. Na2 (purple) is connected to five H$_2$O oxygens and one carboxylate oxygen, whereas Na1 (orange) bonds to four H$_2$O oxygens and two carboxylate oxygens. However, in both cases, Na adopts a six-coordinated configuration.

For the first time, this work elucidated the crystal structure of DIC-Na AH, which crystallizes into an orthorhombic system with the *Pbca* space group, wherein two DIC anions and sodium cations are independent (Figure 5). In contrast to 4.75H and 3.5H, AH does not show an alternating layered structure consisting of a hydrophilic region (Na^+, water, and carboxylate) and hydrophobic region (the main part of DIC) (Figure 6). However, a one-dimensional hydrophilic Na–O chain structure appears along the b-axis in the AH crystal, where [Na–O]$_2$ squares and [Na–OCO(carboxylate)] kites are connected alternately to form an infinite rigid chain (Figure 7). In the crystal structure, each Na^+ ion is coordinated to five carboxylate oxygens (three monodentate carboxylates and one bidentate carboxylate) and adopts a 5-coordinated geometry. To visualize the conformational differences in the two independent DIC anions in the asymmetric unit, they are overlaid in Figure 8, which demonstrates great variation at the carboxylate moiety and the second aromatic ring with chlorine atoms.

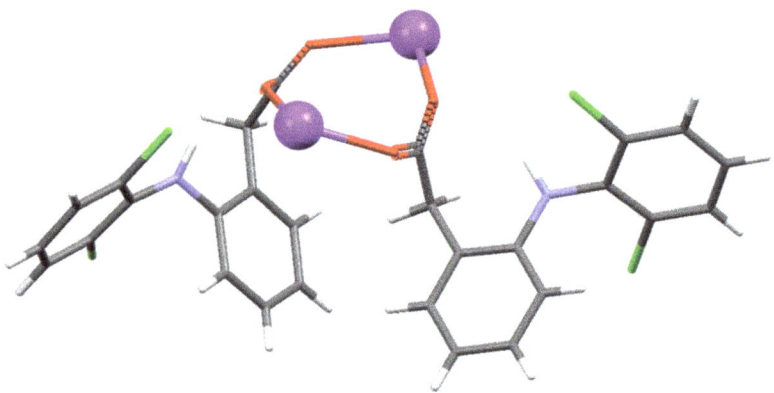

Figure 5. Asymmetric unit of DIC-Na AH.

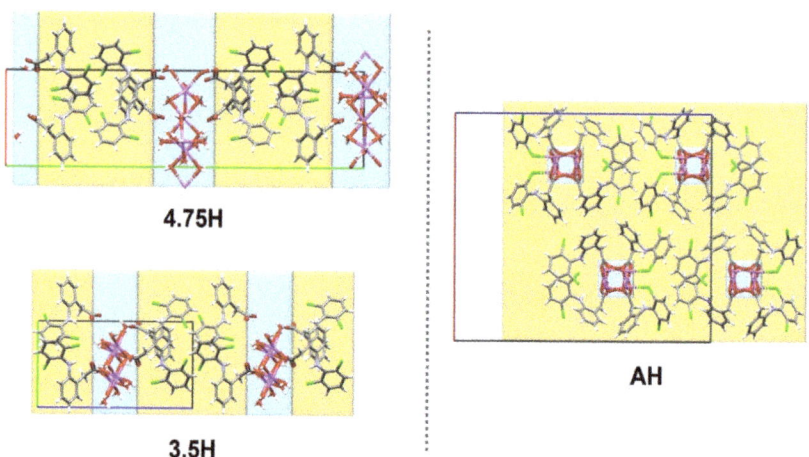

Figure 6. Structural comparison among unit cells of three DIC-Na hydrates.

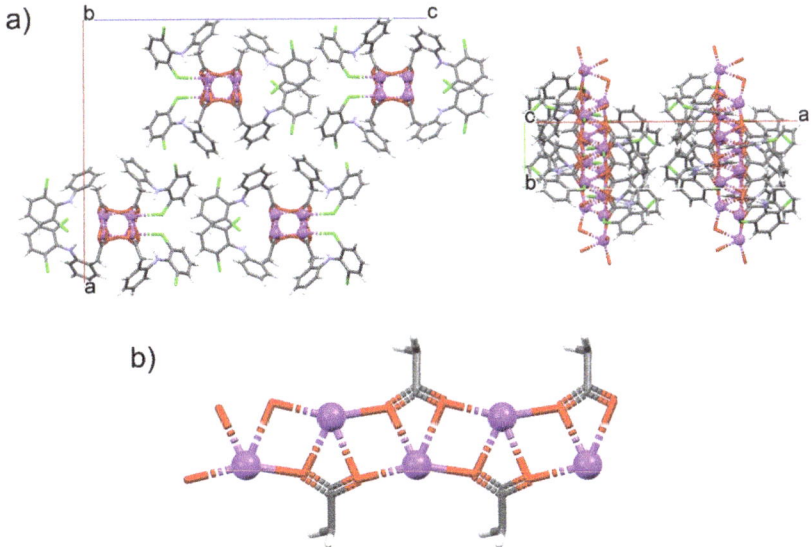

Figure 7. One-dimensional Na–O chain in DIC-Na AH. (**a**) Crystal packing diagrams viewed from the b- (left) and c-axes (right). (**b**) Infinite motif composed of Na–O–Na–O squares and Na–O–C–O kites.

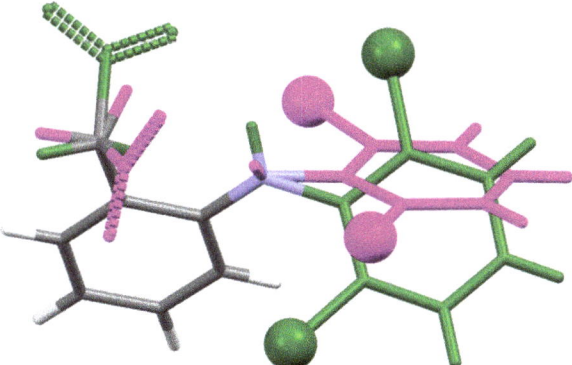

Figure 8. Structural overlay between two independent DIC molecules in DIC-Na AH shown in Figure 5.

The consistency between the powdery materials used in subsequent experiments and the single-crystalline phases was confirmed using their PXRD patterns, and the patterns of the experimental samples were verified to be identical to those calculated from the crystal structure via Mercury 4.3.1 (Figure 9) [43].

3.2. Dehydration Behavior of DIC-Na 4.75H

The dehydration of DIC-Na 4.75H was examined by simultaneous PXRD-DSC measurements, and the results are presented in Figure 10. The preliminary DSC measurement was performed up to 300 °C to show there was no change from the dehydration temperature (108.4 °C) to the melting point of DIC-Na (292.4 °C) (Figure S1). Therefore, the PXRD-DSC and the TG-DTA data (Figure 11) were collected up to 120 °C and 150 °C, respectively. The DSC curve showed two endothermic peaks corresponding to multi-step dehydration transitions. After the first transition, the PXRD pattern changed slightly, indicating the emergence of a hemi-heptahydrate phase (i.e., 3.5H). The second transition led to a distinct pattern derived from an anhydrous phase. Because the second peak bifurcated, the second dehydration may be a multi-step process, and 3.5H may transform into AH via intermediate phases.

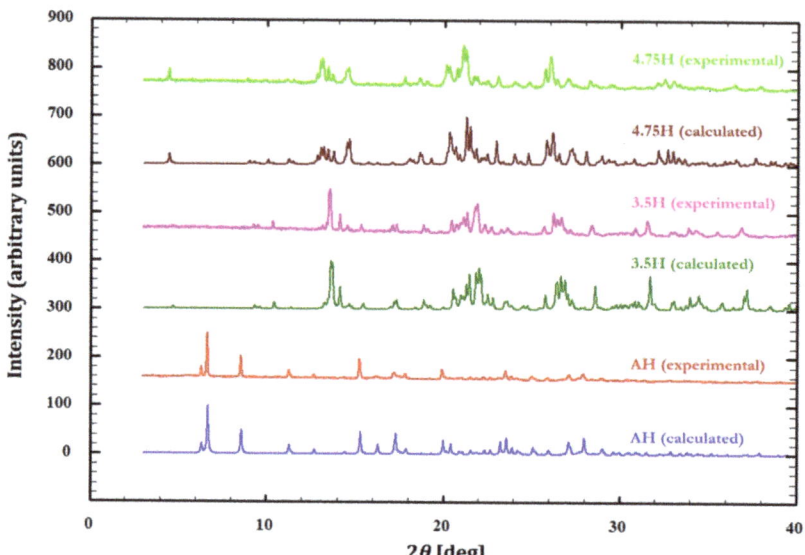

Figure 9. Experimental and calculated powder X-ray diffraction (PXRD) patterns for DIC-Na 4.75H, 3.5H, and AH forms.

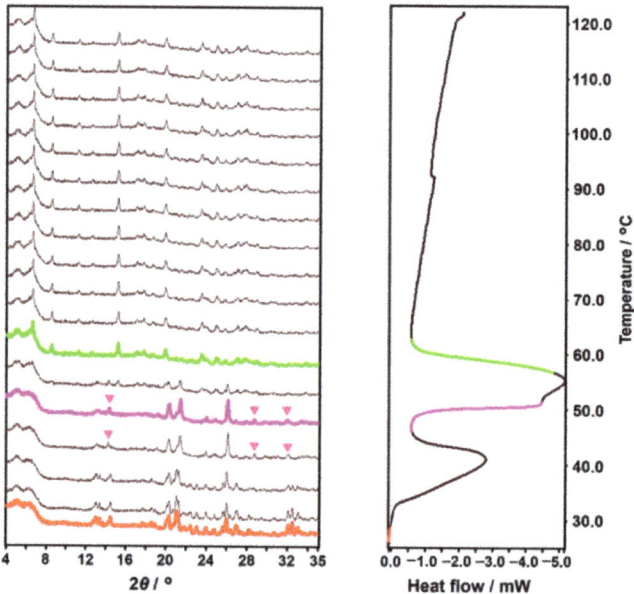

Figure 10. Simultaneously measured variable-temperature powder X-ray diffraction (PXRD) (**left**) and differential scanning calorimetry (DSC) (**right**) diagrams. The colored PXRD patterns and segments in the DSC diagram correspond to the emergence of new phases.

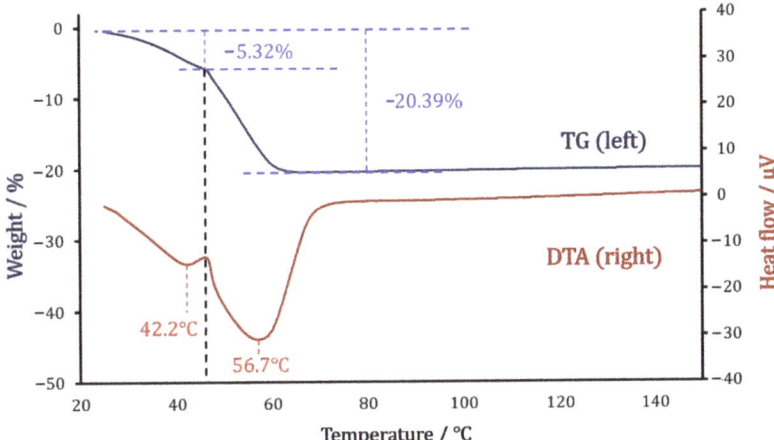

Figure 11. Thermogravimetric (TG) (left axis) and differential thermal analysis (DTA) (right axis) diagrams of DIC-Na 4.75H.

The TG-DTA curves in Figure 11 exhibit the dehydration behavior in further detail. Two DTA endothermic peaks appear. The first peak (42.2 °C) is accompanied by a 5.32% weight decrease, indicating partial dehydration (4.75 to 3.5, calculation: 5.58%), which is followed by the second peak (56.7 °C) with a 15.07% weight decrease, which corresponds to complete dehydration (3.5 to 0, calculation: 16.54%).

The DVS experiments performed at 25 °C revealed hysteresis between the water sorption and desorption processes (Figure 12). During the sorption process, AH started to absorb water at 60% RH and transformed into 4.75H at 65% RH. On the other hand, during the desorption process, 4.75H was almost stable down to 35% RH but started to desorb water at 30% RH and completely changed into AH at 30% RH. The intermediate 3.5H form (simulation: 19.8% mass change) was not observed during the desorption process.

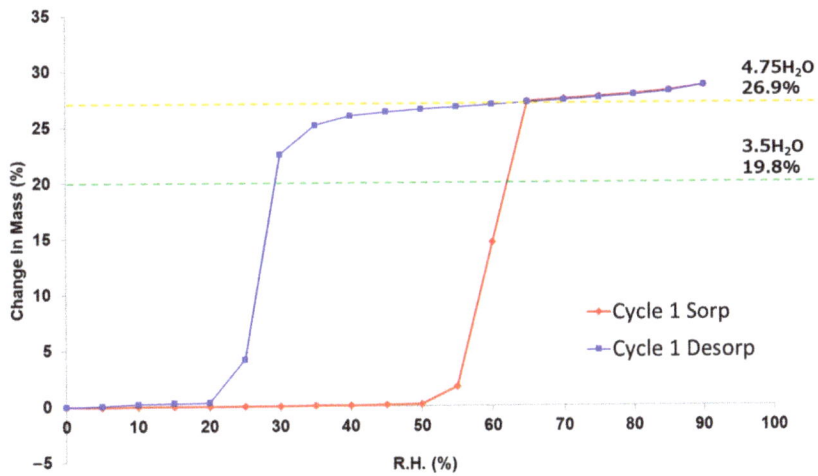

Figure 12. Dynamic vapor sorption (DVS) isotherm plot at 25 °C of DIC-Na anhydrate (AH).

4. Discussion

4.1. Verification of the Validity of the 4.75-Hydrate Crystal Structure

The published crystal structures of pentahydrate, 4.75H, and tetrahydrate have very similar lattice constants but different water contents. Moreover, the space group of 4.75H is $P2_1$, whereas those of the pentahydrate and tetrahydrate forms are both $P2_1/m$ [33,35]. The crystal structure of DIC-Na 4.75H contains a pseudo-mirror plane between two corresponding DIC anions. However, the shape of the cluster of Na$^+$ ions and water molecules is greatly distorted from the mirror symmetry, so it is not suitable to set the mirror plane on this cluster. The published pentahydrate structure was solved in the $P2_1/m$ space group by employing a disordered model at the position of Na$^+$ ions [33]. However, this assignment of the occupancy of disordered water may have been incorrect. The present study revealed that, in one unit cell, four DIC-Na molecules are associated with not 20 but 19 water molecules (4.75 water molecules for one DIC anion) in the hydrated solid state. Notably, the 4.75H structure model reported by Llinàs et al. was validated by a low R factor in their structural refinement [34].

Figure 13 shows the Na–O coordination network observed in the crystal structure of DIC-Na 4.75H. Three 6-coordinated sodium ions (Na1, Na2, and Na3) form a waving [Na–O–Na–O] chain structure, while a 5-coordinated sodium ion (Na4, orange) is connected to the chain via water. The lower panel in Figure 13 displays the chain seen from the direction parallel to the pseudo-mirror plane. Although most atoms have a corresponding atom across the pseudo-mirror plane, one water molecule (red) does not. A different Fourier map exhibited a 0.36 eÅ^{-3} residual electron peak at the corresponding position, which might indicate a water oxygen. However, refining such a model was difficult because the occupancy factor decreased to less than 8%, and the position was unstable. Thus, we concluded that the residual error is not significant, and the phase contains 4.75 water molecules.

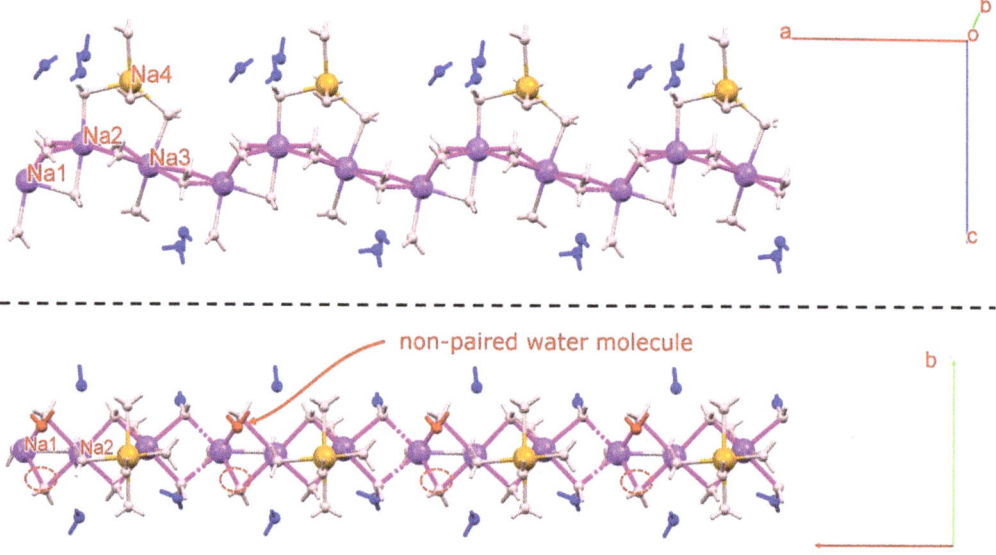

Figure 13. Na–O chain observed in the crystal structure of 4.75H. Three 6-coordinated sodium ions (Na1, Na2, and Na3) form a waving [Na–O–Na–O] chain structure. Red water molecules do not have an associated atom across the pseudo-mirror plane (non-paired water molecule). Figures were drawn with crystallographic a, b, c-axis marks.

4.2. Hydration and Dehydration Mechanism 4.75H Crystal

DIC-Na AH sorbs water molecules and directly transforms into 4.75H, which does not include the 3.5H form. In contrast, DIC-Na 4.75H loses water and transforms first into 3.5H and then into AH. The difference between the hydration and dehydration behaviors can be explained based on the similarity of the crystal structures.

According to the DVS isotherm sorption plot (Figure 12, red), the DIC-Na AH form was stable in a humid environment up to 50% RH. However, it rapidly absorbed water to form DIC-Na 4.75H at 65% RH. The DIC-Na 3.5H form did not appear in the absorption process. This stoichiometric absorption behavior may be due to the large difference in the crystal structures between DIC-Na AH and 4.75H (Figure 6). In fact, the alternating layered structure of hydrophilic and hydrophobic regions in 3.5H and 4.75H forms was not observed in the AH form. Usually, a large hysteresis in the DVS isotherm plot (Figure 12) indicates a large difference in the crystalline structure. The AH form may be kinetically stable owing to such a difference that it did not rapidly change into hydrate phases. The hydration critical RH of 65% RH in the AH form exceeded the stable region of the 3.5H form (30 to 60% RH), which prevented the formation of 3.5H during the hydration of the AH form.

In the case of dehydration, the DVS isotherm desorption plot (Figure 12, blue) reveals that DIC-Na 4.75H was stable down to 65% RH. Then, it gradually released water and transitioned to 3.5H, which was stable between 65% and 30% RH. Below 30% RH, the 3.5H form rapidly when transformed to the AH form. The smooth dehydration from 4.75H to 3.5H can be explained by their similar crystal structure, with analogous hydrophilic/hydrophobic alternating layers (Figure 6). In the TG-DTA curve (Figure 11), which was recorded under flowing dry N_2 gas, a partial stoichiometric weight loss (5.32%) confirmed the presence of 3.5H at approximately 50 °C. Similarly, the simultaneous PXRD-DSC measurements (Figure 10) showed the first dehydration step to generate 3.5H, and a few 2θ diffraction peaks revealing the presence of 3.5H were observed at 14°, 29°, and 32° (indicated by pink markers in Figure 10). Together, these results suggested a mechanistic aspect of this transition, namely that it was not until the crystal lattice of 4.75H could no longer accommodate the void structures formed during dehydration in which another lattice emerged, which corresponded to that of 3.5H. In this manner, the reported "tetrahydrate" structure with the same cell dimensions as 4.75H [35] might arise from the partial decrease in the occupancies of water molecules.

The change in the crystal structure from 4.75H to 3.5H is illustrated in Figure 14. Out of the 19 water molecules in the unit cell of 4.75H, the five that do not interact with Na^+ were released during dehydration to form 3.5H (i.e., the ratio of water/DIC reduced from 19:4 (4.75) to 14:4 (3.5)). Thus, water molecules bonded to their surrounding molecules only through classical OH $\cdots$ O hydrogen bonds were preferentially lost by dehydration. This mechanism is consistent with the previous conjecture by Bartolomei et al. that some water molecules were tightly bound and immobile, while the others were highly mobile [36].

The release of five water molecules during the dehydration changed the coordination environment around Na^+. The number of $Na^+ \cdots$ O interactions is summarized in Table 2 with other crystallographic indices. During dehydration from 4.75H to 3.5H, the number of $Na^+ \cdots$ O(water) interactions decreased, but new $Na^+ \cdots$ O(carboxylate) interactions formed to compensate for this decrease, thereby maintaining either five or six $Na^+ \cdots$ O(all) interactions per one Na^+. This change in the Na^+ coordination environment implies that the coordination of Na^+ with O is flexible, allowing a smooth change in the coordinating atom from O(water) to O(carboxylate). In addition, a coordination number of 5 or 6 around Na^+ in 4.75H is commonly observed, and more than 6-coordination is undesirable owing to steric hindrance [44].

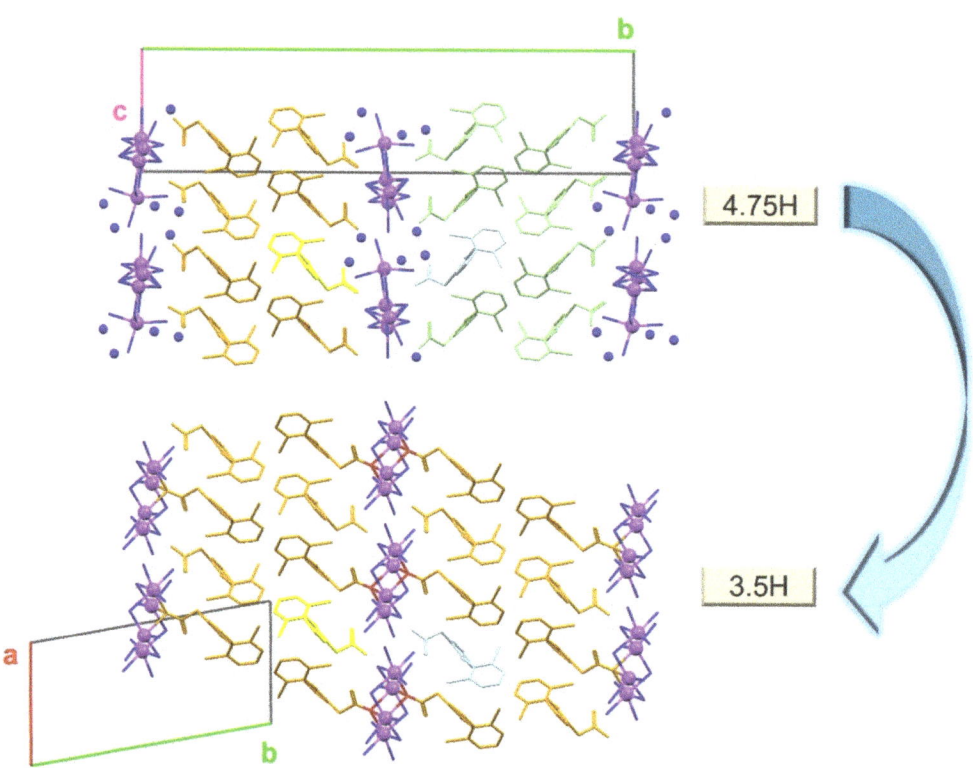

Figure 14. Structural changes during the dehydration from 4.75H to 3.5H. Non-bonded water molecules are represented by blue spheres. Hydrogen atoms are omitted. Figures were drawn with crystallographic a, b, c-axis marks.

During dehydration, the orientation of the DIC molecules changed. Both the 4.75H and 3.5H forms have hydrophobic DIC layer structures, but the directions of these layers differ. Specifically, the alternating layers in the crystal structure of 4.75H are oriented in the opposite direction (orange and light-green in Figure 14), whereas the layers in 3.5H are in the same direction (orange only). This change is highlighted by the yellow and light-blue molecules in Figure 14. During dehydration, the yellow molecule retained the same orientation in both structures, but the light blue one rotated. This rotation may have facilitated the breaking and formation of $Na^+ \cdots O$ (water or carboxylate) interactions associated with structural reconstruction.

A large rearrangement in the crystal structure of the AH form was observed below 30% RH. During this change, the hydrophilic/hydrophobic alternating-layer structure disappeared, and a one-dimensional chain structure of hydrophilic (Na^+ and O) formed along the b-axis (Figure 7). Although this change was large, O(carboxylate) atoms almost maintained the Na^+ coordination number at five. The packing indices (Table 2) were calculated using the PLATON program [40]. The packing index of 4.75H is slightly lower than that of 3.5H, possibly due to a small void space (ca. 5.9 Å^3 × 2), which would explain why the slightly unstable 4.75H starts to dehydrate to 3.5H, even in the high RH region. Meanwhile, compared with AH, the 3.5H form is more efficiently packed, utilizes a greater number of H-bonds, and has more water molecules filling spaces.

Table 2. Number of Na$^+$–O interactions and packing indices.

	4.75H	3.5H	AH
No. of water molecules per four DIC molecules	19	14	0
Na$^+$–O(all) interactions	6 or 5	6	5
Na$^+$–O(water) interactions	6 or 5	5 or 4	0
Na$^+$–O(carboxylate) interactions	0	1 or 2	5
Packing index	70.3	73.3	71.9

5. Conclusions

The novel crystalline phase of DIC-Na AH was revealed by SCXRD. The re-determination of the crystal structure and crystallographic investigation of 4.75H showed that the presence of non-coordinated water molecules caused pseudo-symmetry and structural complexity. The multi-step dehydration mechanism of DIC-Na 4.75H was successfully elucidated using simultaneous PXRD-DSC, TG, and DVS, as well as a comparison of the crystal structures. During the first dehydration step, only water molecules that were not coordinated to Na$^+$ ions were lost, which led to the generation of 3.5H. The second dehydration step into the anhydrous phase (AH) was accompanied by a large structural change. For the first time, this work successfully elucidated the solid-state dehydration transition landscape of DIC-Na, which is a commercially available form of this API, using X-ray crystallographic analysis. These findings help understand the dehydration/hydration mechanism as well as the physicochemical properties of pharmaceutical crystals.

Supplementary Materials: The following are available online at https://www.mdpi.com/article/10.3390/cryst11040412/s1, Figure S1: DSC diagram of DIC-Na 4.75H, Table S1: Crystal structures of diclofenac sodium (DIC-Na) hydrates published thus far.

Author Contributions: Conceptualization, H.O., T.M. and H.U. Structural analysis, H.O. and T.M. Investigation, H.O., T.M. and I.N. Writing—original draft preparation, H.O. and T.M. Writing—review and editing, H.O., A.S. and H.U. Visualization, H.O. Supervision, A.S. and H.U. Project administration, H.U. All authors have read and agreed to the published version of the manuscript.

Funding: Part of this work was supported by JSPS KAKENHI Grant Number JP18H04504 and 20H04661 (H.U.).

Data Availability Statement: CCDC 2065083, 2065085, and 2065086 contains the supplementary crystallographic data for this paper (3.5H, 4.75H, and AH, respectively). These data can be obtained free of charge from The Cambridge Crystallographic Data Centre via www.ccdc.cam.ac.uk/structures.

Acknowledgments: The authors are thankful to Etsuo Yonemochi (Hoshi University) for the DVS measurement.

Conflicts of Interest: The authors declare no conflict of interest.

References

1. Leuner, C.; Dressman, J. Improving drug solubility for oral delivery using solid dispersions. *Eur. J. Pharm. Biopharm.* **2000**, *50*, 47–60. [CrossRef]
2. Ma, X.; Müller, F.; Huang, S.; Lowinger, M.; Liu, X.; Schooler, R.; Williams, R.O., III. Influence of Carbamazepine Dihydrate on the Preparation of Amorphous Solid Dispersions by Hot Melt Extrusion. *Pharmaceutics* **2020**, *12*, 379. [CrossRef] [PubMed]
3. Vikas, Y.; Sandeep, K.; Braham, D.; Manjusha, C.; Budhwar, V. Cyclodextrin complexes: An approach to improve the physicochemical properties of drugs and applications of cyclodextrin complexes. *Asian J. Pharm.* **2018**, *12*, S394.
4. Pang, H.; Sun, Y.-B.; Zhou, J.-W.; Xie, M.-J.; Lin, H.; Yong, Y.; Chen, L.-Z.; Fang, B.-H. Pharmaceutical Salts of Enrofloxacin with Organic Acids. *Crystals* **2020**, *10*, 646. [CrossRef]
5. Karimi-Jafari, M.; Padrela, L.; Walker, G.M.; Croker, D.M. Creating Cocrystals: A Review of Pharmaceutical Cocrystal Preparation Routes and Applications. *Cryst. Growth Des.* **2018**, *18*, 6370–6387. [CrossRef]
6. Childs, S.L.; Chyall, L.J.; Dunlap, J.T.; Smolenskaya, V.N.; Stahly, B.C.; Stahly, G.P. Crystal Engineering Approach to Forming Cocrystals of Amine Hydrochlorides with Organic Acids. Molecular Complexes of Fluoxetine Hydrochloride with Benzoic, Succinic, and Fumaric Acids. *J. Am. Chem. Soc.* **2004**, *126*, 13335–13342. [CrossRef]

7. Takata, N.; Tanida, S.; Nakae, S.; Shiraki, K.; Tozuka, Y.; Ishigai, M. Tofogliflozin Salt Cocrystals with Sodium Acetate and Potassium Acetate. *Chem. Pharm. Bull.* **2018**, *66*, 1035–1040. [CrossRef] [PubMed]
8. Wang, L.-Y.; Bu, F.-Z.; Li, Y.-T.; Wu, Z.-Y.; Yan, C.-W. A Sulfathiazole–Amantadine Hydrochloride Cocrystal: The First Codrug Simultaneously Comprising Antiviral and Antibacterial Components. *Cryst. Growth Des.* **2020**, *20*, 3236–3246. [CrossRef]
9. Gould, P.L. Salt selection for basic drugs. *Int. J. Pharm.* **1986**, *33*, 201–217. [CrossRef]
10. Serajuddin, A.T.M. Salt formation to improve drug solubility. *Adv. Drug Deliv. Rev.* **2007**, *59*, 603–616. [CrossRef]
11. Paulekuhn, G.S.; Dressman, J.B.; Saal, C. Trends in Active Pharmaceutical Ingredient Salt Selection based on Analysis of the Orange Book Database. *J. Med. Chem.* **2007**, *50*, 6665–6672. [CrossRef] [PubMed]
12. Dzidic, I.; Kebarle, P. Hydration of the alkali ions in the gas phase. Enthalpies and entropies of reactions $M^+(H_2O)_{n-1} + H_2O = M^+(H_2O)_n$. *J. Phys. Chem.* **1970**, *74*, 1466–1474. [CrossRef]
13. Stephenson, G.A.; Diseroad, B.A. Structural relationship and desolvation behavior of cromolyn, cefazolin and fenoprofen sodium hydrates. *Int. J. Pharm.* **2000**, *198*, 167–177. [CrossRef]
14. Banerjee, R.; Bhatt, P.M.; Kirchner, M.T.; Desiraju, G.R. Structural studies of the system Na(saccharinate)·nH_2O: A model for crystallization. *Angew. Chem. Int. Ed.* **2005**, *44*, 2515–2520. [CrossRef]
15. Bond, A.D.; Cornett, C.; Larsen, F.H.; Qu, H.; Raijada, D.; Rantanen, J. Structural basis for the transformation pathways of the sodium naproxen anhydrate-hydrate system. *IUCrJ* **2014**, *1*, 328–337. [CrossRef]
16. Dračínský, M.; Šála, M.; Hodgkinson, P. Dynamics of water molecules and sodium ions in solid hydrates of nucleotides. *CrystEngComm* **2014**, *16*, 6756–6764. [CrossRef]
17. Spielberg, E.T.; Campbell, P.S.; Szeto, K.C.; Mallick, B.; Schaumann, J.; Mudring, A. Sodium Salicylate: An In-Depth Thermal and Photophysical Study. *Chem. Eur. J.* **2018**, *24*, 15638–15648. [CrossRef] [PubMed]
18. Shah, H.S.; Chaturvedi, K.; Zeller, M.; Bates, S.; Morris, K. A threefold superstructure of the anti-epileptic drug phenytoin sodium as a mixed methanol solvate hydrate. *Acta Cryst.* **2019**, *C75*, 1213–1219. [CrossRef] [PubMed]
19. Ding, Z.; Su, W.; Huang, X.; Tian, B.; Cheng, X.; Mao, Y.; Li, G.; Liu, H.; Hao, H. Understanding the Role of Water in Different Solid Forms of Avibactam Sodium and Its Affecting Mechanism. *Cryst. Growth Des.* **2020**, *20*, 1150–1161. [CrossRef]
20. Fujii, K.; Aoki, M.; Uekusa, H. Solid-State Hydration/Dehydration of Erythromycin an Investigated by ab Initio Powder X-ray Diffraction Analysis: Stoichiometric and Nonstoichiometric Dehydrated Hydrate. *Cryst. Growth Des.* **2013**, *13*, 2060–2066. [CrossRef]
21. Mizoguchi, R.; Uekusa, H. Elucidating the Dehydration Mechanism of Ondansetron Hydrochloride Dihydrate with a Crystal Structure. *Cryst. Growth Des.* **2018**, *18*, 6142–6149. [CrossRef]
22. Griesser, U.J. The Importance of Solvates. In *Polymorphism in the Pharmaceutical Industry*; Wiley: Weinheim, Germany, 2006; pp. 211–233.
23. Jurczak, E.; Mazurek, A.H.; Szeleszczuk, Ł.; Pisklak, D.M.; Zielińska-Pisklak, M. Pharmaceutical Hydrates Analysis—Overview of Methods and Recent Advances. *Pharmaceutics* **2020**, *12*, 959. [CrossRef] [PubMed]
24. Rietveld, I.B.; Céolin, R. Rotigotine: Unexpected Polymorphism with Predictable Overall Monotropic Behavior. *J. Pharm. Sci.* **2015**, *104*, 4117–4122. [CrossRef] [PubMed]
25. Fujii, K.; Uekusa, H.; Itoda, N.; Hasegawa, G.; Yonemochi, E.; Terada, K.; Pan, Z.; Harris, K.D.M. Physicochemical under-standing of polymorphism and solid-state dehydration/rehydration processes for the pharmaceutical material acrinol, by ab initio powder X-ray diffraction analysis and other techniques. *J. Phys. Chem.* **2010**, *114*, 580–586.
26. Suzuki, T.; Terada, K. Elucidation of the crystal structure-physicochemical property relationship among polymorphs and hydrates of sitafloxacin, a novel fluoroquinolone antibiotic. *Int. J. Pharm.* **2012**, *422*, 1–8. [CrossRef]
27. Khomane, K.S.; More, P.K.; Raghavendra, G.; Bansal, A.K. Molecular understanding of the compaction behavior of indo-methacin polymorphs. *Mol. Pharm.* **2013**, *10*, 631–639. [CrossRef]
28. Datta, S.; Grant, D.J.W. Crystal structures of drugs: Advances in determination, prediction and engineering. *Nat. Rev. Drug Discov.* **2004**, *3*, 42–57. [CrossRef]
29. Sakon, A.; Sekine, A.; Uekusa, H. Powder Structure Analysis of Vapochromic Quinolone Antibacterial Agent Crystals. *Cryst. Growth Des.* **2016**, *16*, 4635–4645. [CrossRef]
30. Putra, O.D.; Pettersen, A.; Yonemochi, E.; Uekusa, H. Structural origin of physicochemical properties differences upon dehydration and polymorphic transformation of ciprofloxacin hydrochloride revealed by structure determination from powder X-ray diffraction data. *Cryst. Eng. Comm.* **2020**, *22*, 7272–7279. [CrossRef]
31. Skomski, D.; Varsolona, R.J.; Su, Y.; Zhang, J.; Teller, R.; Forster, S.P.; Barrett, S.E.; Xu, W. Islatravir Case Study for Enhanced Screening of Thermodynamically Stable Crystalline Anhydrate Phases in Pharmaceutical Process Development by Hot Melt Extrusion. *Mol. Pharm.* **2020**, *17*, 2874–2881. [CrossRef]
32. Takagi, T.; Ramachandran, C.; Bermejo, M.; Yamashita, S.; Yu, L.X.; Amidon, G.L. A provisional biopharmaceutical classification of the top 200 oral drug products in the United States, Great Britain, Spain and Japan. *Mol. Pharm.* **2006**, *3*, 631–643. [CrossRef]
33. Muangsin, N.; Prajaubsook, M.; Chaichit, N.; Siritaedmukul, K.; Hannongbua, S. Crystal Structure of a Unique Sodium Distorted Linkage in Diclofenac Sodium Pentahydrate. *Anal. Sci.* **2002**, *18*, 967–968. [CrossRef]
34. Llinàs, A.; Burley, J.C.; Box, K.J.; Glen, R.C.; Goodman, J.M. Diclofenac Solubility: Independent Determination of the Intrinsic Solubility of Three Crystal Forms. *J. Med. Chem.* **2007**, *50*, 979–983. [CrossRef]

35. Reck, G.; Faust, G.; Dietz, G. X-ray crystallographic studies of diclofenac-sodium—Structural analysis of diclofenac-sodium tetrahydrate. *Die Pharm.* **1988**, *43*, 771–774.
36. Bartolomei, M.; Rodomonte, A.; Antoniella, E.; Minelli, G.; Bertocchi, P. Hydrate modifications of the non-steroidal anti-inflammatory drug diclofenac sodium: Solid-state characterisation of a trihydrate form. *J. Pharm. Biochem. Anal.* **2007**, *45*, 443–449. [CrossRef]
37. Nieto, I.A.; Bernès, S.; Pérez-Benítez, A. Crystal structure of a new hydrate form of the NSAID sodium diclofenac. *Acta Crystallogr. Sect. E Crystallogr. Commun.* **2020**, *76*, 1846–1850. [CrossRef]
38. Shah, S.R.; Shah, Z.; Khan, A.; Ahmed, A.; Sohani; Hussain, J.; Csuk, R.; Anwar, M.U.; Al-Harrasi, A. Sodium, Potassium, and Lithium Complexes of Phenanthroline and Diclofenac: First Report on Anticancer Studies. *ACS Omega* **2019**, *25*, 21559–21566. [CrossRef] [PubMed]
39. Nugrahani, I.; Kumalasari, R.A.; Auli, W.N.; Horikawa, A.; Uekusa, H. Salt Cocrystal of Diclofenac Sodium-L-proline: Structural, Pseudopolymorphism, and Pharmaceutics Performance Study. *Pharmaceutics* **2020**, *12*, 690. [CrossRef]
40. Spek, A.L. Structure validation in chemical crystallography. *Acta Crystallogr. Sect. D Biol. Crystallogr.* **2009**, *D65*, 148–155. [CrossRef] [PubMed]
41. Sheldrick, G.M. SHELXT—Integrated space-group and crystal-structure determination. *Acta Cryst.* **2015**, *A71*, 3–8. [CrossRef] [PubMed]
42. Sheldrick, G.M. Crystal structure refinement with SHELXL. *Acta Cryst.* **2015**, *C71*, 3–8. [CrossRef]
43. Macrae, C.F.; Sovago, I.; Cottrell, S.J.; Galek, P.T.A.; McCabe, P.; Pidcock, E.; Platings, M.; Shields, G.P.; Stevens, J.S.; Towler, M.; et al. Mercury 4.0: From visualization to analysis, design and prediction. *J. Appl. Crystallogr.* **2020**, *53*, 226–235. [CrossRef] [PubMed]
44. Fifen, J.J.; Agmon, N. Structure and Spectroscopy of Hydrated Sodium Ions at Different Temperatures and the Cluster Stability Rules. *J. Chem. Theory Comput.* **2016**, *12*, 1656–1673. [CrossRef] [PubMed]

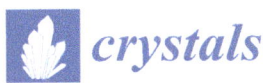

Article

Crystal Structures of Antiarrhythmic Drug Disopyramide and Its Salt with Phthalic Acid

Majid Ismail Tamboli [1,†], Yushi Okamoto [1], Yohei Utsumi [1], Takayuki Furuishi [1,†], Siran Wang [1], Daiki Umeda [1], Okky Dwichandra Putra [1,*], Kaori Fukuzawa [1], Hidehiro Uekusa [2] and Etsuo Yonemochi [1,*]

[1] Department of Physical Chemistry, School of Pharmacy and Pharmaceutical Sciences, Hoshi University, 2-4-41 Ebara, Shinagawa-ku, Tokyo 142-8501, Japan; t-majid@hoshi.ac.jp (M.I.T.); m1903@hoshi.ac.jp (Y.O.); s172504@hoshi.ac.jp (Y.U.); t-furuishi@hoshi.ac.jp (T.F.); m1936@hoshi.ac.jp (S.W.); m1802@hoshi.ac.jp (D.U.); k-fukuzawa@hoshi.ac.jp (K.F.)

[2] Department of Chemistry, School of Science, Tokyo Institute of Technology, Tokyo 152-8551, Japan; uekusa@chem.titech.ac.jp

* Correspondence: dwichandraputra@yahoo.com (O.D.P.); e-yonemochi@hoshi.ac.jp (E.Y.); Tel.: +81-3-5498-5148 (O.D.P.); +81-3-5498-5048 (E.Y.)

† Co-first author, these authors contributed equally to this work.

Abstract: Disopyramide (DPA) is as a class IA antiarrhythmic drug and its crystallization from cyclohexane at ambient condition yields lower melting form crystals which belong to the monoclinic centrosymmetric space group $P2_1/n$, having two molecules in an asymmetric unit. Crystal structure analysis of pure DPA revealed closely associated DPA molecules aggregates via amide–amide dimer synthon through the N–H···O hydrogen bond whereas the second amide hydrogen N–H engaged in an intramolecular N–H···N hydrogen bond with N-nitrogen of 2-pyridine moieties. Crystallization of DPA and phthalic acid (PA) in 1: 1 stoichiometric molar ratio from acetone at ambient condition yielded block shape crystals of 1:1 DPA_PA salt. Its X-ray single crystal structure revealed the formation of salt by transfer of acidic proton from one of the carboxylic acidic groups of PA to the tertiary amino group of chain moiety (N3-nitrogen atom) of DPA molecules. DPA_PA salt crystals belong to the monoclinic centrosymmetric space group $P2_1/n$, comprising one protonated DPA and one PA⁻ anion (hydrogen phthalate counterion) in an asymmetric unit and linked by N–H···O and C–H···O hydrogen bonds. Pure DPA and DPA_PA salt were further characterized by differential calorimetric analysis, thermal gravimetric analysis, powder x-ray diffraction and infrared spectroscopy.

Keywords: disopyramide; phthalic acid; salt; crystal structure; metastable

Citation: Tamboli, M.I.; Okamoto, Y.; Utsumi, Y.; Furuishi, T.; Wang, S.; Umeda, D.; Putra, O.D.; Fukuzawa, K.; Uekusa, H.; Yonemochi, E. Crystal Structures of Antiarrhythmic Drug Disopyramide and Its Salt with Phthalic Acid. *Crystals* **2021**, *11*, 379. https://doi.org/10.3390/cryst11040379

Academic Editor: Duane Choquesillo-Lazarte

Received: 27 February 2021
Accepted: 30 March 2021
Published: 6 April 2021

Publisher's Note: MDPI stays neutral with regard to jurisdictional claims in published maps and institutional affiliations.

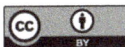

Copyright: © 2021 by the authors. Licensee MDPI, Basel, Switzerland. This article is an open access article distributed under the terms and conditions of the Creative Commons Attribution (CC BY) license (https://creativecommons.org/licenses/by/4.0/).

1. Introduction

Recent past literature related to crystal engineering revealed that there is an intensification of interest in the preparation, crystallization, solid-state characterization and the studying of the X-ray single-crystal structure of active pharmaceutical ingredients (APIs) and their novel solid forms that includes polymorph [1–5], multi-component crystal such as cocrystals [6–8], salt [9], and solvate [10–14] due to their potential applications in the improvement of physicochemical properties of APIs such as solubility [15–17], stability [18–20], hygroscopicity [21], bioavailability [22–24] and so on. Further, advancement in this research area directed towards the understanding crystal–structure, studying supramolecular synthons, hydrogen/halogen bonding interaction and other various non-covalent interactions within them [25–27] as well as correlating structure with the physicochemical properties [28–32]. These structure-property relation studies are helpful and encourage many researchers towards designing and synthesis of new functional molecular solids, and multi-component complexes of APIs, and other molecular entities with desirable and specific chemical or physical properties [33–38].

Disopyramide (2-diisopropylaminoethyl)-phenyl-2-pyridineacetamide (DPA) was developed [39] as a class IA antiarrhythmic drug with a pharmacological profile of action similar to that of quinidine and procainamide in that targets sodium channels to inhibit conduction [40,41]. Currently, DPA and $[C_{21}H_{30}N_3O]^+[H_2PO_4]^-$ disopyramide dihydrogen phosphate are intravenously and orally administrated for clinical use. DPA displaying polymorphism behavior and two solid forms were reported in the literature and named as a low-melting type crystal (85–87 °C) and a high-melting type crystal (95–98 °C) [42]. Of the two crystal forms, the high melting point type crystal is thermodynamically stable, and the low melting point type crystal is easily converted to the high melting point type crystal [42]. However, single-crystal X-ray data of either of crystal form were not present in the Cambridge Structural Database (CSD), whereas the crystal structure of $[C_{21}H_{30}N_3O]^+[H_2PO_4]^-$ disopyramide dihydrogen phosphate has been reported by Kawamura and Hirayama in 2011 [43]. Furthermore, X-single crystal structure of (+)-disopyramide (2R,3R)-bitartrate salt was reported in 1980 for determining the absolute configuration of disopyramide by Burke and Nelson [44], and the structure was not present in the CSD. Moreover, to the best knowledge of the authors, not much research has been carried out with respect to creating the novel salt form of DPA.

DPA has asymmetric carbon marked by a star that is connected to four different groups shown in Figure 1a. It has a flexible molecular framework as well as the presence of a hydrogen bond donor and acceptor site, and hence there will be a high possibility to form multicomponent crystals. Thus, it could be the potential candidate in exploring its different conformational modification by obtaining X-ray single crystal structures of different solid forms of DPA.

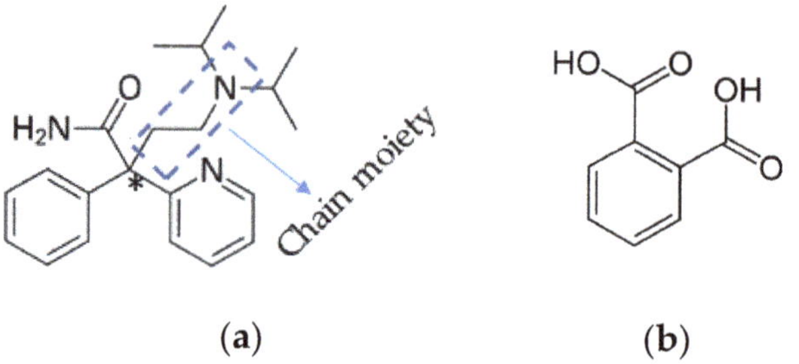

Figure 1. Structures of (**a**) racemic disopyramide (DPA) and (**b**) phthalic acid (PA).

We are going to focus on the crystallization and crystal engineering research on active pharmaceutical ingredients (APIs), particularly on improving the physicochemical properties of drug molecules by undertaking polymorphic study [45], making multicomponent crystals [46], such as its solvates [47], cocrystals [48], and salts [49]. In this report, we discuss the X-ray single-crystal structure of the lower melting temperature form of DPA and novel DPA_PA salt [Phthalic acid (PA), Figure 1b], detailed crystal structure analysis and its characterization.

2. Materials and Methods

2.1. Materials

DPA and PA were purchased from Tokyo Chemical Industry Co. Ltd. (Tokyo, Japan). All other analytical-grade solvents and reagents were commercially obtained and used without further purification.

2.2. Crystallization

2.2.1. DPA

The minimum amount of solvent cyclohexane was used to dissolve the DPA by sonication at 25 °C; it was then immediately filtered and the resulting solution was maintained at ambient temperature for 1–2 days, yielding a colorless block-shaped crystal.

2.2.2. DPA_PA Salt for Single X-ray Crystal Structure Analysis

DPA and PA were each taken in a molar ratio of 1:1, suspended in diethyl ether and stirred at 25 °C and 170 rpm (IKA Plate_RCT 4, IKA, IKA® Japan K.K., Osaka, Japan) for 5 days. After that, the precipitated material was recrystallized in acetone, yielding a colorless block-shaped crystal.

2.2.3. DPA_PA Salt for Characterization (PXRD, DSC, IR, and TG)

DPA (0.5 mmole) and PA (0.5 mmole) in a 1:1 molar ratio was grinded in a mortar and pestle for about 10 min to become a fine powder, then a few drops of acetone were added to it, then again grinded for 10–15 min to obtain powder. From this grinded material, 150 mg was used for the crystallization experiment. Colorless crystals were obtained on the side wall of the vial by upon dissolving the 150 mg grinded material in 20 mL acetone under sonication at a temperature 30 °C for 10 min; the resulting solution obtained after filtration was left for slow evaporation at ambient condition for 3–4 days.

2.3. Single-Crystal X-ray Diffraction

The single-crystal X-ray diffraction data for DPA and DPA_PA salt were collected at 93 K. The measurements were carried out in ω-scan mode with an R-AXIS RAPID II (Rigaku Co., Tokyo, Japan) using the Cu-Kα X-ray obtained from rotating the anode source with a graphite monochromator. The integrated and scaled data were empirically corrected for absorption effects using ABSCOR [50,51]. The initial structure was solved using the direct method with SIR 2004 and refined on F^2 with SHELXL 2014 [52,53]. All non-hydrogen atoms were refined anisotropically. The hydrogen atom attached to the nitrogen N2 and N5 atom in pure DPA and the hydrogen atom attached to the nitrogen N2 as well as hydrogen H5A present in between the O3 and O5 oxygen in the DPA_PA salt were located using the differential Fourier map and refined isotropically. All other hydrogen atom positions were calculated geometrically and included in the calculation using the riding atom model; the calculations were performed for all the hydrogen atoms. Moreover, in the DPA_PA salt, protonated DPA molecules display disordered structure in which two molecules with opposite configuration share the same site. Their occupancies were fixed to 0.5.

The molecular graphics were produced using Mercury 4.1.0 software [54]. CCDC 2065231 contains the supplementary crystallographic data for the DPA and CCDC 2065230 contains the supplementary crystallographic data for the DPA_PA salt, and can be obtained free of charge from the Cambridge Crystallographic Data Centre via www.ccdc.cam.ac.uk/data_request/cif (accessed on 2 April 2021).

2.4. Powder X-ray Diffraction (PXRD)

The PXRD patterns of all samples were measured in the reflectance mode using a SmartLab diffractometer (Cu Kα source (40 kV and 200 mA), D/teX ultra-high-speed position-sensitive detector, Rigaku). Diffraction patterns (2θ) were collected from 5° to 40° at 25 °C with a step of 0.01° and a scan speed of 20°/min.

2.5. Differential Scanning Calorimetry (DSC) and Thermogravimetric (TG) Measurements

DSC and TG measurements were carried out with the Thermo plus EVO2-DSC 8230 and the Thermo plus EVO2-TG8120 TG-DTA, respectively (Rigaku). The DSC sample (~3 mg) was placed in an aluminum-crimped pan, measured at a speed of 5 °C/min from 25 to 250 °C under nitrogen gas (flow rate = 50 mL/min. The TG sample (~10 mg) was placed into an aluminum-open pan, respectively, and measured at a speed of 5 °C/min from 25 to 250 °C under nitrogen gas (flow rate = 50 mL/min for DPA, PA and 100 mL/min for DPA_PA salt).

2.6. Fourier Transform Infrared Spectroscopy (FT-IR)

The infrared spectra of samples were obtained using FT-IR (FT-IR-4200 spectrometer, JASCO Co., Tokyo, Japan) with an attenuated total reflection (ATR) unit (ATR-PRO 670H-S, JASCO Co.). The spectrum recorded represents an average of 64 scans obtained with a resolution of 4 cm^{-1} at room temperature. The spectra were collected in the wavenumber ranging from 4000 to 400 cm^{-1}. The internal reflectance element used in this study was a diamond trapezoid having 45° entrance and exit faces.

3. Results and Discussion

3.1. Crystal Structure of DPA

Suitable crystals of DPA were grown from the cyclohexane solvent by slow evaporation at ambient conditions. Its structure was determined by single crystal X-ray diffraction and showed that it crystallized in monoclinic centrosymmetric space group $P2_1/n$, containing two symmetry independent molecules (designated as A and B molecules) in the asymmetric unit and which have opposite configuration. The Oak Ridge Thermal Ellipsoid Plot (ORTEP) of DPA is shown in Figure 2a. In the structural overlay studies two conformers which, having similar configuration, are used and reveal a minor conformational difference at the amide group, phenyl and 2-pyridine moieties, whereas difference at *iso*-propyl moiety was found to be more as shown in Figure 2b. Furthermore, interestingly in both molecules A and B of DPA, the phenyl ring moiety is nearly coplanar with the chain moiety (excluding the *iso*-propyl moiety) whereas the 2-pyridine moiety is oriented nearly perpendicular to the planar part as shown in Figure 2b. The crystallographic information and geometrical parameters for the hydrogen bonding interaction are summarized in Tables 1 and 2.

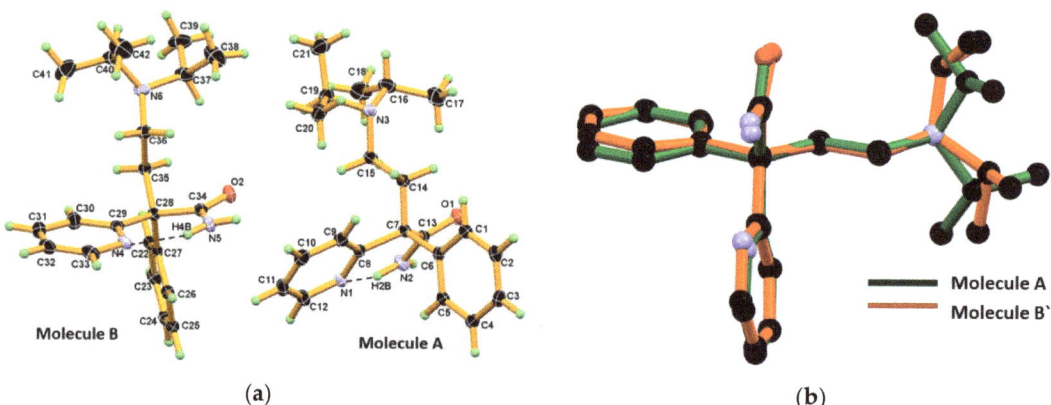

Figure 2. (a) The Oak Ridge Thermal Ellipsoid Plot (ORTEP) diagram of Molecule A and Molecule B of DPA, showing the atom numbering scheme in. Thermal ellipsoid drawn at 50% probability level, and H-atoms are shown as small spheres with arbitrary radii. Both symmetry independent molecules A and B in the asymmetric unit display the N–H···N intramolecular hydrogen bond in $S^1_1(6)$ motif; (b) Structural overlay of two conformers in DPA which, having similar configuration, reveal considerable conformational differences at the *iso*-propyl moiety present on the tertiary N-atom of chain moiety. Molecule B' is inversion symmetry related to Molecule B.

Table 1. Crystallographic data table for the DPA and DPA_PA salt.

Parameters	DPA	DPA_PA
Empirical formula	$C_{21}H_{29}N_3O$	$C_{29}H_{35}N_3O_5$
Formula weight	339.47	505.60
Temperature [K]	93(2)	93(2)
Wavelength [Å]	1.54187	1.54187
Crystal system	Monoclinic	Monoclinic
Space group	$P2_1/n$	$P2_1/n$
Unit cell dimensions		
a [Å]	17.2970 (3)	14.2741 (4)
b [Å]	10.7861 (2)	7.8827 (2)
c [Å]	21.4831 (4)	23.5355 (7)
α [°]	90	90
β [°]	99.385 (7)	91.428 (6)
γ [°]	90	90
Volume [Å^3]	3954.39 (15)	2647.35 (13)
Z and Z'	4, 2	4, 1
Density (calculated) [g/cm^3]	1.140	1.269
Absorption coefficient [mm^{-1}]	0.552	0.705
F (000)	1472	1080.0
Crystal size [mm x mm x mm]	0.247 × 0.231 × 0.221	0.49 × 0.47 × 0.23
Theta range for data collection [°]	3.048 to 68.192	3.582 to 68.188
Index ranges	$-20 <= h <= 20, -12 <= k <= 12, -25 <= l <= 25$	$-17 <= h <= 17, -9 <= k <= 9, -28 <= l <= 28$
Reflections collected	44379	29013
Independent reflections	7200 [R_{int} = 0.0215, R_{sigma} = 0.0129]	4847 [R_{int} = 0.0412, R_{sigma} = 0.0326]
Completeness to theta = 67.687°	99.9%	100%
Absorption correction	Semi-empirical from equivalents	Semi-empirical from equivalents
Max. and min. transmission	0.873 and 0.711	0.850, 0.513
Refinement method	Full-matrix least-squares on F^2	Full-matrix least-squares on F^2
Data/restraints/parameters	7200/0/475	4847/0/350
Goodness-of-fit on F^2	1.052	1.079
Final R indices [I>2sigma(I)]	R_1 = 0.0416, wR_2 = 0.1024	R_1 = 0.0434, wR_2 = 0.1123
R indices (all data)	R_1 = 0.0435, wR_2 = 0.1040	R_1 = 0.0489, wR_2 = 0.11659
$\Delta\rho_{max}$, $\Delta\rho_{min}$ (e·Å^{-3})	0.424 and $-$0.215	0.265/$-$0.171

Table 2. Geometrical parameters of the hydrogen bond interaction in DPA and DPA_PA salt.

D-H···A	D-H (Å)	H···A (Å)	D···A (Å)	D-H···A (°)	Symmetry Codes
			DPA		
N2-H2B···N1	0.887 (17)	1.965 (17)	2.7006 (16)	139.5 (14)	Intramolecular
N2-H2A···O2	0.890 (16)	2.025 (16)	2.8959 (15)	166.2 (14)	$-x + 3/2, y - 1/2, -z+1/2$
N5-H4B···N4	0.887 (17)	1.970 (17)	2.7035 (16)	139.1 (14)	Intramolecular
N5-H4A···O1	0.890 (17)	2.046 (17)	2.9286 (14)	171.1 (14)	$-x + 3/2, y + 1/2, -z+1/2$
C2-H2···O2	0.95	2.677	3.605	165.71	$-x + 3/2, y - 1/2, -z+1/2$
C10-H10···O2	0.95	2.62	3.3855(15)	138	x, y, z
C11-H11···C$_g$4	0.95	2.98	3.7910(13)	145	x, y, z
C32-H32···C$_g$2	0.95	2.90	3.7631(13)	152	$-1 + x, y, z$
C42-H42A···C$_g$4	0.98	2.93	3.6320(18)	129	$1/2 - x, 1/2 + y, 1/2 - z$

C$_g$2 centroid of the ring (C1-C2-C3-C4-C5-C6), C$_g$4 centroid of the ring (C22-C23-C24-C25-C26-C27) of molecule A and molecule B of DPA respectively

Table 2. Cont.

D-H···A	D-H (Å)	H···A (Å)	D···A (Å)	D-H···A (°)	Symmetry Codes
		DPA_PA salt			
N2-H2A···O4	0.88 (2)	2.02 (2)	2.895 (2)	174 (19)	x, y, z
N2-H2B···O1	0.920 (18)	2.071 (18)	2.9910 (17)	177.8 (18)	−x, 2 − y, 1 − z
N3-H3A···O2	1.00	1.72	2.7159 (16)	173	−1/2 + x, 3/2 − y, 1/2 +z
O5-H5A···O3	1.11(2)	1.30 (2)	2.4047 (19)	172 (2)	Intramolecular
C2-H2···O1	0.95	2.52	3.4269 (19)	159	−x, 1 − y, 1 − z
C9-H9···O4	0.95	2.36	3.294 (2)	167	x, y, z
C15-H15B···N1	0.99	2.57	3.078 (2)	112	Intramolecular
C17-H17C···O1	0.98	2.54	3.4952 (19)	166	Intramolecular
C22-H22···O2	0.95	2.33	2.674 (2)	101	Intramolecular
C25-H25···O4	0.95	2.33	2.688 (2)	101	Intramolecular
C17-H17A···O2	0.98	2.685	3.359 (2)	126.23	−1/2 + x, 3/2 − y,1/2 + z
C14-H14B···O2	0.99	2.603	3.0812(18)	109.73	−1/2 + x,3/2 − y, 1/2 + z
C11-H11···O2	0.95	2.711	3.519	143.35	1 − x, 2 − y, 1 − z
C18-H18A···C_g5	0.98	2.93	3.6222(18)	129	−x, 1 − y, 1 − z
C29-O4··· C_g2		3.4808 (16)		146.59 (14)	x, y, z
C29-O4··· C_g3		3.4808 (16)		146.59 (14)	x; y, z

C_g2 centroid of the ring (C1-C3-C2-C1A-C6-C5), C_g3 centroid of the ring (N1-C2-C3-C1-C5-C6) of disordered protonated DPA, C_g5 centroid of the ring (C22-C23-C24-C25-C26-C27) of PA$^-$ anion in the DPA_PA salt

In the crystal structure of pure DPA, two closely associated DPA molecules, that is, molecules A and B aggregate via amide homodimer through N–H···O hydrogen bonds, namely N2-H2A···O2, N5-H4A···O1 hydrogen bonds involving amide hydrogen N–H and amide C=O oxygen from both DPA molecules resulting $R^2_2(8)$ ring motifs involving two donor and two acceptor atoms. Whereas second amide hydrogen N–H in both symmetry independent DPA molecules formed an intramolecular N-H···N hydrogen bond with the N-nitrogen atom of 2-pyridine moiety in $S^1_1(6)$ motif, namely N2-H2B···N1 and N5-H4B···N4, and hence it controls orientation of 2-pyridine moiety of DPA molecules in the crystal structure as shown in the Figure 3.

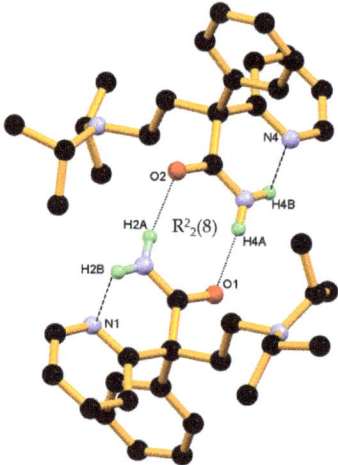

Figure 3. Two closely associated molecules of DPA, that is, molecules A and B involved in ring formation (basic dimeric unit) through an N–H···O hydrogen bond and the resulting $R^2_2(8)$ ring motifs. A second amide hydrogen N–H engaged in intramolecular hydrogen bonding with the N-atom of the 2-pyridine moiety in $S^1_1(6)$ motif. Dotted lines indicate the non-covalent interaction (hydrogen atoms not involved in the hydrogen bonding were removed for clarity).

Packing of the dimeric unit down the *c*-axis, resulting in a 1-D chain of the dimeric unit along the *ab*-diagonal, wherein dimeric units of DPA are linked through C-H···O and C-H···π interaction, containing alternate arrangements of vertically and horizontally oriented dimeric units. In this association C10-H10, C11-H11 hydrogen of 2-pyridine moiety of molecule A and C32-H32 hydrogen of 2-pyridine moiety, and C42-H42A hydrogen of *iso*-propyl moiety of molecules B are involved in the alternate C10-H10···O2, C11-H11···C_g4, and C32-H32···C_g2, C42-H42A···C_g4 interaction shown Figure 4a. The dimeric unit assembled helically along the *b*-axis to form a helical chain of the dimeric unit as shown in Figure 4b and dimeric unit along the *b*-axis linked through longer and roughly linear C2-H2···O2 (H2···O2, 2.67 Å, Angle 165.71°) interaction.

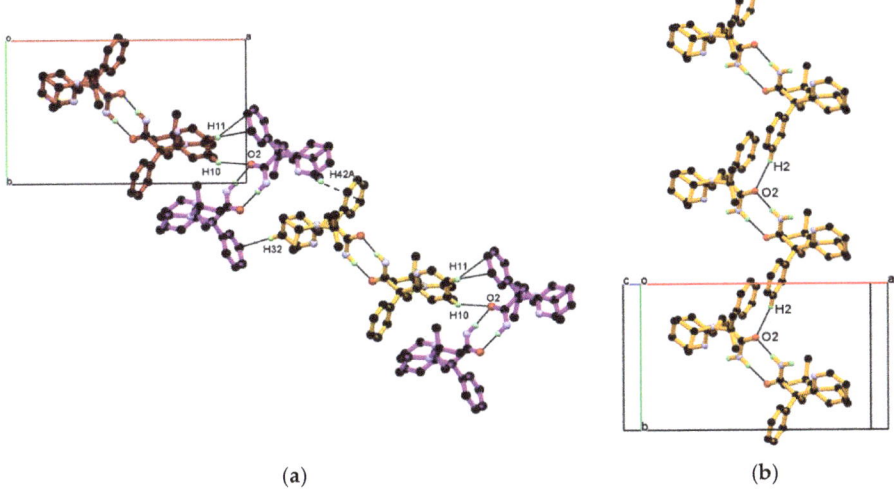

Figure 4. (a) Packing view of the dimeric unit down the *c*-axis, resulting in a 1-D chain of dimeric unit containing an alternate arrangement of vertically and horizontally oriented dimeric unit along the *ab*-diagonal; they are associated through alternate C10-H10···O2, C11-H11···C_g4, and C32-H32···C_g2, C42-H42A···C_g4 interaction and (b) Packing of dimeric unit along the *b*-axis resulting in a helical chain of the dimeric unit, linked through C2-H2···O2 interaction.

Combining the above mentioned packings resulted in the 2-D packing of the dimeric unit in the *ab*-plane, as shown Figure 5. In this packing, the neighboring helical chain of the dimeric unit packed in the *ab*-plane through the alternate C10-H10···O2 C11-H11···C_g4, and C32-H32···C_g2, C42-H42A···C_g4 interaction generate the 2-D packing of the dimeric unit in the *ab*-plane, as shown in Figure 5.

Furthermore, such 2-dimensional structure of the dimeric unit assembled loosely due to the absence of strong interaction along the *c*-axis. In this direction, that is, along the *c*-axis, the 2-D network of dimeric units interact with each other by weak non-covalent interactions and hydrophobic forces between adjacent phenyl and *iso*-propyl groups and such packing of dimeric unit in the *ac*-plane creates a solvent assessable void of size 54.85 Å^3 per unit cell and 1.4% of unit cell volume, calculated by using contact surface from Mercury 2020, 2.0 software [54] shown in Figure 6. Crystal with assessable solvent void is recently reported in [55].

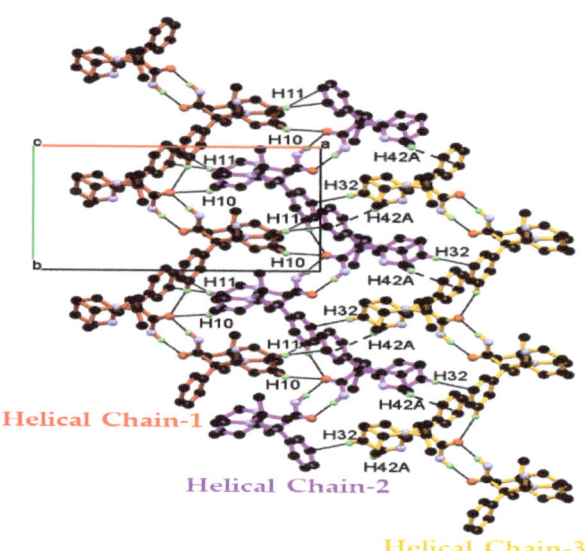

Figure 5. Helical 1-D chain of dimeric unit of DPA is assembled in the *ab*-plane resulting in 2-D packing. In this packing, the central 1-D dimeric unit chain of DPA molecules is associated with the neighboring dimeric chain via C–H···O and C–H···π interaction and the resulting tight packing in the *ab*-plane.

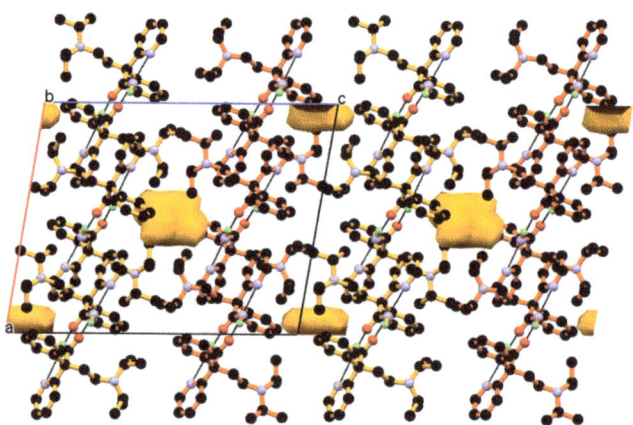

Figure 6. Neighboring 2-dimensional network of dimeric units of DPA assembled loosely via relatively weak non-covalent interaction and hydrophobic forces along the *c*-axis, resulting in 3-dimensional packing; such packing creates a solvent accessible void between them.

3.2. Crystal Structure of DPA_PA Salt

DPA and PA in the 1: 1 stoichiometric molar ratio were crystallized from acetone at ambient condition to obtain a colorless block shape crystal. The ΔpKa difference between DPA (pka: 8.36) and coformer PA (pKa: 2.94, 5.41) is more than 3 and salt formation was expected based on the basic rule of three [56]. The X-ray single-crystal structure confirmed the formation of DPA_PA salt with approximately similar C–O bond lengths C28-O2, 1.2438 (18), C28-O3, 1.2676 (19) Å) of the (COO$^-$) carboxylate group of PA. These approximate similarities in the bond length of C–O confirmed the transfer of an acidic proton from one of the carboxylic acidic group of PA to the N3-nitrogen atom of the tertiary amino group (chain moiety) of DPA. DPA_PA salt crystalized in the monoclinic centrosymmetric $P2_1/n$ space group comprising one protonated DPA and one PA$^-$ anion in an asymmetric unit, revealing the molecular salt in the 1:1 molar ratio. In the crystal structure of DPA_PA salt, protonated DPA molecules displayed positional disorder and ratio fixed 0.5/0.5 for the two disordered components. DPA is a racemic compound consisting of R and S configurations. These two racemic components R and S are found to occupy the same site with 0.5 and 0.5 occupancy in DPA_PA. In this disorder model, phenyl and pyridine ring were exchanged between R and S, and the other part of DPA molecule was completely overlapped in DPA_PA salt. (Figure 7a).

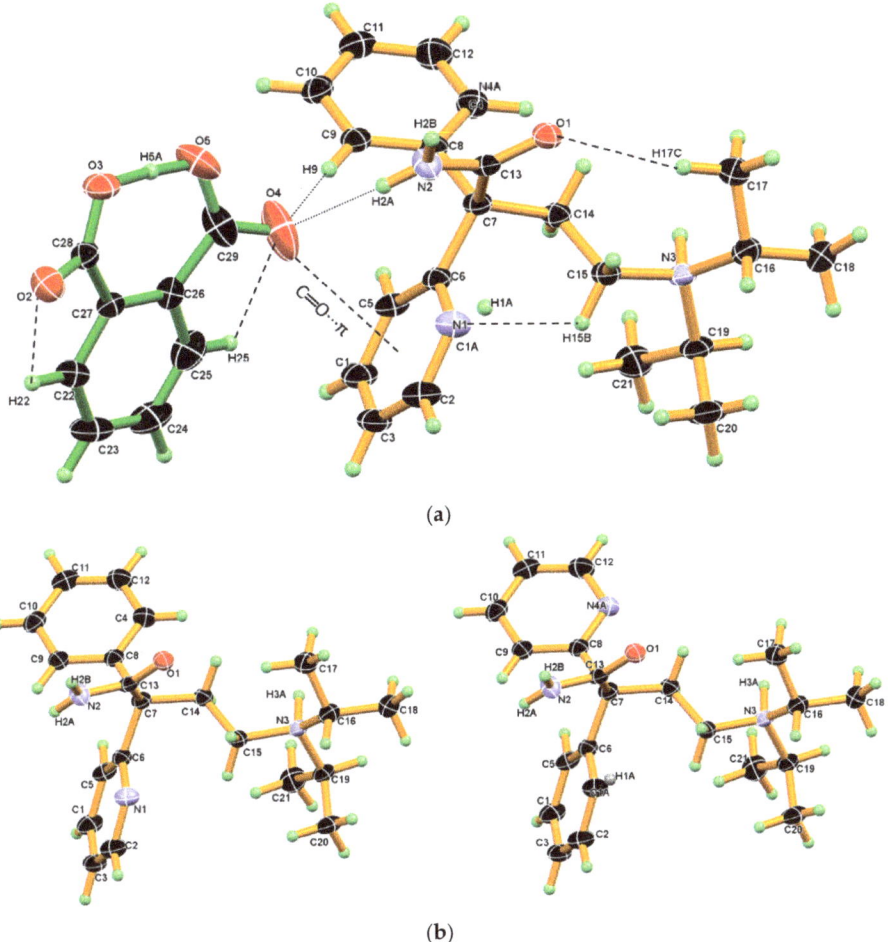

Figure 7. (a) ORTEP diagram of DPA_PA salt, showing the atom numbering scheme wherein C1, N4A and N1, and C1A share the same position. Thermal ellipsoid drawn at 50% probability level, and H-atoms are shown as small spheres with arbitrary radii. DPA_PA salts, displaying intramolecular hydrogen bonds O5-H5A···O3, C17-H17C···O1, C22-H22···O2, C25-H25···O4 C15-H15B···N1 and intermolecular hydrogen bonds N2–H2A···O4 and C9–H9···O4, C=O4···π between the salt pair. (b) The disordered DPA molecule in salt crystal. R and S configuration molecules occupied the same site with 0.5 and 0.5 occupancy.

A similar phenomenon was also observed in the crystal structure of ketoconazole [57]. Interestingly, in the one configuration, the phenyl ring is roughly coplanar with chain moiety (excluding the *iso*-propyl moiety), whereas in other configuration, the 2-pyridine moiety is roughly coplanar with the chain moiety (excluding the *iso*-propyl moiety). (Figure 7b).

Both the component in the asymmetric unit, that is, protonated DPA and PA$^-$ anion linked by strong N2–H2A···O4 hydrogen bond and C9–H9···O4 hydrogen bonds and such assembly in salt facilitated the formation C=O···π interaction between the carboxyl C=O4 of PA$^-$ anion and phenyl ring Cg2 in one configuration/2-pyridine ring Cg3- in other configuration. In the crystal structure of salt, PA$^-$ displaying an intramolecular strong O5-H5A···O3 hydrogen bond in which hydroxyl (O5-H5A) of the carboxyl group of the PA$^-$ anion donates H5A hydrogen intramolecularly to an O3-oxygen atom of the carboxylate group of the PA$^-$ anion and other C-H···O intramolecular hydrogen bonds namely, C22-H22···O2, C25-H25···O4 present in PA$^-$ anion and C17-H17C···O1, C15-H15B···N1 in protonated DPA which stabilize the conformation the salt as shown in Figure 7a. The crystallographic information and geometrical parameters for the hydrogen bonding interaction are summarized in Tables 1 and 2.

Hereafter, one conformer of disordered protonated DPA molecule used for discussion of crystal structure and packing of DPA_PA salt. Crystal structure of DPA_PA salt reveals the presence of a dimeric association between the protonated DPA molecule through the N–H···O hydrogen bond like DPA alone with different symmetry operation (Table 2 and Figure 8a). There is no direct association between the PA$^-$-PA$^-$ anion observed in DPA_PA salt. However the protonated DPA molecule linked PA$^-$ anions alternatively through N–H···O, and charge assisted the N$^+$–H···O$^-$ hydrogen bond shown in Figure 8b, in which one PA$^-$ anion associated with the protonated DPA molecule by forming the N–H···O hydrogen bond involving carbonyl C=O4 oxygen of the carboxyl group of PA$^-$ anion and amide N-H2A hydrogen of protonated DPA. Whereas the other PA$^-$ anion associated by forming a charge assisted N$^+$–H···O$^-$ hydrogen bond by using carboxylate (COO$^-$) O2-oxygen of the PA anion and the protonated tertiary amino group N3$^+$-H3A hydrogen of protonated DPA; both associations were supported by C–H···O interaction as shown in Figure 8b.

In the crystal structure of DPA_PA salt, two inversion-symmetry related protonated DPA molecules form amide homodimer, via a pair of strong N2–H2B···O1 hydrogen bonds in R$^2_2$(8) ring motif that involve two acceptor and two donor atoms. In this association, protonated DPA donates amide hydrogen N2–H2B to amide carbonyl (C=O1) oxygen of inversion-symmetry related protonated DPA molecules in dimeric N2–H2B···O1 hydrogen bonding interaction. Further, this amide homodimer of protonated DPA molecule linked to two PA anions through N2–H2A···O4 hydrogen bonding interaction between the second hydrogen of amide N2–H2A and carbonyl (C=O4) oxygen of the carboxyl group of the PA$^-$ anion and further supported by C9–H9···O4 interaction, between C9–H9 hydrogen of the phenyl ring of protonated DPA and carbonyl (C=O4) oxygen of the carboxyl group of the PA$^-$ anion resulting basic dimeric unit shown in Figure 9.

The dimeric unit linked to four *n*-glide related neighboring dimeric units through charge assisted strong and linear N$^+$–H···O$^-$ hydrogen bonding interaction and supported by two longer and non-linear C–H ···O$^-$ interactions, namely C17–H17A ···O2$^-$, C14–H14B ···O2$^-$ resulting 2-D packing. In this association, the carboxylate (COO$^-$) O2-oxygen of PA$^-$ anion is made hydrogen bond with N3$^+$–H3A (protonated tertiary amino nitrogen) hydrogen of protonated DPA via the charge assisted strong N3$^+$–H3A···O2$^-$ hydrogen bond; such association was further supported by longer and non-linear C–H···O$^-$ interaction, namely C17–H17A···O2$^-$, C14–H14B···O2$^-$ interactions and resulting packing view down the *a*-axis is shown in Figure 10a (above). In this packing, the dimeric unit assembled along the *b*-axis through the short C2–H2···O1 hydrogen bond between amide carbonyl (C=O1) oxygen and C2-H2 hydrogen of 2-pyridine moieties of the next dimeric unit along the *b*-axis and supported by weak C18-H18A···C$_g$5 interaction between the C18–H18A hydrogen of *iso*-propyl moieties of protonated DPA and the π cloud of the aromatic ring (C22-C23-C24-C25-C26-C27) of PA⁻ anion; the resulting association is shown in Figure 10a (down). Similar packing views in the *ac*-plane, reveal that the neighboring dimeric unit assembled along the *ac*-diagonal through hydrogen bonding, wherein there is an alternate arrangement of protonated DPA amide dimer and PA⁻ anion as shown in Figure 10b.

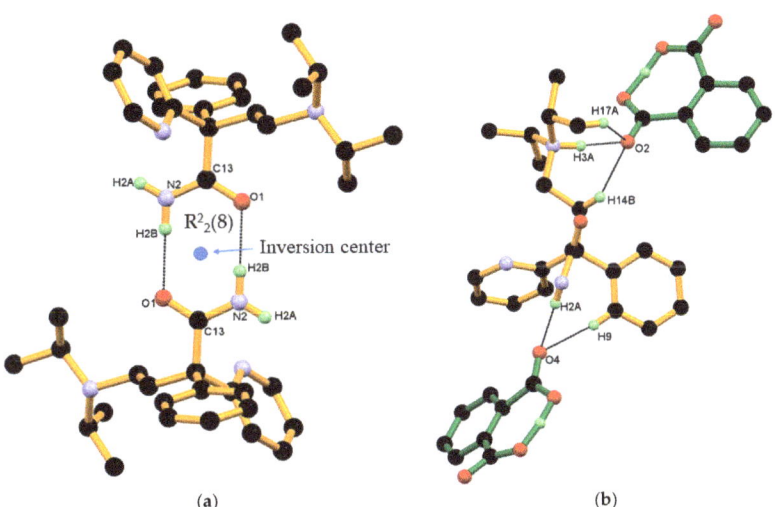

Figure 8. (**a**) Association between protonated DPA molecules through a pair of strong N–H···O hydrogen bonds in $R^2_2(8)$ ring motif; and(**b**) Association between the protonated DPA and PA⁻ anions in DPA_PA salt, hereby protonated DPA molecules engaging both carboxylate and carboxyl groups of the PA⁻ anion alternatively through a strong N–H···O and charge assisted N⁺–H···O⁻ hydrogen bond and further supported by C–H···O interaction.

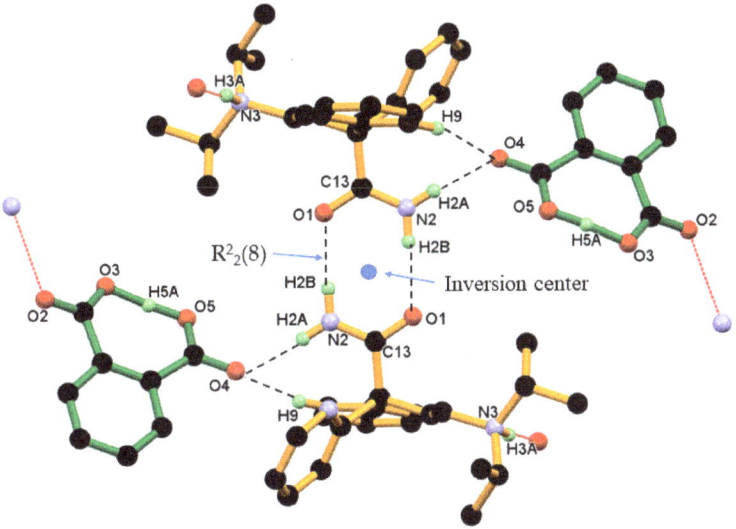

Figure 9. Dimeric unit of DPA_PA salt in crystal. Dotted lines indicate the non-covalent interaction (hydrogen atoms not involved in the hydrogen bonding were removed for clarity).

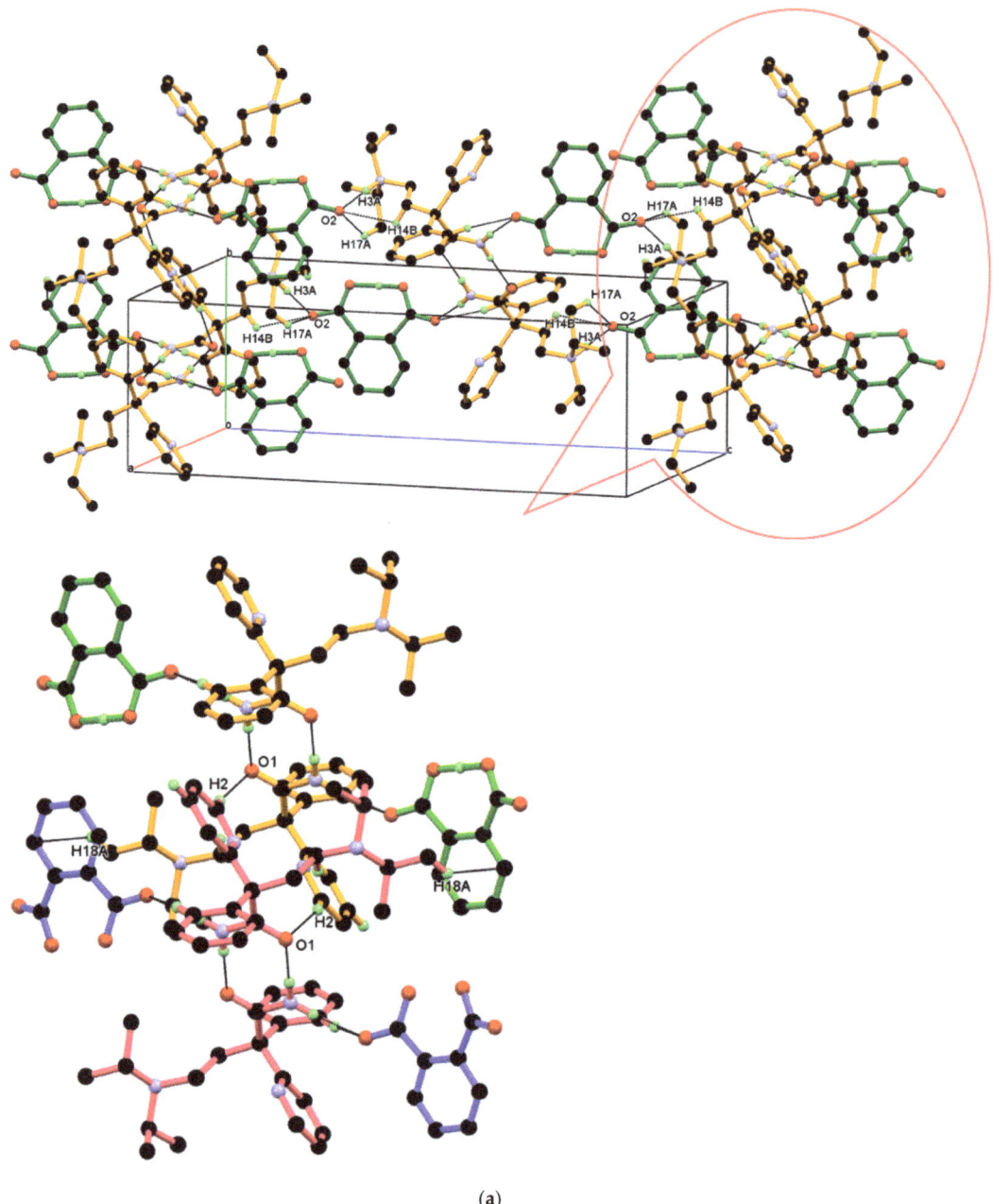

(a)

Figure 10. *Cont.*

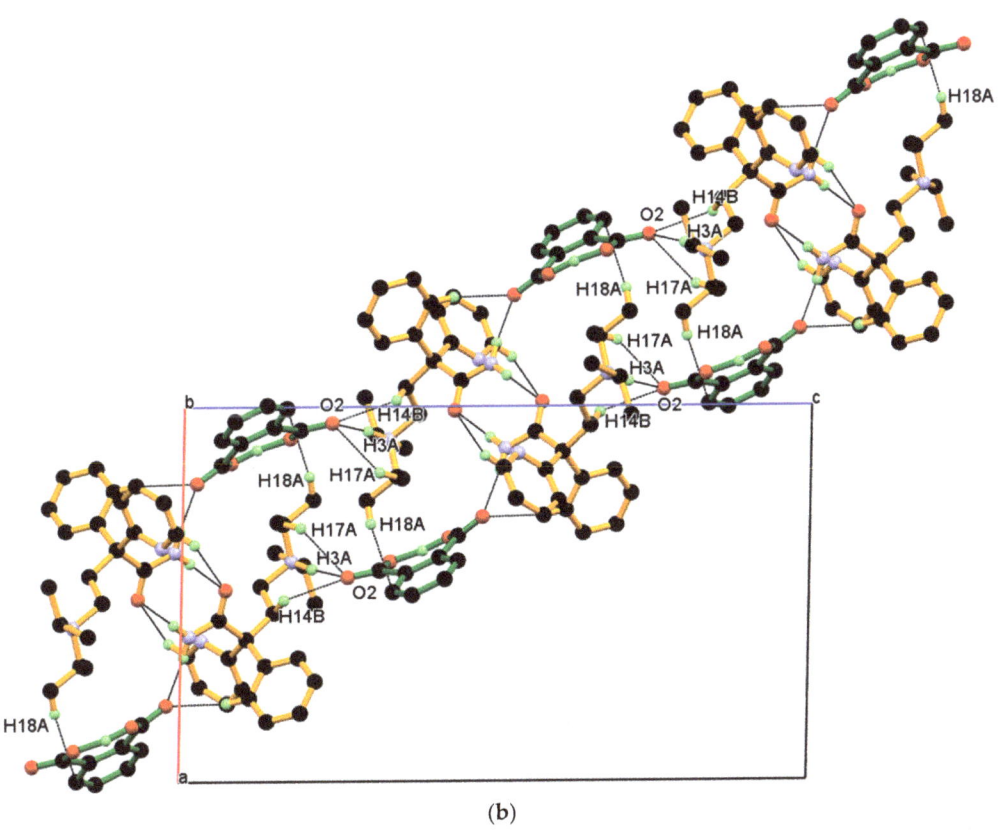

Figure 10. (a) Packing view down the *a*-axis, with each dimeric unit linked to four *n*-glide related neighboring dimeric units, resulting in 2-D packing (above). The inset shows the association between the neighboring dimeric unit shown in different colors through C2–H2···O1 interaction and supported by C18-H18A···C_g5 along the *b*-axis. (down) (b) Similar packing view in the *ac*-plane.

Further, such a two-dimensional network of dimeric unit assembled centrosymmetrically along the *a*-axis (parallel to the *ac*-diagonal) through longer and weak C11–H11···O2$^-$ interaction between C11-H11 hydrogen of the phenyl ring of protonated DPA and carboxylate (COO$^-$) O2-oxygen of PA$^-$ anions resulting in three-dimensional packing of the dimeric unit in the *ac*-plane, as shown in Figure 11.

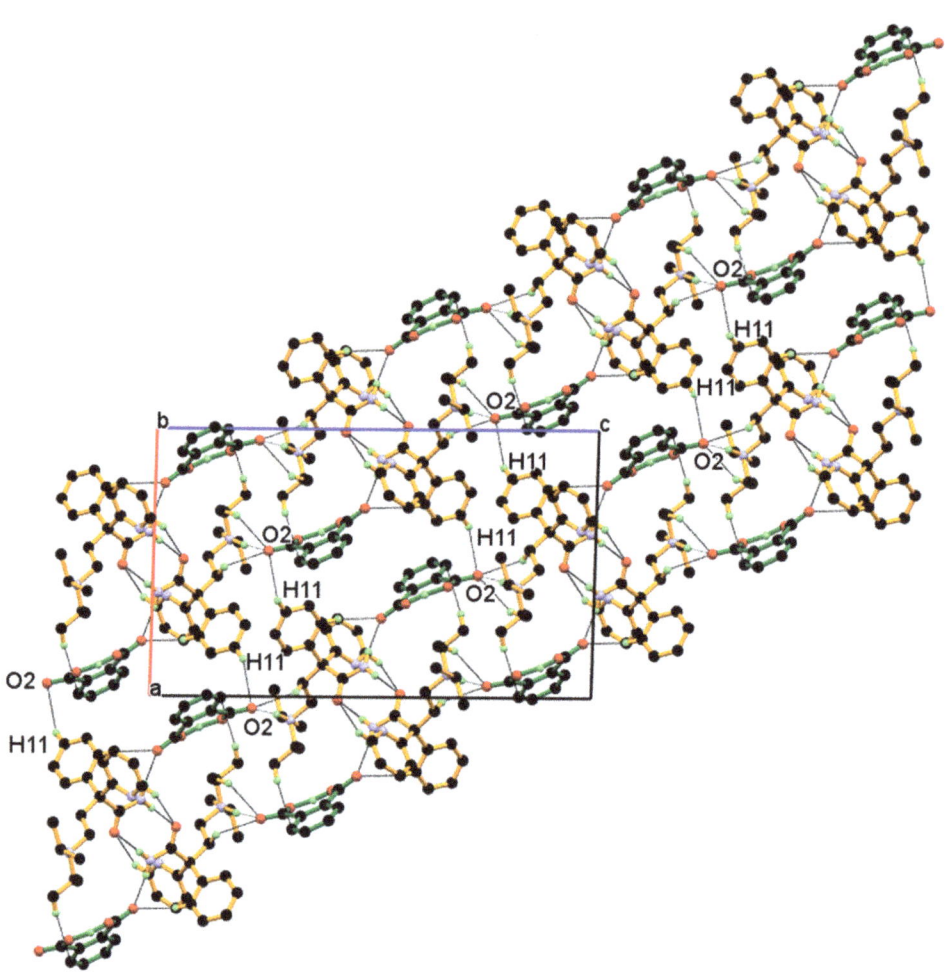

Figure 11. 2-Dimentonal network of dimeric unit assembled centrosymmetric fashion through weak and longer C11-H11⋯O2⁻ interaction resulting in 3-D packing of dimeric unit in the *ac*-plane.

3.3. Structural Overlay

DPA (Figure 12a), has freely rotatable groups connected to asymmetric carbon marked by a star and anticipated to display conformational or orientational changes in its solid forms. The structural overlay of the DPA molecule by overlapping the (C-C-C-N) backbone chain, shown in Figure 12b, reveals conformational and orientational differences owing to rotational freedom around the C—C, C-N bonds. Conformational difference in both solid forms could be characterized by torsion angles τ_1, τ_2, τ_3 and τ_4 as shown in Figure 12a, and the dihedral angle between the phenyl and 2-pyridine moieties and values listed in Table 3. In pure DPA crystal structure, both conformers in the pure DPA crystal display slight difference in torsion angles τ_1 (−179.78, −171.37), while values of τ_2 (177.67, 177.17) and τ_3 (−1.01, 3.01) are comparable and indicate that the (C-C-C-N) backbone chain moiety connecting to the phenyl ring are nearly coplanar in molecule A, while there is a slight deviation observed in coplanarity in B molecules. On the other hand, the 2-pyridine ring is roughly perpendicular to the planar part of A and B molecules. The dihedral angle between the phenyl and 2-pyridine rings is 87.16° and 79.83° in molecules A and B, respectively. In DPA_PA salt crystal structure, the torsion angles τ_1 and τ_2 are −177.58°, −175.47° suggesting coplanarity in the backbone chain as pure DPA, whereas torsion angles τ_3 −16.81° indicate deviation in coplanarity in backbone chain moiety and the phenyl ring. Further, the dihedral angle between the phenyl and 2-pyridine moiety is significantly changed to 59.43° and such deviation in orientation of 2-pyridine and phenyl moiety could be due to the association of salt former (PA) with drug (DPA) through hydrogen bond in this direction. However, the torsional value τ_4 is for the orientation of the amide group with a planar part; it is nearly similar for both conformers in pure DPA, and such orientation of the amide group brings 2-pyridine moiety close enough to facilitate an intramolecular hydrogen bond between amide N-H hydrogen and N-atom of 2-pyridine moiety. Whereas in the DPA_PA salt a conformational twist is observed at amide group as shown in Figure 12b to facilitate the intermolecular hydrogen bond between amide N-H hydrogen of protonated DPA and carbonyl oxygen (C=O) of the carboxyl group PA⁻ anion. Moreover, *iso*-propyl moiety present on tertiary nitrogen in all molecules shows conformational/orientational difference.

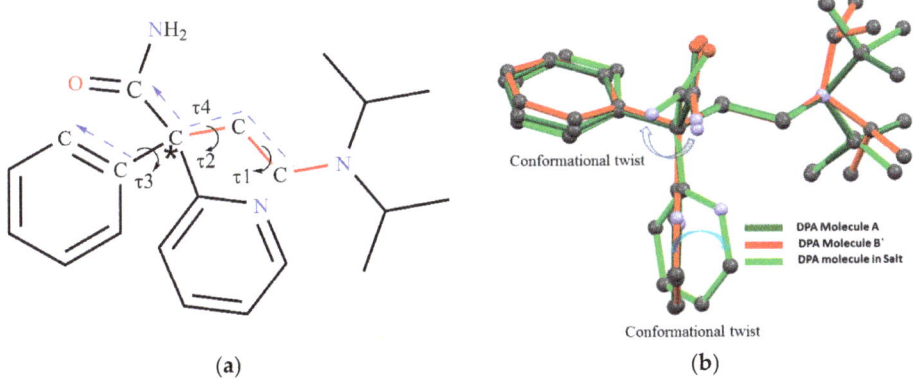

Figure 12. (a) Chemical structure of DPA, in which the (C-C-C-N) backbone chain is marked by a red color bond and (b) Structural overlay of DPA molecules in both solid forms showing significant conformational variation; Green-Molecule A, Red-Molecule B' in DPA, Light green-DPA molecules from DPA_PA salt.

Table 3. Torsional/dihedral angle in DPA and DPA_PA.

	τ_1 °	τ_2 °	τ_3 °	τ_4 °	Dihedral Angle °
DPA Molecule A	−179.78	177.67	−1.01	63.83	87.16(6)
DPA Molecule B'	−171.37	177.17	3.12	63.90	79.83(6)
DPA from Salt	−177.60	−175.45	−16.81	69.39	59.43(7)

In DPA Molecule A: τ_1—C7-C14-C15-N3, τ_2—C6-C7-C14-C15, τ_3—C1-C6-C7-C14, τ_4—C13-C7-C14-C15; In DPA Molecule B': τ_1—C28-C35-C36-N6, τ_2—C27-C28-C35-C36, τ_3—C22-C27-C28-C35, τ_4—C34-C28-C35-C36; DPA from Salt: τ_1—C7-C14-C15-N3, τ_2—C8-C7-C14-C15, τ_3—C4-C8-C7-C14, τ_4—C13-C7-C14-C15. The dihedral angle is the angle between planes of the phenyl and 2-pyridine ring in DPA.

Crystal structure analysis showed that the drug–drug amide homosynthon retained in salt as in pure DPA (differed in symmetry operation). Further, the density of DPA alone and its salt DPA_PA calculated from single crystal X-ray diffraction were found to increase from 1.140 g/cm³ in DPA to 1.269 g/cm³ in the salt, indicating denser packing in salt.

3.4. Characterization of DPA and DPA_PA Salt

3.4.1. PXRD

The PXRD pattern recorded for commercially available DPA, DPA crystals, DPA_PA salt and PA. The PXRD pattern of the commercially available DPA and DPA crystal is matched to reveal that both are in the same crystalline phase. Further PXRD patterns of the salt are different from individual components, suggesting formation of a new crystalline phase in the solid-state. (Figure S1). Furthermore, the overlapping of the experimental PXRD pattern of these crystals matched well the simulated PXRD pattern obtained from the single-crystal X-ray data, confirming the homogeneity of the sample.

3.4.2. FT-IR Spectrum

Considered as a reasonable and reliable technique to detect the formation of the multi-component crystal, Fourier transform infrared (FT-IR) spectroscopy is a very important tool to determine typical carboxylate anion and confirm the proton transfer when carboxylic acid is used as a coformer.

FT-IR spectra were obtained for commercial DPA, prepared DPA crystal, PA and DPA_PA salt (Figure S2). FT-IR spectrum of commercial DPA and prepared DPA crystal showed same characteristic peaks, which were observed as amide N-H stretching at 3263 cm^{-1}, amide C=O stretching and NH_2 deformation overlap peak at 1664 cm^{-1}, whereas in DPA_PA amide N-H stretching was observed at 3354.57 cm^{-1}, amide C=O stretch and NH_2 deformation at 1680, 1625 cm^{-1}, respectively [58]. The blue shift of amide-derived peaks suggests the possible changes in the hydrogen bonding interaction between molecules due to the formation of a new solid form [59,60]. In general, for tertiary amine salts, a broad band at 2300–2700 cm^{-1} was due to the NH^+ stretching, which was also observed in DPA-PA salt, revealing the protonation of tertiary amine in DPA [60,61]. In addition, the peaks at 1590 and 1568 cm^{-1} in DPA were probably attributed to benzene and pyridine rings. It was observed that similar peaks appeared with minor differences in DPA_PA salt. Hence, it appears there is no chemical interaction on benzene and pyridine rings.

Due to the hydrogen bond of the PA dimer, pure PA existed over a broad band around 2800 cm^{-1}, attributed to the OH group, which shifts to 3191 cm^{-1} in DPA_PA salt. The carbonyl stretches of two carboxylic acid groups of PA were observed at 1666 and 1583 cm^{-1}, which appeared at 1679 cm^{-1} for the COOH group and 1556 cm^{-1} for the COO^- group in DPA-PA salt [62].

In short, the appearance of a broad band at 2300–2700 cm^{-1} and a peak at 1556 cm^{-1}, where the ionized tertiary amine and carboxylate group could be observed, respectively, indicate a proton transfer from the salt former PA to DPA, confirming the salt formation between DPA and PA.

3.4.3. Thermal Properties

The thermal properties of the DPA and DPA_PA salt were evaluated by DSC and TG measurements. DSC revealed a single sharp endotherm at 84 °C in agreement with a reported metastable form at 85 °C. In the DSC curve of the DPA_PA salt, the endothermic peak at around 161 °C is the melting point of salt, which is significantly different from DPA (84 °C) and PA (216 °C) (Figure S3). TG data of the DPA single crystal revealed that no weight loss before melting confirmed the absence of any solvent or hydrate in the crystal lattice as same as that of DPA commercial. Also, the thermal stability and decomposition processes of DPA_PA salt have been shown, measured by simultaneous TG in flowing air. The DPA_PA salt is stable until 160 °C (Figure S4). There are no thermal moments for all crystals before the melting process, indicating that these crystals are unsolvated.

4. Conclusions

Pure DPA and its 1:1 DPA_PA salt crystals have been obtained from the slow solvent evaporation method and both belong to the centrosymmetric monoclinic crystal system having a $P2_1/n$ space group. The asymmetric unit of pure DPA contains two molecules while 1:1 DPA_ PA salt contains one protonated DPA and one PA^- anion.

Crystal structure analysis of pure DPA showed two closely associated molecules formed amide–amide dimer through an N-H···O hydrogen bond and resulting in the $R^2_2(8)$

ring motifs. Dimeric units were assembled in the *ab*-plane through C-H···O and C-H···π interaction, whereas it packed loosely along the *c*-axis via weak non-covalent interaction. Crystal structure analysis of 1: 1 DPA_ PA salt showed a strong association between the drug and the salt former leading to compact molecular packing, with an increase in crystal density compared to DPA alone. In salt, two inversion symmetry related protonated DPA molecules formed amide homodimer through an N-H···O hydrogen bond in $R^2{}_2(8)$ ring motifs and such dimer is hydrogen bonded to two PA$^-$ anions through N-H···O and C-H···O hydrogen bonds to form the basic dimeric unit comprising two protonated DPA and two PA$^-$ anion. Furthermore, dimeric units linked to four *n*-glide related neighboring dimeric units through a strong N$^+$–H···O$^-$ hydrogen bond resulted in a 2-Dimentional packing network. Such a 2-D network assembled in centrosymmetric fashion along the *a*-axis through weak C-H···O interaction resulting 3-D packing in the *ac*-plane.

Supplementary Materials: The following are available online at https://www.mdpi.com/article/10.3390/cryst11040379/s1, Figure S1. PXRD patterns of (**a**) commercial DPA; (**b**) DPA crystal, (**c**) simulated DPA, (**d**) PA, (**e**) DPA_PA salt and (**f**) simulated DPA_PA salt, Figure S2. FT-IR spectra of (**a**) commercial DPA; (**b**) DPA crystal, (**c**) PA, (**d**) DPA_PA salt, Figure S3. DSC profiles of (**a**) commercial DPA, (**b**) DPA crystal, (**c**) PA, (**d**) DPA_PA, Figure S4. TG curves of commercial DPA (yellow), DPA crystal (gray), PA (orange), DPA_PA salt (blue).

Author Contributions: Conceptualization, Y.O., D.U., and O.D.P.; formal analysis, M.I.T., Y.O., D.U., O.D.P. and H.U.; investigation, Y.O., Y.U. and D.U.; writing of original draft preparation, M.I.T., T.F. and S.W.; writing of review and editing; T.F., O.D.P. and E.Y.; visualization, M.I.T., T.F., Y.U. and S.W.; supervision, T.F., O.D.P., K.F., H.U. and E.Y.; project administration, T.F., K.F. and E.Y. All authors have read and agreed to the published version of the manuscript.

Funding: Part of this work was supported by the Mochida Memorial Foundation for Medical and Pharmaceutical Research 2019–2020 (to T.F.) and JSPS KAKENHI Grant Number JP18H04504 and 20H04661 (to H.U.).

Acknowledgments: The authors are thankful to Takashi Kikuchi (Rigaku Corporation) for refining and solving the disorder in DPA_PA salt.

Conflicts of Interest: The authors declare no conflict of interest.

References

1. Brittain, H.G. *Polymorphism in Pharmaceutical Solids*; Taylor & Francis: London, UK, 1999.
2. Hilfiker, R.; von Raumer, M. *Polymorphism in the Pharmaceutical Industry: Solid Form and Drug Development*; Wiley: Hoboken, NJ, USA, 2019.
3. SeethaLekshmi, S.; Guru Row, T.N. Conformational Polymorphism in a Non-steroidal Anti-inflammatory Drug, Mefenamic Acid. *Cryst. Growth Des.* **2012**, *12*, 4283–4289. [CrossRef]
4. Babu, N.J.; Cherukuvada, S.; Thakuria, R.; Nangia, A. Conformational and Synthon Polymorphism in Furosemide (Lasix). *Cryst. Growth Des.* **2010**, *10*, 1979–1989. [CrossRef]
5. Li, L.; Yin, X.H.; Diao, K.S. Improving the Solubility and Bioavailability of Pemafibrate via a New Polymorph Form II. *ACS Omega* **2020**, *5*, 26245–26252. [CrossRef] [PubMed]
6. Karimi-Jafari, M.; Padrela, L.; Walker, G.M.; Croker, D.M. Creating Cocrystals: A Review of Pharmaceutical Cocrystal Preparation Routes and Applications. *Cryst. Growth Des.* **2018**, *18*, 6370–6387. [CrossRef]
7. Schultheiss, N.; Newman, A. Pharmaceutical Cocrystals and Their Physicochemical Properties. *Cryst. Growth Des.* **2009**, *9*, 2950–2967. [CrossRef] [PubMed]
8. Yousef, M.A.E.; Vangala, V.R. Pharmaceutical Cocrystals: Molecules, Crystals, Formulations, Medicines. *Cryst. Growth Des.* **2019**, *19*, 7420–7438. [CrossRef]
9. Gunnam, A.; Nangia, A.K. High-Solubility Salts of the Multiple Sclerosis Drug Teriflunomide. *Cryst. Growth Des.* **2019**, *19*, 5407–5417. [CrossRef]
10. Bezerra, B.P.; Pogoda, D.; Perry, M.L.; Vidal, L.M.T.; Zaworotko, M.J.; Ayala, A.P. Cocrystal Polymorphs and Solvates of the Anti-Trypanosoma cruzi Drug Benznidazole with Improved Dissolution Performance. *Cryst. Growth Des.* **2020**, *20*, 4707–4718. [CrossRef]
11. Berziņš, A.; Skarbulis, E.; Rekis, T.; Actiņš, A. On the Formation of Droperidol Solvates: Characterization of Structure and Properties. *Cryst. Growth Des.* **2014**, *14*, 2654–2664. [CrossRef]
12. Zvoníček, V.; Skořepová, E.; Dušek, M.; Babor, M.; Žvátora, P.; Šóóš, M. First Crystal Structures of Pharmaceutical Ibrutinib: Systematic Solvate Screening and Characterization. *Cryst. Growth Des.* **2017**, *17*, 3116–3127. [CrossRef]

13. Zhang, G.; Xiao, X.; Zhang, L.; Ren, G.; Zhang, S. Hydrates and Solvates of Acotiamide Hydrochloride: Crystallization, Structure, Stability, and Solubility. *Cryst. Growth Des.* **2018**, *19*, 768–779. [CrossRef]
14. Wang, K.; Wang, C.; Sun, C.C. Structural Insights into the Distinct Solid-State Properties and Interconversion of Celecoxib N-Methyl-2-pyrrolidone Solvates. *Cryst. Growth Des.* **2020**, *21*, 277–286. [CrossRef]
15. Sathisaran, I.; Dalvi, S.V. Engineering Cocrystals of PoorlyWater-Soluble Drugs to Enhance Dissolution in Aqueous Medium. *Pharmaceutics* **2018**, *10*, 108. [CrossRef] [PubMed]
16. Banerjee, R.; Bhatt, P.M.; Ravindra, N.V.; Desiraju, G.R. Saccharin Salts of Active Pharmaceutical Ingredients, Their Crystal Structures, and Increased Water Solubilities. *Cryst. Growth Des.* **2005**, *5*, 2299–2309. [CrossRef]
17. Shan, N.; Perry, M.L.; Weyna, D.R.; Zaworotko, M.J. Impact of pharmaceutical cocrystals: The effects on drug pharmacokinetics. *Expert Opin. Drug Metab. Toxicol.* **2014**, *10*, 1255–1271. [CrossRef]
18. Swapna, B.; Maddileti, D.; Nangia, A. Cocrystals of the Tuberculosis Drug Isoniazid: Polymorphism, Isostructurality, and Stability. *Cryst. Growth Des.* **2014**, *14*, 5991–6005. [CrossRef]
19. Guo, C.; Zhang, Q.; Zhu, B.; Zhang, Z.; Bao, J.; Ding, Q.; Ren, G.; Mei, X. Pharmaceutical Cocrystals of Nicorandil with Enhanced Chemical Stability and Sustained Release. *Cryst. Growth Des.* **2020**, *20*, 6995–7005. [CrossRef]
20. Nechipadappu, S.K.; Reddy, I.R.; Tarafder, K.; Trivedi, D.R. Salt/Cocrystal of Anti-Fibrinolytic Hemostatic Drug Tranexamic acid: Structural, DFT, and Stability Study of Salt/Cocrystal with GRAS Molecules. *Cryst. Growth Des.* **2018**, *19*, 347–361. [CrossRef]
21. Thakur, T.S.; Thakuria, R. Crystalline Multicomponent Solids: An Alternative for Addressing the Hygroscopicity Issue in Pharmaceutical Materials. *Cryst. Growth Des.* **2020**, *20*, 6245–6265. [CrossRef]
22. Chen, Y.; Li, L.; Yao, J.; Ma, Y.-Y.; Chen, J.-M.; Lu, T.-B. Improving the Solubility and Bioavailability of Apixaban via Apixaban–Oxalic Acid Cocrystal. *Cryst. Growth Des.* **2016**, *16*, 2923–2930. [CrossRef]
23. Zhu, B.; Zhang, Q.; Wang, J.-R.; Mei, X. Cocrystals of Baicalein with Higher Solubility and Enhanced Bioavailability. *Cryst. Growth Des.* **2017**, *17*, 1893–1901. [CrossRef]
24. Mannava, M.K.C.; Suresh, K.; Nangia, A. Enhanced Bioavailability in the Oxalate Salt of the Anti-Tuberculosis Drug Ethionamide. *Cryst. Growth Des.* **2016**, *16*, 1591–1598. [CrossRef]
25. Desiraju, G.R. Supramolecular Synthons in Crystal Engineering—A New Organic Synthesis. *Angew. Chem. Int. Ed. Engl.* **1995**, *34*, 2311–2327. [CrossRef]
26. Corpinot, M.K.; Bučar, D.-K. A Practical Guide to the Design of Molecular Crystals. *Cryst. Growth Des.* **2018**, *19*, 1426–1453. [CrossRef]
27. Desiraju, G.R. *Crystal Engineering: The Design of Organic Solids*; Elsevier: Amsterdam, The Netherlands, 1989.
28. Berry, D.J.; Steed, J.W. Pharmaceutical cocrystals, salts and multicomponent systems; intermolecular interactions and property based design. *Adv. Drug Deliv. Rev.* **2017**, *117*, 3–24. [CrossRef] [PubMed]
29. Martins, I.C.B.; Sardo, M.; Santos, S.M.; Fernandes, A.; Antunes, A.; André, V.; Mafra, L.; Duarte, M.T. Packing Interactions and Physicochemical Properties of Novel Multicomponent Crystal Forms of the Anti-Inflammatory Azelaic Acid Studied by X-ray and Solid-State NMR. *Cryst. Growth Des.* **2015**, *16*, 154–166. [CrossRef]
30. Lin, B.; Liu, Y.; Wang, M.; Wang, Y.; Du, S.; Gong, J.; Wu, S. Intermolecular Interactions and Solubility Behavior of Multicomponent Crystal Forms of Orotic Acid: Prediction and Experiments. *Cryst. Growth Des.* **2021**. [CrossRef]
31. Rajput, L.; Sanphui, P.; Desiraju, G.R. New Solid Forms of the Anti-HIV Drug Etravirine: Salts, Cocrystals, and Solubility. *Cryst. Growth Des.* **2013**, *13*, 3681–3690. [CrossRef]
32. George, C.P.; Thorat, S.H.; Shaligram, P.S.; Gonnade, R.G. Drug–drug cocrystals of anticancer drugs erlotinib–furosemide and gefitinib–mefenamic acid for alternative multi-drug treatment. *Cryst. Eng. Comm.* **2020**, *22*, 6137–6151. [CrossRef]
33. Nangia, A.K.; Desiraju, G.R. Crystal Engineering: An Outlook for the Future. *Angew. Chem. Int. Ed. Engl.* **2019**, *58*, 4100–4107. [CrossRef]
34. Desiraju, G.R. Crystal engineering: From molecule to crystal. *J. Am. Chem. Soc.* **2013**, *135*, 9952–9967. [CrossRef]
35. Mir, N.A.; Dubey, R.; Desiraju, G.R. Strategy and Methodology in the Synthesis of Multicomponent Molecular Solids: The Quest for Higher Cocrystals. *Acc. Chem. Res.* **2019**, *52*, 2210–2220. [CrossRef]
36. Sarkar, N.; Sinha, A.S.; Aakeröy, C.B. Systematic investigation of hydrogen-bond propensities for informing co-crystal design and assembly. *Cryst. Eng. Comm.* **2019**, *21*, 6048–6055. [CrossRef]
37. Chu, Q.; Duncan, A.J.E.; Papaefstathiou, G.S.; Hamilton, T.D.; Atkinson, M.B.J.; Mariappan, S.V.S.; MacGillivray, L.R. Putting Cocrystal Stoichiometry to Work: A Reactive Hydrogen-Bonded "Superassembly" Enables Nanoscale Enlargement of a Metal-Organic Rhomboid via a Solid-State Photocycloaddition. *J. Am. Chem. Soc.* **2018**, *140*, 4940–4944. [CrossRef]
38. Ericson, D.P.; Zurfluh-Cunningham, Z.P.; Groeneman, R.H.; Elacqua, E.; Reinheimer, E.W.; Noll, B.C.; MacGillivray, L.R. Regiocontrol of the [2 + 2] Photodimerization in the Solid State Using Isosteric Resorcinols: Head-to-Tail Cyclobutane Formation via Unexpected Embraced Assemblies. *Cryst. Growth Des.* **2015**, *15*, 5744–5748. [CrossRef]
39. Katz, M.J.; Meyer, C.E.; El-Etr, A.; Slodki, S.J. Clinical evaluation of a new anti-arrhythmic agent, SC-7031. *Curr. Ther. Res. Clin. Exp.* **1963**, *5*, 343–350.
40. Rizos, I.; Brachmann, J.; Lengfelder, W.; Schmitt, C.; von Olshausen, K.; Kubler, W.; Senges, J. Effects of intravenous disopyramide and quinidine on normal myocardium and on the characteristics of arrhythmias: Intraindividual comparison in patients with sustained ventricular tachycardia. *Eur. Heart J.* **1987**, *8*, 154–163. [CrossRef]

41. Kim, S.Y.; Benowitz, N.L. Poisoning due to class IA antiarrhythmic drugs. Quinidine, procainamide and disopyramide. *Drug Saf.* **1990**, *5*, 393–420. [CrossRef]
42. Gunning, S.R.; Freeman, M.; Stead, J.A. Polymorphism of disopyramide. *J. Pharm. Pharmacol.* **1976**, *28*, 758–761. [CrossRef] [PubMed]
43. Kawamura, T.; Hirayama, N. Crystal structure of α-diisopropylaminoethyl-α-phenylpyridine-2-Acetamide phosphate, [C21H30N3O] [H2PO4]. *Z. Krist. N. Cryst. Struct.* **2011**, *226*, 479. [CrossRef]
44. Burke, T.R., Jr.; Nelson, W.L.; Mangion, M.; Hite, G.J.; Mokler, C.M.; Ruenitz, P.C. Resolution, absolute configuration, and antiarrhythmic properties of the enantiomers of disopyramide, 4-(diisopropylamino)-2-(2-pyridyl)-2-phenylbutyramide. *J. Med. Chem.* **1980**, *23*, 1044–1048. [CrossRef] [PubMed]
45. Putra, O.D.; Pettersen, A.; Nilsson Lill, S.O.; Umeda, D.; Yonemochi, E.; Nugraha, Y.P.; Uekusa, H. Capturing a new hydrate polymorph of amodiaquine dihydrochloride dihydrate via heterogeneous crystallisation. *Cryst. Eng. Comm.* **2019**, *21*, 2053–2057. [CrossRef]
46. Putra, O.D.; Furuishi, T.; Yonemochi, E.; Terada, K.; Uekusa, H. Drug–Drug Multicomponent Crystals as an Effective Technique to Overcome Weaknesses in Parent Drugs. *Cryst. Growth Des.* **2016**, *16*, 3577–3581. [CrossRef]
47. Nagase, H.; Kobayashi, M.; Ueda, H.; Furuishi, T.; Gunji, M.; Endo, T.; Yonemochi, E. Crystal Structure of an Epalrestat Dimethanol Solvate. *X Ray Struct. Anal. Online* **2016**, *32*, 7–9. [CrossRef]
48. Putra, O.D.; Umeda, D.; Nugraha, Y.P.; Furuishi, T.; Nagase, H.; Fukuzawa, K.; Uekusa, H.; Yonemochi, E. Solubility improvement of epalrestat by layered structure formation via cocrystallization. *Cryst. Eng. Comm.* **2017**, *19*, 2614–2622. [CrossRef]
49. Hata, N.; Furuishi, T.; Tamboli, M.I.; Ishizaki, M.; Umeda, D.; Fukuzawa, K.; Yonemochi, E. Crystal Structural Analysis of DL-Mandelate Salt of Carvedilol and Its Correlation with Physicochemical Properties. *Crystals* **2020**, *10*, 53. [CrossRef]
50. Higashi, T. *Calculated Using ABSCOR. Empirical Absorption Correction Based on Fourier Series Approximation*; Rigaku: The Woodland, TX, USA, 1994.
51. Messerschmidt, A.; Schneider, M.; Huber, R. ABSCOR: A scaling and absorption correction program for the FAST area detector diffractometer. *J. Appl. Crystallogr.* **1990**, *23*, 436–439. [CrossRef]
52. Burla, M.C.; Caliandro, R.; Camalli, M.; Carrozzini, B.; Cascarano, G.L.; De Caro, L.; Giacovazzo, C.; Polidori, G.; Spagna, R. SIR2004: An improved tool for crystal structure determination and refinement. *J. Appl. Crystallogr.* **2005**, *38*, 381–388. [CrossRef]
53. Sheldrick, G.M. A short history of SHELX. *Acta Crystallographica. Sect. Found. Crystallogr.* **2008**, *64*, 112–122. [CrossRef]
54. Macrae, C.F.; Bruno, I.J.; Chisholm, J.A.; Edgington, P.R.; McCabe, P.; Pidcock, E.; Rodriguez-Monge, L.; Taylor, R.; van de Streek, J.; Wood, P.A. Mercury CSD 2.0–New features for the visualization and investigation of crystal structures. *J. Appl. Crystallogr.* **2008**, *41*, 466–470. [CrossRef]
55. Mittapalli, S.; Mannava, M.K.C.; Sahoo, R.; Nangia, A. Cocrystals, Salts, and Supramolecular Gels of Nonsteroidal Anti-Inflammatory Drug Niflumic Acid. *Cryst. Growth Des.* **2018**, *19*, 219–230. [CrossRef]
56. Kavanagh, O.N.; Walker, G.; Lusi, M. Graph-Set Analysis Helps to Understand Charge Transfer in a Novel Ionic Cocrystal When the ΔpKa Rule Fails. *Cryst. Growth Des.* **2019**, *19*, 5308–5313. [CrossRef]
57. Chen, X.; Li, D.; Deng, Z.; Zhang, H. Ketoconazole: Solving the Poor Solubility via Cocrystal Formation with Phenolic Acids. *Cryst. Growth Des.* **2020**, *20*, 6973–6982. [CrossRef]
58. Wickman, A.; Finnegan, P. Disopyramide Phosphate. In *Analytical Profiles of Drug Substances*; Florey, K., Ed.; Academic Press: New York, NY, USA, 1984; Volume 13, pp. 183–209.
59. Brittain, H.G. Vibrational Spectroscopic Studies of Cocrystals and Salts. 1. The Benzamide−Benzoic Acid System. *Crystal Growth Des.* **2009**, *9*, 2492–2499. [CrossRef]
60. Brittain, H.G. Vibrational Spectroscopic Studies of Cocrystals and Salts. 2. The Benzylamine−Benzoic Acid System. *Cryst. Growth Des.* **2009**, *9*, 3497–3503. [CrossRef]
61. Smith, B.C. Organic nitrogen compounds V: Amine salts. *Spectroscopy* **2019**, *34*, 30–37.
62. Kundu, S.; Kumari, N.; Soni, S.R.; Ranjan, S.; Kumar, R.; Sharon, A.; Ghosh, A. Enhanced Solubility of Telmisartan Phthalic Acid Cocrystals within the pH Range of a Systemic Absorption Site. *ACS Omega* **2018**, *3*, 15380–15388. [CrossRef] [PubMed]

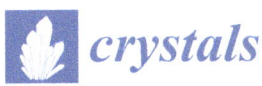

Article

Crystal Structure of Novel Terephthalate Salt of Antiarrhythmic Drug Disopyramide

Majid Ismail Tamboli [†], Yohei Utusmi [†], Takayuki Furuishi *, Kaori Fukuzawa and Etsuo Yonemochi *

Department of Physical Chemistry, School of Pharmacy and Pharmaceutical Sciences, Hoshi University, 2-4-41 Ebara, Shinagawa-ku, Tokyo 142-8501, Japan; t-majid@hoshi.ac.jp (M.I.T.); s172504@hoshi.ac.jp (Y.U.); k-fukuzawa@hoshi.ac.jp (K.F.)
* Correspondence: t-furuishi@hoshi.ac.jp (T.F.); e-yonemochi@hoshi.ac.jp (E.Y.); Tel.: +81-3-5498-5159 (T.F.); +81-3-5498-5048 (E.Y.)
† Co-first author, these authors contributed equally to this work.

Abstract: 1:1 salt of Disopyramide (DPA) with Terephthalic acid (TA) was obtained by the slow solvent evaporation and the slurry crystallization methods. X-ray single crystal diffraction of DPA:TA confirmed the formation of salt by the transfer of an acidic proton from one of the carboxylic acidic groups of TA to the tertiary amino group of the chain moiety (N3-nitrogen atom) of the DPA molecules. DPA:TA salt crystals crystalize in the triclinic system with space group P-1. The asymmetric unit, comprising one protonated DPA and one TA anion, are linked by a strong charge assisted N^+–H$\cdots$O$^-$ hydrogen bond and a C–H$\cdots$O$^-$ hydrogen bond. Moreover, structural characterization of DPA:TA salt was carried out using Fourier transform infrared spectroscopy, differential scanning calorimeter, thermogravimetric analysis, and powder X-ray diffraction techniques

Keywords: Disopyramide; Terephthalic acid; salt; crystal structure; molecular packing; slurry crystallization

Citation: Tamboli, M.I.; Utusmi, Y.; Furuishi, T.; Fukuzawa, K.; Yonemochi, E. Crystal Structure of Novel Terephthalate Salt of Antiarrhythmic Drug Disopyramide. *Crystals* **2021**, *11*, 368. https://doi.org/10.3390/cryst11040368

Academic Editor: Sławomir J. Grabowski

Received: 28 February 2021
Accepted: 28 March 2021
Published: 31 March 2021

Publisher's Note: MDPI stays neutral with regard to jurisdictional claims in published maps and institutional affiliations.

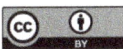

Copyright: © 2021 by the authors. Licensee MDPI, Basel, Switzerland. This article is an open access article distributed under the terms and conditions of the Creative Commons Attribution (CC BY) license (https:// creativecommons.org/licenses/by/ 4.0/).

1. Introduction

Crystal engineering deals with the study of non-covalent interactions within crystals, the understanding of crystal structures, and the design and synthesis of new solids with desired and specific properties by utilizing the hydrogen bond, supramolecular synthon strategy [1–5]. Crystal engineering approaches have been used in the preparation of novel solid active forms of pharmaceutical ingredients (APIs), for improving the physicochemical properties of drug molecules by making multi-component crystals, such as solvates [6], cocrystals [7–9], and salts [10]. In the supramolecular synthon strategy in the pharmaceutical field, salt formation of APIs remains a potential method to improve the solubility and stability of native APIs.

Disopyramide (2-diisopropylaminoethyl)-phenyl-2-pyridineacetamide) (DPA) is a class IA antiarrhythmic drug [11] that shows polymorphism behavior [12]. Disopyramide and its phosphate salt are intravenously and orally administrated for clinical use [13,14]. There is very limited research on the crystal engineering of DPA available in the literature [15], and there are only limited DPA phosphate salt [16] crystal structures of solid forms of DPA to be found in the Cambridge Structural Database (CSD). DPA has a basic nature and is likely to form salts/cocrystal adduct with different cofomers that have acid functionality. Moreover, DPA has a flexible molecular framework, with a hydrogen bond donor and acceptor site, and can adopt different orientations or conformations in the novel solid form; hence, from a crystal engineering viewpoint, DPA could be a molecules that has the potential for the exploration of different solid forms by the use of crystal engineering principles.

With this in mind, our intention is to explore the novel solid form of DPA by using different acidic coformers and to see their effect on the conformation of DPA and molecular packing in crystal structures, because there is only one crystal structure of DPA phosphate salt reported by Kawamura and Hirayama [16] in the CSD. In the current study, we have selected Terephthalic acid (TA) as the salt former, which has a para disubstituted carboxyl group on the benzene ring (Figure 1). In this article, we discuss the preparation method of DPA:TA salt and carry out X-ray single-crystal structural analysis; the obtained new salt was further evaluated by solid-state characterization.

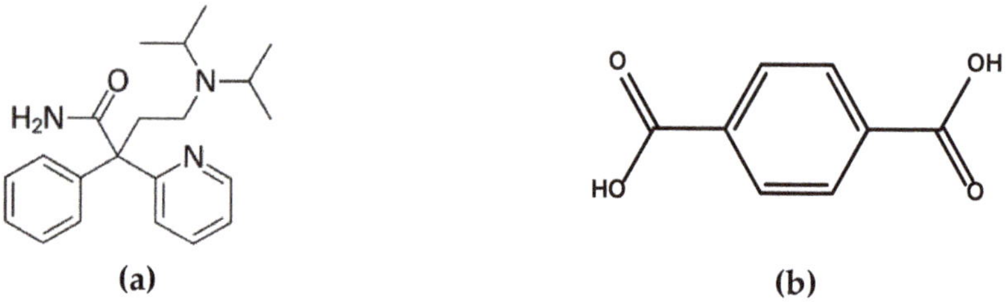

Figure 1. Structures of (**a**) racemic Disopyramide (DPA) and (**b**) Terephthalic acid (TA).

2. Materials and Methods

2.1. Materials

DPA and TA were purchased from Tokyo Chemical Industry Co. Ltd. (Tokyo, Japan). All other analytical-grade solvents and reagents were commercially obtained and used without further purification.

2.2. Crystallization of DPA:TA Salt

2.2.1. Slow Evaporation Method

For X-ray single-crystal structure analysis, DPA (0.5 mmole) and TA (0.5 mmole) in a 1:1 molar ratio were ground in a mortar and pestle for 10 min to obtain a fine powder, then a few drops of ethanol were added to it, before grinding again for 10–15 min to obtain a powder. From this, 50 mg was used for the crystallization experiment. Colorless single crystals suitable for single crystal X-ray diffraction were obtained by dissolving the 50 mg of ground material in 15 mL acetonitrile and 5 mL ethanol under sonication at a temperature of 50 °C for 1h. The resulting solution, obtained after filtration, was left for slow evaporation at ambient conditions for 4–6 weeks to obtain a long plate-like crystal, which was stuck on the wall of the flask.

2.2.2. Slurry Method

Reproducing the salt crystal was found to be difficult, so another method for crystallization was used. Luckily, similar solid salt is easily obtained by the slurry method. One mmole each of DPA and TA were weighed at a molar ratio of 1:1 and suspended in 50 mL acetonitrile in a 250 mL conical flask. The resulting suspension was stirred in a magnetic stirrer at 25 °C, 500 rpm for about 36 h until a white solid material precipitated out. The resulting suspension was filtered to isolate the white solid, which was then air dried for 5–6 days at ambient conditions before being used for further analysis. Powder X-ray diffraction (PXRD) patterns of the isolated solids matched the simulated PXRD pattern obtained from single crystal data DPA:TA, suggesting that both were the same solid form.

2.3. Single-Crystal X-ray Diffraction

The single-crystal X-ray diffraction data for DPA:TA salt was collected at 93 K. The measurements were carried out in ω-scan mode with an R-AXIS RAPID II (Rigaku Co., Tokyo, Japan) with the Cu-Kα X-ray obtained from rotating the anode source with a graphite monochromator. The integrated and scaled data were empirically corrected for absorption effects using ABSCOR [17,18]. The structures were solved by direct methods using SHELXS and refinement was carried out by full-matrix least-squares technique using SHELXL [19,20]. All non-hydrogen atoms were refined anisotropically. The hydrogen atom attached to the nitrogen N2, N3, and O4 atoms in the DPA:TA salt were located using the differential Fourier map and refined isotropically. All other hydrogen atom positions were calculated geometrically and included in the calculation using the riding atom model.

The molecular figures were produced and prepared using Mercury 4.1.0 software [21]. CCDC 2065287 contains the supplementary crystallographic data for the DPA:TA salt and can be obtained free of charge from the Cambridge Crystallographic Data Centre via www.ccdc.cam.ac.uk/data_request/cif (accessed on 28 March 2021).

2.4. PXRD

The PXRD patterns of the DPA:TA samples were measured in the reflectance mode using a SmartLab diffractometer (Cu Kα source (40 kV and 200 mA), D/teX ultra-high-speed position-sensitive detector, Rigaku, Tokyo, Japan). Diffraction patterns (2θ) were collected from 5° to 40° at 25°C with a step of 0.01° and a scan speed of 20°/min.

2.5. Fourier Transform Infrared Spectroscopy (FT-IR)

The infrared spectra of all samples were measured using FT-IR (FT-IR- 4200 spectrometer, JASCO Co., Tokyo, Japan) with an attenuated total reflection (ATR) unit (ATR-PRO 670H-S, JASCO Co., Tokyo, Japan). The recorded spectrum represents an average of 64 scans obtained with a resolution of 4 cm^{-1} at room temperature. The spectra were collected in wavenumbers ranging from 4000 to 400 cm^{-1}. The internal reflectance element used in this study was a diamond trapezoid having 45° entrance and exit faces.

2.6. Differential Scanning Calorimetry (DSC) and Thermogravimetric (TG) Measurements

DSC and TG measurements were recorded with a Thermo plus EVO2-DSC 8230 and a Thermo plus EVO2-TG8120 TG-DTA, respectively (Rigaku Co., Tokyo, Japan). The DSC sample (~3 mg) was placed into an aluminum-crimped pan and the TG sample (~4–5 mg) was placed into an aluminum-open pan, and both were measured at a speed of 5°C/min from 25 to 300°C under nitrogen gas (flow rate = 50 and 100 L/min, respectively).

3. Results and Discussion

3.1. Crystal Structure of DPA:TA Salt

TA and DPA in a 1:1 molar ratio were crystallized from acetonitrile and ethanol mixtures at ambient condition by slow solvent evaporation to obtain a colorless long plate crystal suitable for X-ray analysis. The X-ray single-crystal structure confirmed the formation of DPA:TA salt with approximately similar C–O bond lengths of C28-O2, 1.2538 (19), C28-O3, 1.268 (2), Å of the (COO$^-$) carboxylate group of TA (Figure 2a). These similarities in the bond length of C–O confirmed the transfer of an acidic proton from one of the carboxylic acidic group of TA to the N3-nitrogen atom of the tertiary amino group (chain moiety) of DPA.

DPA:TA salt crystallized in the centrosymmetric triclinic P-1 space group containing one protonated DPA and one TA anion in the asymmetric unit revealed that the molecular salt is in the 1:1 molar ratio. The salt pair, i.e., the protonated DPA and TA anion in the asymmetric unit linked by a strong charge, assisted the N3$^+$–H3A···O2$^-$ hydrogen bond and the C9–H9···O3$^-$ hydrogen bond. In the crystal structure of DPA:TA salt, protonated DPA displays an intramolecular N2-H2A···N1 hydrogen bond by donating second amide hydrogen N–H to the N-atom of 2-pyridine moiety in the $S^1_1(6)$ ring motif, along with other C-H···O intramolecular interactions, namely C15-H15B···O1 and C17-H17B···O1, which stabilize the conformation protonated DPA molecules in the salt, as shown in Figure 2a. The crystallographic information and geometrical parameters for the hydrogen bonding interaction are summarized in Tables 1 and 2.

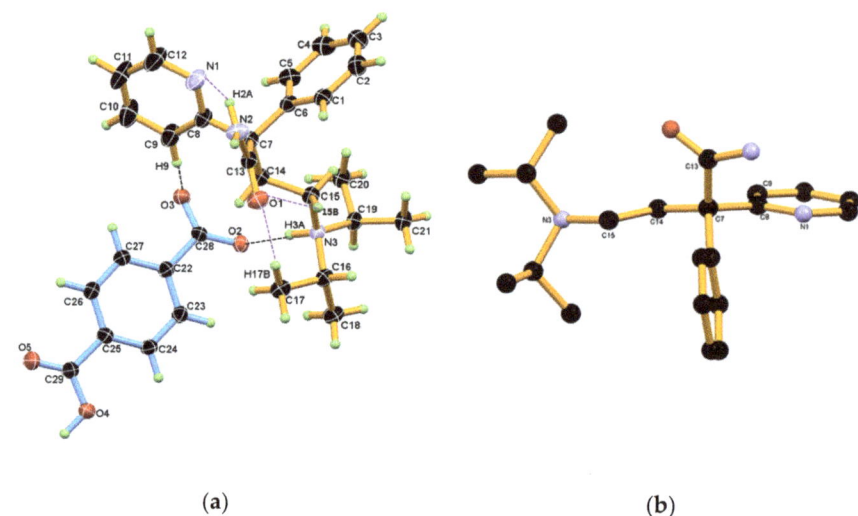

(a) (b)

Figure 2. (**a**) ORTEP diagram of DPA:TA salt showing the atom numbering scheme. The thermal ellipsoid is drawn at 50% probability level, and H-atoms are shown as small spheres with arbitrary radii. The association between the salt pair in the asymmetric unit of DPA:TA salt is shown by the black dotted line and, in this association, only the carboxylate group of TA is involved. Protonated DPA in salt displaying the intramolecular N2-H2A···N1, C15-H15B···O1, C17-H17B···O1 hydrogen bond is shown by the purple dotted line. (**b**) Conformation of protonated DPA in salt and torsional angle τ_1—C7-C14-C15-N3, τ_2—C8-C7-C14-C15, τ_3 –C9-C8-C7-C14, τ_4—C13-C7-C14-C15.

Table 1. Crystallographic data table for the DPA:TA salt.

Parameters	DPA:TA
Empirical formula	$C_{29}H_{35}N_3O_5$
Formula weight	505.60
Temperature	93(2) K
Wavelength	1.54187 Å
Crystal system	Triclinic
Space group	P-1
Unit cell dimensions	a = 8.6855(2) Å, α = 100.640(7) °.
	b = 9.7036(3) Å, β = 103.230(7) °
	c = 17.1705(4) Å, γ = 91.205(6) °
Volume	1381.48(8) Å^3
Z, Z'	2.1
Density (calculated)	1.215 g/cm^3
Absorption coefficient	0.676 mm^{-1}
F (000)	540.0
Crystal size	0.460 × 0.420 × 0.220 mm^3
Theta range for data collection	4.647 to 68.224°.
Index ranges	$-10 \leq h \leq 10, -11 \leq k \leq 11, -20 \leq l \leq 20$
Reflections collected	16230
Independent reflections	4955 [R_{int} = 0.0307, R_{sigma} = 0.0411]
Completeness to theta = 67.687°	98.1 %
Absorption correction	Semi-empirical from equivalents
Max. and min. transmission	0.862 and 0.67
Refinement method	Full-matrix least-squares on F^2
Data/restraints/parameters	4955/0/354
Goodness-of-fit on F^2	1.078
Final R indices [I>2sigma(I)]	R_1 = 0.0478, wR_2 = 0.1280
R indices (all data)	R_1 = 0.0555, wR_2 = 0.1337
$\Delta\rho_{max}, \Delta\rho_{min}$	0.32/−0.25e. Å^{-3}

Table 2. Geometrical parameters of the hydrogen bond interaction in DPA:TA salt.

D-H···A	D-H (Å)	H···A (Å)	D···A (Å)	D-H···A (°)	Symmetry Codes
N2-H2A···N1	0.934(19)	2.076(18)	2.783(3)	131.4(16)	Intramolecular
N2-H2B···O1	0.88(2)	2.00(2)	2.876(2)	176(2)	$2-x, 1-y, 1-z$
N3-H3A···O2	0.946(18)	1.821(18)	2.7617(18)	172.5(17)	x, y, z
O4-H4A···O3	0.96(3)	1.57(3)	2.5211(18)	176(2)	$x, -1+y, z$
C9-H9···O3	0.95	2.58	3.389(2)	143	x, y, z
C15-H15B···O1	0.99	2.41	3.008(2)	118	Intramolecular
C16-H16···O3	1.00	2.50	3.499(2)	176	$1+x, y, z$
C17-H17B···O1	0.98	2.49	3.469(2)	173	Intramolecular
C20-H20B···O4	0.98	2.48	3.344(2)	147	$x, 1+y, z$
C21-H21C···O5	0.98	2.57	3.478(2)	154	$1+x, 1+y, z$
C19-H19···O2	1.00	2.609	3.2976(18)	126.02	$1-x, 1-y, -z$
C20-H20C···O2	0.98	2.693	3.3375(19)	123.65	$1-x, 1-y, -z$

In the DPA:TA salt, DPA adopts conformation, where the 2-pyridine ring moiety is roughly coplanar with the chain moiety (excluding the iso-propyl moiety), and the phenyl moiety is oriented roughly perpendicular to the planar part, as shown in Figure 2b. In the DPA:TA salt, the torsional angle τ_1 179.38, τ_2 170.70 suggests planarity in the backbone chain, and torsional angle τ_3 (12.75) suggests slight twist in the coplanarity between the chain moiety and the 2-pyridine moiety.

The dihedral angle between the phenyl and pyridine rings is 78.76(10) in DPA:TA salt, suggesting a nearly perpendicular orientation. However, the torsional value τ_4 (−71.52) is for the orientation of the amide group, with the planar part also being roughly perpendicular.

In the crystal structure of DPA:TA salt, two inversion-symmetry related protonated DPA molecules form an amide homodimer synthon via a pair of strong N-H···O hydrogen bonds in the $R^2_2(8)$ ring motif, and they are listed in Table 2. In this dimeric association, protonated DPA donates amide hydrogen N2–H2B to the amide C=O1 oxygen of inversion-symmetry related protonated DPA molecules in the dimeric N2–H2B···O1 hydrogen bond, whereas the second hydrogen of amide N2–H2A engaged in the intramolecular N2–H2A···N1 nitrogen bonds with the N1-atom of the 2-pyridine moiety in the $S^1_1(6)$ ring motif. This homodimer of protonated DPA molecules were linked to two TA anion via a strong charge assisted $N3^+$–H3A···$O2^−$ hydrogen bond and the C9–H9···$O3^−$ interaction to form a centrosymmetric dimeric unit comprising two protonated DPA and two TA anion, as shown in Figure 3a. In this association, N^+3–H3A (protonated tertiary amino nitrogen) hydrogen of the protonated DPA donates hydrogen to carboxylate ($COO^−$) O2-oxygen of the TA anion in the $N3^+$–H3A···$O2^−$ hydrogen bond, and the C9–H9 Hydrogen of the 2-pyridine moiety donates hydrogen to carboxylate ($COO^−$) O3-oxygen of the TA anion in the C9–H9···O3 interaction. Thus, in this association, both carboxylate ($COO^−$) O2-, O3-oxygen of TA anion are engaged in hydrogen bonding with protonated DPA molecules, as shown in Figure 3a. The closely associated TA anion forms a one-dimensional (1D) chain using a linear and strong O4–H4A···$O3^−$ hydrogen bond, as shown in Figure 3b.

Such dimeric units are extended through linear and strong O4–H4A···$O3^−$ and short and non-linear C20–H20B···O4 hydrogen bonds with the neighboring unit translated dimeric units along the b-axis to generate a ladder-like network where the protonated DPA dimer units join the 1D chains of the TA anion, as shown in Figure 4. In this association, the $O3^−$ oxygen atom of the carboxylate anion of TA accepts hydrogen from the carboxyl OH (O4–H4A) of the neighboring unit translated TA anion in the O4–H4A···$O3^−$ hydrogen bond along the b-axis. Whereas, in turn, carboxyl hydroxyl (O4–H4A) O4-oxygen accept C20–H20B hydrogen of unit translated protonated DPA molecules in short and non-linear C20–H20B···O4 hydrogen bonds.

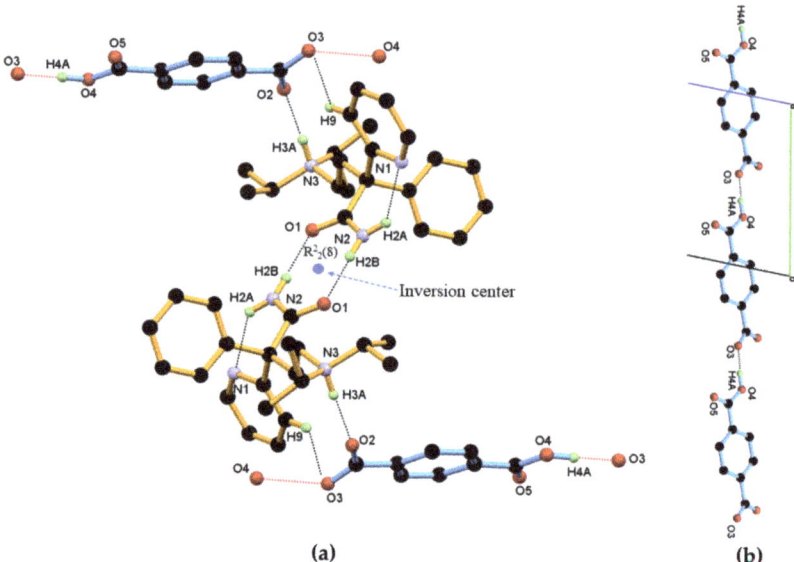

Figure 3. (**a**) Dimeric unit of DPA:TA salt. In this, the inversion center related asymmetric unit of DPA:TA extends through the N−H···O hydrogen bond in the $R^2_2(8)$ ring motif in *ac*-diagonally. (**b**) TA anion linked to neighboring unit translated TA anion through a strong and linear O4−H4A···O3$^-$ hydrogen bond to form a one-dimensional (1D) chain of TA anion alon the *b*-axis. Dotted lines indicate the non-covalent interaction (hydrogen atoms not involved in the hydrogen bonding were removed for clarity).

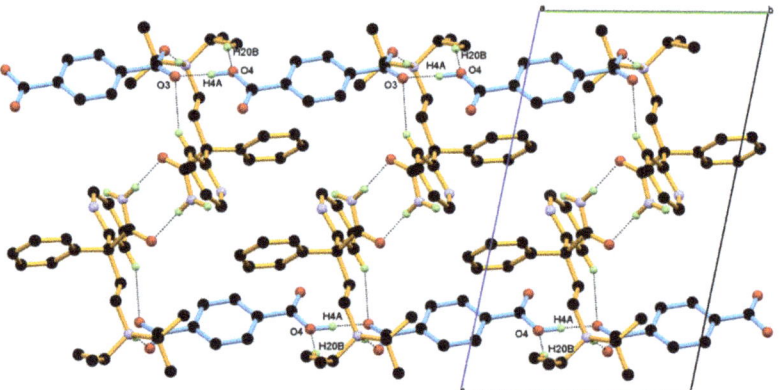

Figure 4. Linking of neighboring unit translated dimeric units along the *b*-axis through O4−H4···O3$^-$ and C20−H20B···O4 hydrogen bonding interaction to form a ladder structure along the *b*-axis. In this packing, the protonated DPA dimer is held between the 1D chain of the TA anion.

Such 1D chains of dimeric units (ladder-like structures), assembled along the *a*-axis to generate two-dimensional (2D) layer packing through C16−H16···O3$^-$, C21−H21C···O5 interaction, generate a 2D layer. In this association, the *iso*-propyl moiety of protonated DPA molecules are involved in C−H···O hydrogen bonding by donating C16−H16 and C21−H21 hydrogen to the carboxylate oxygen O3 and carboxyl (C=O5) oxygen of the neighboring 1D chain of dimeric units along the *a*-axis, as shown in Figure 5a. Whereas the packing of such 1D chains of dimeric units (ladder-like structures) along the *ac*-diagonal are done through relatively weak and longer C−H···O interaction by donating C19−H19 and C20–H20 hydrogen of the *iso*-propyl moiety of protonated DPA molecules to the carboxylate oxygen O2 of the TA anion from the neighboring 1D chain of dimeric units through C19–H19···O2⁻ and C20–H20C···O2⁻ interaction, as shown in Figure 5b.

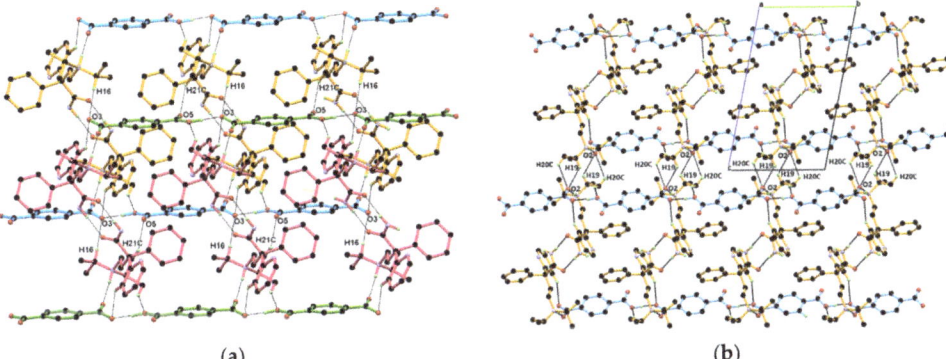

Figure 5. Packing of the 1D dimeric unit chain (**a**) along the *a*-axis through C16–H16···O3⁻, C21–H21C···O5 interaction to generate a two-dimensional (2D) layer (**b**) along the *ac*-diagonal through C19–H19···O2⁻ and C20–H20C···O2⁻ interaction to generate a 2D layer.

Packing the view down the *b*-axis, in this packing, the dimeric unit is associated with the neighboring dimeric unit along the *a*-axis (parallel to the *ac*-diagonal) through short C16–H16···O3⁻ interaction; in this association, the *iso*-propyl moiety of the protonated DPA donates C16–H16 hydrogen to the carboxylate O3-oxygen of the TA anion of the neighboring dimeric unit. Whereas, along the *ac*-diagonal dimeric unit, the DPA:TA associated centrosymmetric combine with the neighboring dimeric unit through relatively weaker and longer C–H···O interactions by donating C19–H19 and C20–H20C hydrogen of the *iso*-propyl moiety of the protonated DPA molecules to the carboxylate O2-oxygen of the TA anion from the neighboring dimeric unit through C19–H19···O2⁻ and C20–H20C···O2⁻ interactions, as shown in Figure 6. Packing of the 1D chain of dimeric units in the *ac*-plane creates a solvent assessable void and void space ~22 Å³ per molecule (asymmetric unit) in the unit cell, calculated by using the contact surface from Mercury 2020, 2.0 software.

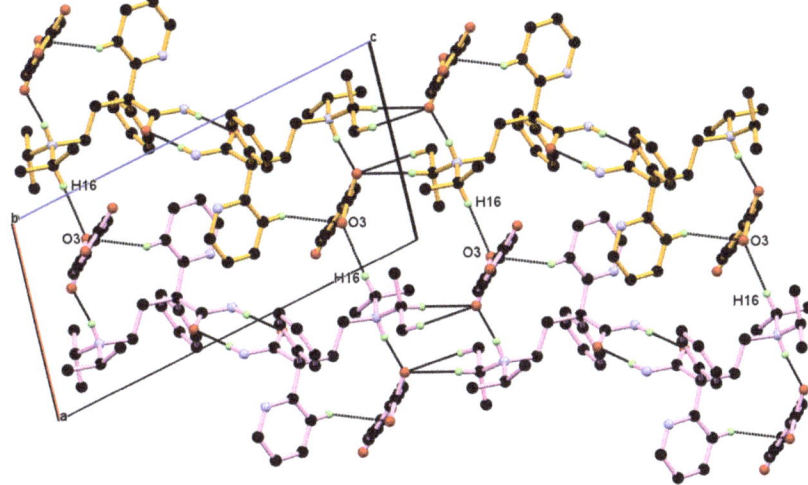

Figure 6. Packing of dimeric unit view down the *b*-axis. The neighboring dimeric unit is associated through C–H···O interaction.

3.2. Characterization of DPA:TA Salt

3.2.1. PXRD

The PXRD patterns were recorded for commercially available DPA, TA, and DPA:TA crystals obtained from slow solvent evaporation and DPA:TA salt obtained from the slurry method. The PXRD pattern of the salt is different from the DPA component, suggesting the formation of a new crystalline phase in the solid-state. (Figure 7). Furthermore, the peak position of the experimental PXRD pattern obtained from the slow solvent evaporation and the slurry method matched well with the simulated PXRD pattern obtained from the single-crystal X-ray structure, confirming the homogeneity of the sample and ruling out the presence of another phase. It also confirms that the single-crystal structure is representative of the bulk and that there is no phase transition between 93 K (at which the single-crystal structure was determined) and room temperature (at which the powder pattern was measured). The subtle differences could be due to the different data collection temperatures (for powder and a single crystal). Thus, a PXRD analysis of samples obtained by the slurring of DPA and TA in acetonitrile at 25 °C is matched very well to the DPA:TA salt obtained from the slow evaporation methods, which indicated a similar solid form of salt DPA:TA obtained from both methods.

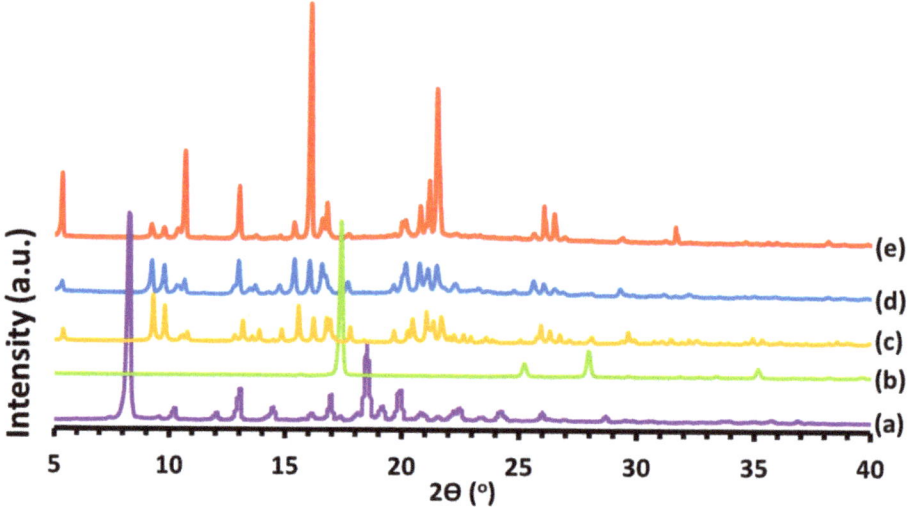

Figure 7. Powder X-ray diffraction (PXRD) patterns of (**a**) commercial DPA, (**b**) TA, (**c**) simulated DPA:TA, (**d**) DPA:TA salt obtained from slurry method, and (**e**) DPA:TA salt obtained from slow solvent evaporation.

3.2.2. FT-IR Spectrum

FT-IR is a very important and useful techniques for detecting the formation of salt by the typical carboxylate anion present in spectra (Figure 8). Due to changes in the hydrogen bonding patterns of a molecule in salt or a co-crystal, there are resulting changes in the IR frequencies of vibrations associated with the functional groups. The changes in IR frequencies suggest changes in hydrogen bonding pattern. Examination of FT-IR spectra could confirm salt formation due to the transfer of acidic hydrogen TA to DPA.

FT-IR spectra were obtained for commercially pure DPA, prepared DPA:TA crystal, pure TA, and DPA:TA salt obtained from the slurry method. Commercially pure DPA demonstrated characteristic peaks, amide N-H stretching at 3263 cm^{-1}, amide C=O stretching, and NH$_2$ deformation overlap peak at 1664 cm^{-1}, and in TA spectra presently peak at 1671 due to C=O stretching and broad band around 2800 cm^{-1}, attributed to the carboxylic OH group [22]. Whereas the spectra of salt give many characteristic peaks as 3350, 3149,

1679, and 1589 cm^{-1} that are different from the starting component DPA and TA shown in Figure 8.

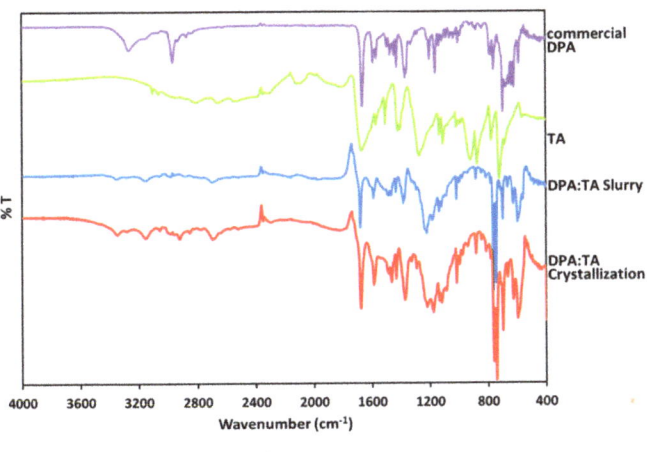

(a)

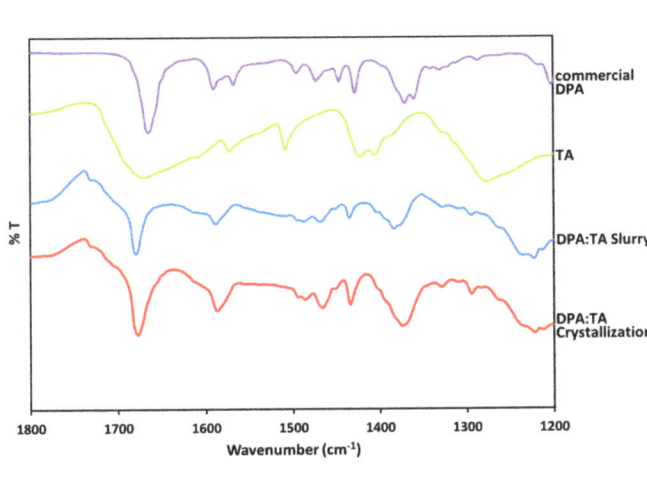

(b)

Figure 8. FT-IR spectra, (**a**) 4000–400 cm^{-1} and (**b**) 1800–1200 cm^{-1}, of commercial DPA, TA, and DPA:TA salt obtained from the slurry method and DPA:TA salt obtained from the slow evaporation method.

Thus, in DPA:TA salt, the spectrum peaks at 1589 cm^{-1}; where the carboxylate group is observed respectively and is not present in the spectrum of the individual components, which indicates a proton transfer from the salt former TA to DPA, confirming salt formation between DPA and TA.

3.2.3. Thermal Properties

The thermal behavior of the DPA:TA was measured by DSG and TG. DPA:TA salt, exhibits a sharp, single endothermic peak at around 181 °C, corresponding to melting point of salt in DSC (Figure 9). It has been reported that there are two melting points of DPA; a low-melting type crystal (85–87 °C) and a high-melting type crystal (95–98 °C) [12], and TA melted with sublimation at around 350 °C [23–25]. DPA:TA showed a different melting point from each starting materials, suggesting that DPA:TA is a novel salt. TG data of DPA:TA revealed that there was no weight loss before melting, which confirmed the absence of any solvent or hydrate in the crystal lattice, as per the single crystal data.

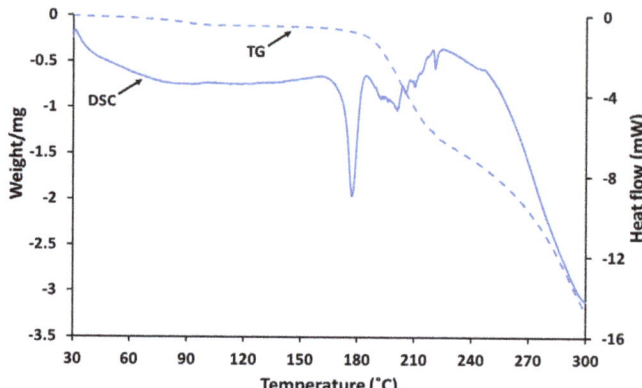

Figure 9. DSC and TG profiles of DPA:TA salt obtained from the slow evaporation method.

4. Conclusions

1:1 DPA:TA salt crystals were obtained from the slow evaporation method, and its crystal structure belongs to the triclinic P-1 space group. The asymmetric unit of 1:1 DPA:TA salt contains one protonated DPA and one TA anion.

In the crystal structure of DPA:TA salt, two inversion symmetry related protonated DPA molecules formed an amide homodimer through a N-H···O hydrogen bond in the $R^2_2(8)$ ring motifs, and such a dimer is hydrogen bonded to two TA anions through charge assisted N^+-H···O^- and C-H···O^- hydrogen bonds to form a basic centrosymmetric dimeric unit, comprising two protonated DPA and two TA anions. Furthermore, such a dimeric unit linked to a unit translated neighboring dimeric unit along the b-axis through an $O3^-$···H4-O4 hydrogen bond between carboxylate O3-oxygen and the carboxyl (O-H) of the next TA anion along the b-axis results in a one-dimensional chain, which is further supported by C20-H20B···O4 interaction between DPA and TA. Such a 1D chain assembled along the a-axis through C16-H16···$O3^-$ and C21-H21C···O5 interaction generates a two-dimensional structure. Such a 2D layer structure, assembled centrosymmetrically along the c-axis through relatively weaker C-H···O interactions, results in a 3D layer in the ac-plane.

Author Contributions: Conceptualization, M.I.T.; formal analysis, M.I.T. and Y.U.; investigation, M.I.T. and Y.U.; writing–original draft preparation, M.I.T. and T.F.; writing–review and editing, T.F. and E.Y.; visualization, M.I.T., Y.U., and T.F.; funding acquisition, T.F.; supervision, K.F. and E.Y.; project administration, T.F., K.F., and E.Y. All authors have read and agreed to the published version of the manuscript.

Funding: This study was supported by the Mochida Memorial Foundation for Medical and Pharmaceutical Research 2019-2020 (to T.F.).

Conflicts of Interest: The authors declare no conflict of interest.

References

1. Desiraju, G.R. Supramolecular Synthons in Crystal Engineering—A New Organic Synthesis. *Angew. Chem. Int. Ed. Engl.* **1995**, *34*, 2311–2327. [CrossRef]
2. Berry, D.J.; Steed, J.W. Pharmaceutical cocrystals, salts and multicomponent systems; intermolecular interactions and property based design. *Adv. Drug Deliv. Rev.* **2017**, *117*, 3–24. [CrossRef]

3. Martins, I.C.B.; Sardo, M.; Santos, S.M.; Fernandes, A.; Antunes, A.; André, V.; Mafra, L.; Duarte, M.T. Packing Interactions and Physicochemical Properties of Novel Multicomponent Crystal Forms of the Anti-Inflammatory Azelaic Acid Studied by X-ray and Solid-State NMR. *Cryst. Growth Des.* **2015**, *16*, 154–166. [CrossRef]
4. Corpinot, M.K.; Bučar, D.-K. A Practical Guide to the Design of Molecular Crystals. *Cryst. Growth Des.* **2018**, *19*, 1426–1453. [CrossRef]
5. Desiraju, G.R. *Crystal Engineering: The Design of Organic Solids*; Elsevier: Amsterdam, The Netherlands; New York, NY, USA, 1989.
6. Bezerra, B.P.; Pogoda, D.; Perry, M.L.; Vidal, L.M.T.; Zaworotko, M.J.; Ayala, A.P. Cocrystal Polymorphs and Solvates of the Anti-Trypanosoma cruzi Drug Benznidazole with Improved Dissolution Performance. *Cryst. Growth Des.* **2020**, *20*, 4707–4718. [CrossRef]
7. Karimi-Jafari, M.; Padrela, L.; Walker, G.M.; Croker, D.M. Creating Cocrystals: A Review of Pharmaceutical Cocrystal Preparation Routes and Applications. *Cryst. Growth Des.* **2018**, *18*, 6370–6387. [CrossRef]
8. Schultheiss, N.; Newman, A. Pharmaceutical Cocrystals and Their Physicochemical Properties. *Cryst. Growth Des.* **2009**, *9*, 2950–2967. [CrossRef]
9. Yousef, M.A.E.; Vangala, V.R. Pharmaceutical Cocrystals: Molecules, Crystals, Formulations, Medicines. *Cryst. Growth Des.* **2019**, *19*, 7420–7438. [CrossRef]
10. Gunnam, A.; Nangia, A.K. High-Solubility Salts of the Multiple Sclerosis Drug Teriflunomide. *Cryst. Growth Des.* **2019**, *19*, 5407–5417. [CrossRef]
11. Katz, M.J.; Meyer, C.E.; El-Etr, A.; Slodki, S.J. Clinical evaluation of a new anti-arrhythmic agent, SC-7031. *Curr. Ther. Res. Clin. Exp.* **1963**, *5*, 343–350. [PubMed]
12. Gunning, S.R.; Freeman, M.; Stead, J.A. Polymorphism of disopyramide. *J. Pharm Pharm.* **1976**, *28*, 758–761. [CrossRef]
13. Rizos, I.; Brachmann, J.; Lengfelder, W.; Schmitt, C.; von Olshausen, K.; Kubler, W.; Senges, J. Effects of intravenous disopyramide and quinidine on normal myocardium and on the characteristics of arrhythmias: Intraindividual comparison in patients with sustained ventricular tachycardia. *Eur. Heart J.* **1987**, *8*, 154–163. [CrossRef]
14. Kim, S.Y.; Benowitz, N.L. Poisoning due to class IA antiarrhythmic drugs. Quinidine, procainamide and disopyramide. *Drug Saf.* **1990**, *5*, 393–420. [CrossRef] [PubMed]
15. Burke, T.R., Jr.; Nelson, W.L.; Mangion, M.; Hite, G.J.; Mokler, C.M.; Ruenitz, P.C. Resolution, absolute configuration, and antiarrhythmic properties of the enantiomers of disopyramide, 4-(diisopropylamino)-2-(2-pyridyl)-2-phenylbutyramide. *J. Med. Chem.* **1980**, *23*, 1044–1048. [CrossRef]
16. Kawamura, T.; Hirayama, N. Crystal structure of α-diisopropylaminoethyl-α-phenylpyridine-2-acetamide phosphate, [C21H30N3O][H2PO4]. *Z. Krist. New Cryst. Struct.* **2011**, *226*, 479. [CrossRef]
17. Higashi, T. *Calculated Using ABSCOR: Empirical Absorption Correction Based on Fourier Series Approximation*; Rigaku: The Woodland, TX, USA, 1994.
18. Messerschmidt, A.; Schneider, M.; Huber, R. ABSCOR: A scaling and absorption correction program for the FAST area detector diffractometer. *J. Appl. Crystallogr.* **1990**, *23*, 436–439. [CrossRef]
19. Sheldrick, G.M. SHELXT—Integrated space-group and crystal-structure determination. *Acta Cryst. A Found. Adv.* **2015**, *71*, 3–8. [CrossRef]
20. Sheldrick, G.M. Crystal structure refinement with SHELXL. *Acta Cryst. C Struct. Chem* **2015**, *71*, 3–8. [CrossRef]
21. Macrae, C.F.; Bruno, I.J.; Chisholm, J.A.; Edgington, P.R.; McCabe, P.; Pidcock, E.; Rodriguez-Monge, L.; Taylor, R.; van de Streek, J.; Wood, P.A. Mercury CSD 2.0– new features for the visualization and investigation of crystal structures. *J. Appl. Crystallogr.* **2008**, *41*, 466–470. [CrossRef]
22. Pavia, D.L.; Lampman, G.M.; Kriz, G.S.; Vyvyan, J.A. *Introduction to Spectroscopy*; Cengage Learning: Boston, MA, USA, 2014.
23. Elmas Kimyonok, A.B.; Ulutürk, M. Determination of the Thermal Decomposition Products of Terephthalic Acid by Using Curie-Point Pyrolyzer. *J. Energetic Mater.* **2015**, *34*, 113–122. [CrossRef]
24. Machado Cruz, R.; Boleslavska, T.; Beranek, J.; Tieger, E.; Twamley, B.; Santos-Martinez, M.J.; Dammer, O.; Tajber, L. Identification and Pharmaceutical Characterization of a New Itraconazole Terephthalic Acid Cocrystal. *Pharmaceutics* **2020**, *12*, 741. [CrossRef] [PubMed]
25. Ma, Y.-H.; Ge, S.-W.; Wang, W.; Sun, B.-W. Studies on the synthesis, structural characterization, Hirshfeld analysis and stability of apovincamine (API) and its co-crystal (terephthalic acid: Apovincamine=1:2). *J. Mol. Struct.* **2015**, *1097*, 87–97. [CrossRef]

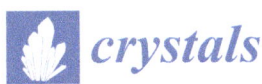

Article

New Crystal Forms for Biologically Active Compounds. Part 2: Anastrozole as N-Substituted 1,2,4-Triazole in Halogen Bonding and Lp-π Interactions with 1,4-Diiodotetrafluorobenzene

Mariya A. Kryukova, Alexander V. Sapegin, Alexander S. Novikov, Mikhail Krasavin and Daniil M. Ivanov *

Institute of Chemistry, Saint Petersburg State University, Universitetskaya Nab. 7/9, 199034 Saint Petersburg, Russia; mary_kryukova@mail.ru (M.A.K.); sapegin_yar@mail.ru (A.V.S.); ja2-88@mail.ru (A.S.N.); krasavintm@gmail.com (M.K.)
* Correspondence: st024644@student.spbu.ru

Received: 28 March 2020; Accepted: 2 May 2020; Published: 5 May 2020

Abstract: For an active pharmaceutical ingredient, it is important to stabilize its specific crystal polymorph. If the potential interconversion of various polymorphs is not carefully controlled, it may lead to deterioration of the drug's physicochemical profile and, ultimately, its therapeutic efficacy. The desired polymorph stabilization can be achieved via co-crystallization with appropriate crystallophoric excipients. In this work, we identified an opportunity for co-crystallization of anastrozole (**ASZ**), a well-known aromatase inhibitor useful in second-line therapy of estrogen-dependent breast cancer, with a classical XB donor, 1,2,4,5-tetrafluoro-3,6-diiodobenzene (**1,4-FIB**). In the X-ray structures of **ASZ**·1.5 (**1,4-FIB**) co-crystal, different non-covalent interactions involving hydrogen and halogen atoms were detected and studied by quantum chemical calculations and QTAIM analysis at the ωB97XD/DZP-DKH level of theory.

Keywords: anastrozole; non-covalent interactions; halogen bonding; lp-π interactions; DFT; QTAIM

1. Introduction

The generation of a new salt form is a proven way to modify the physical and chemical properties of an active pharmaceutical ingredient (API) [1]. To be able to give rise to a new salt form, however, the API in question should be ionizable. For non-ionizable APIs, co-crystallization with a crystallophoric excipient (non-API component of the solid drug form) has become an alternative, proven way of accessing a broad range of solid forms and thus modifying various physicochemical properties and increasing API's stability [2–4]. An overwhelming majority of API co-crystals reported today are based on hydrogen bonding as the principal means of constructing the crystalline form. However, halogen bonds have emerged as an equally promising basis for designing new co-crystalline API forms [5–12]. However, despite the emergence of this intriguing supramolecular interaction, halogen-bonded API co-crystals remain relatively scarce. This may have to do with the limited range of pharmaceutically acceptable excipients containing polarized halogen atoms [13]. In continuation of our efforts to identify new crystalline forms for APIs that would be stabilized by halogen bonding [14,15], we turned our attention to screening of crystallization conditions for the title compound, anastrozole (IUPAC name 2,2′-(5-((1H-1,2,4-triazol-1-yl)methyl)-1,3-phenylene)bis(2-methylpropanenitrile), abbreviated as **ASZ**), which is an aromatase inhibitor useful in second-line therapy of estrogen-dependent breast cancer [16–18].

We choose this API as a potential recipient of XB due to its 1,2,4-triazole moiety, containing at least two nucleophilic $N_{sp}2$ atoms as potential XB acceptor centers. One of them is a hydrogen bond [19] (HB) acceptor in the crystal structure of ASZ itself (Figure 1) [20].

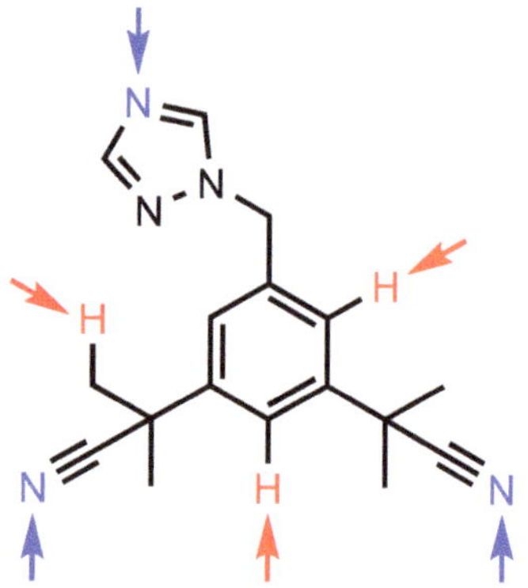

Figure 1. Structure of anastrozole with assigned hydrogen bond donor (red) and hydrogen bond acceptor centers (blue) found in its crystal structure (SATHOL) [20].

Previously, we successfully cocrystallized another API, nevirapine, with classic XB donor, 1,2,4,5-tetrafluoro-3,6-diiodobenzene (also known as 1,4-diiodotetrafluorobenzene, **1,4-FIB**). Noticeably, **1,4-FIB** has already been employed in the co-crystal formation for a number of biologically active compounds including nicotine [21], pyrazinamide, lidocaine, and pentoxifylline [22]. It should be noted, however, that in these studies (as well as in present work), **1,4-FIB** is employed as an exploratory co-crystallization partner. For its use as an excipient for the design of solid drug forms, a further clinical investigation will be required. In this work, we found ASZ can also be cocrystallized with **1,4-FIB** from their solution in MeOH, forming the 2:3 adduct. Herein, we present the results of combined single-crystal XRD experimental and theoretical studies of the adduct and noncovalent interactions found in it.

2. Materials and Methods

2.1. Materials

Anastrozole, 1,2,4,5-tetrafluoro-3,6-diiodobenzene, and MeOH were obtained from a commercial source and used as received.

2.2. X-ray Structure Determination

Crystal of **ASZ**·1.5(**1,4-FIB**) was investigated on an Xcalibur, Eos diffractometer at 100 K (monochromated MoKα radiation with λ = 0.71073 Å). The structure was solved by the direct methods (SHELX program [23]) in the OLEX2 program package [24]. The carbon-bound H atom positions were calculated and included in the refinement in the 'riding' model approximation. U_{iso}(H) were set to 1.5U_{eq}(C) (for CH_3 groups) or 1.2U_{eq}(C) (for CH_2 and CH groups). The C–H bond lengths are 0.98 Å for CH_3 groups, 0.99 Å for CH_2 groups, and 0.95 Å for CH groups. Empirical absorption correction was applied in the CrysAlisPro [25] program. For crystallographic data and refinement parameters see Supplementary material (Table S3). Supplementary crystallographic data was deposited at Cambridge Crystallographic Data Centre (CCDC 1960975) and can be obtained free of charge via www.ccdc.cam.ac.uk/data_request/cif.

2.3. Powder X-ray Diffraction Experiments

The X-ray diffraction of powder samples was measured at room temperature on a D8 Discover high-resolution diffractometer using monochromated CuKα (λ = 1.54184 Å) radiation.

2.4. Computational Details

The single point calculations based on the experimental X-ray geometry of (**ASZ**)$_3$·(**1,4-FIB**)$_4$ have been carried out at the DFT level of theory using the dispersion-corrected hybrid functional ωB97XD [26] with the help of the Gaussian-09 [27] program package. The Douglas–Kroll–Hess 2nd order scalar relativistic calculations requested relativistic core Hamiltonian were carried out using the DZP-DKH basis sets [28–31] for all atoms. The topological analysis of the electron density distribution with the help of the atoms in molecules (QTAIM) method developed by Bader [32] has been performed by using the Multiwfn program [33]. The Cartesian atomic coordinates of a model supramolecular cluster are presented in Supporting Information, Table S4.

3. Results and Discussion

3.1. Halogen Bonding in ASZ·1.5(1,4-FIB)

Slow evaporation of a MeOH solution of **ASZ** with **1,4-FIB** taken in a 1:1 ratio leads to the formation on single crystals of **ASZ**·1.5(**1,4-FIB**) suitable for the X-ray diffraction experiment. It is notable that we also tried to synthesize the **ASZ**·1.5(**1,4-FIB**) pure phase both by mechanical grinding of 2:3 **ASZ** + **1,4-FIB** mixture with MeOH additions during the process or by crystallization of the same 2:3 mixture from methanol with the following grinding of obtained crystalline material. Powder X-ray diffraction experiments for both cases show that **ASZ**·1.5(**1,4-FIB**) coexists with some other unidentified phases (see Figures S3 and S4 in SI). For details on the powder x-ray diffraction experiments see also Section 2.3.

According to the single-crystal XRD data, the cocrystallization of **ASZ** with **1,4-FIB** does not lead to any relevant changes, considering the 3σ criterion, in covalent bond lengths of **ASZ** [20] and **1,4-FIB** [34].

As expected, the C–I···N contacts were found in **ASZ**·1.5(**1,4-FIB**) (Figure 2), which can be interpreted as halogen bonding [35]. In accordance with their geometrical parameters (Table 1), the theoretically estimated energies of these contacts are 4.6–5.3 kcal/mol (I3S···N2) and 4.8–6.0 kcal/mol (I1S···N3), which is comparable with a lower limit for strength of "moderate" hydrogen bonding according to Jeffrey's classification ("strong": 40–15 kcal/mol; "moderate": 15–4 kcal/mol; "weak": <4 kcal/mol) [36]. For **1,4-FIB**, the molecular electrostatic potential calculations were reported [37–39], which confirm the σ-hole electrophilicity [40,41] of iodine atoms in this molecule.

Table 1. Parameters of the C–I···X XBs in **ASZ**·1.5(**1,4-FIB**).

C–I···X	d(I···X), Å	R_{IX} [b]	∠(C–I···X),°
C8S–I3S···N2	2.913 (6)	0.83	175.3 (2)
C1S–I1S···N3	2.883 (7)	0.82	169.3 (2)
C4S–I2S···F6S	3.390 (5)	0.98	149.97 (19)
C4S–I2S···I3S	3.8529 (8)	0.97	157.68 (18)
Comparison [a]	3.53 (I···N)		
	3.45 (I···F)	1.00	180
	3.96 (I···I)		

[a] Comparison is the vdW radii sum [42] for distances and classic XB angle. [b] $R_{IX} = d(I···X)/(R_{vdW}(I) + R_{vdW}(X))$.

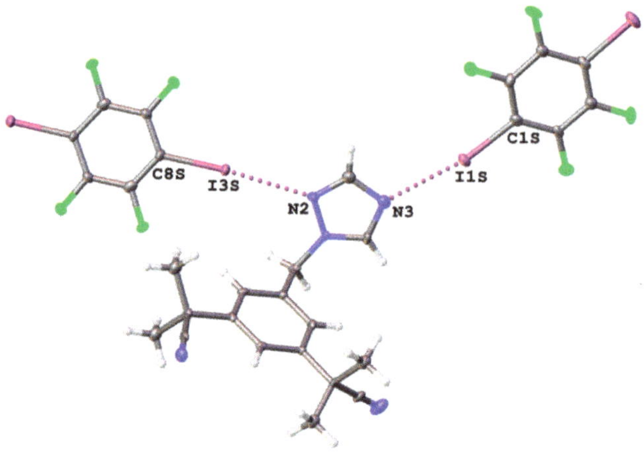

Figure 2. The C–I···N XBs in anastrozole **(ASZ)**·1.5(**1,4-FIB**). Hereinafter noncovalent interactions were assigned by dotted lines and ellipsoids are drawn with 50% probability.

Previously, the C–I···N XBs including 1,2,4-triazole moiety was mentioned only in two metal-organic frameworks (FALNEN [43] and UMOTOG [44]) and one free 4H-1,2,4-triazole (FARCIN01 [45]). We analyzed all the structures containing the C–I···N XBs with 1,2,4-triazoles in CCDC and found 9 more structures [44,46–52]. It is notable that in all corresponding works, these interactions were not even mentioned. The I···N distances are in the range of 2.839 (4)–3.378 (3) Å, and the ∠(C–I···N) angles vary from 157.18 (17) to 177.57 (8)° (for details see Table S1 in supplementary materials). In **ASZ**·1.5 (**1,4-FIB**), both distances (2.883 (7) and 2.913 (6) Å) are shorter than in most previously published structures, which can be explained by the electron-withdrawing I substituent in **1,4-FIB**. Noticeably, the C–Cl···N [53–55] and C–Br···N [45,53,56–58] XBs including 1,2,4-triazole moiety are also mentioned in the literature.

Halogen bonding was also found between **1,4-FIB** molecules, represented by bifurcated C–I···(I,F) contact (Figure 3). Both distances are less than vdW sums, and both angles are around 150° (Table 1) and fall into an acceptable value for XBs. These non-covalent interactions are weak, viz. 1.3 kcal/mol in the case of I2S···F6S and 1.6 kcal/mol in the case of I2S···I3S.

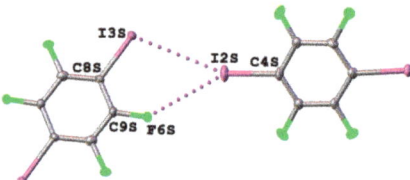

Figure 3. Bifurcated C–I···(I,F) halogen bonding between **1,4-FIB** molecules in **ASZ**·1.5(**1,4-FIB**).

A resembling feature can be found in the structure KUWRAX [59], where both I···F and I···I distances are less than the corresponding vdW sums (3.6889 (7) vs 3.96 Å and 3.409 (3) vs 3.45 Å), however, in this structure, the corresponding ∠(C–I···F) angle (125.09 (13)°) is not high enough to recognize this interaction as halogen bonding. Thus, **ASZ**·1.5(**1,4-FIB**) demonstrates the first example of bifurcated C–I···(I,F) halogen bonding between **1,4-FIB** molecules.

3.2. Lone-Pair···π Interactions in ASZ·1.5(1,4-FIB)

Besides the expected C–I···N halogen bonding, the C···I–C contacts (Table 2) were identified between **ASZ** and **1,4-FIB** molecules in **ASZ**·1.5 (**1,4-FIB**) (Figure 4). According to the ∠(C···I–C) angle, which is close to 90° (Table 2), this interaction can be interpreted as lp(I)···π(C) interaction [60]. Their theoretically estimated strength is 1.6 kcal/mol.

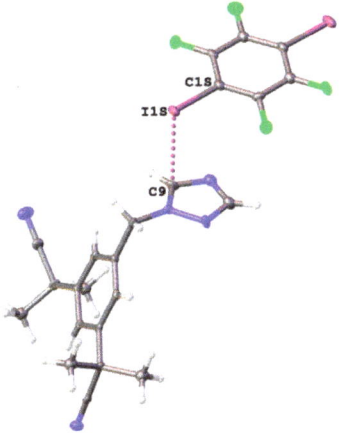

Figure 4. The lp(I)···π(C) interaction between **ASZ** and **1,4-FIB** molecules in **ASZ**·1.5(**1,4-FIB**).

Table 2. Parameters of the lp(I)···π(C) interactions in **ASZ**·1.5(**1,4-FIB**).

C···I–C	d(C···I), Å	R_{CI} [b]	∠(C···I–C),°
C9···I1S–C1S	3.528 (8)	0.96	86.6(3)
C9S···I2S–C4S	3.686 (8)	1.00	92.9(3)
Comparison [a]	3.68	1.00	90

[a] Comparison is the vdW radii sum [42] for distances and classic XB acceptor angle. [b] $R_{CI} = d(C···I)/(R_{vdW}(I) + R_{vdW}(C))$.

Previously, the lp(I)···π(C) interactions including 1,2,4-triazole moiety were discussed only for five 1,2,4-triazolium iodides [61,62], where these interactions are interionic. We analyzed the CCDC data and identified 23 more structures with the C···I interactions including 1,2,4-triazoles. 1,2,4-triazolium iodides [20,63–70] were also found in 15 structures. The C···I–M interactions [71–76] in 1,2,4-triazole-containing MOFs were detected in 6 structures. Structure XIWGOC contains the C···I⁻ interactions between the cationic Ir[III] complex and iodide counterion [77]. Only in the IDIFEH structure was another example of the C···I–C interactions between neutral isolated molecules [78] identified. The C···I distances vary from 3.4363(2) to 3.670 (3) Å (for details see Table S2), and the C9···I1S distance (3.528 (8) Å) in **ASZ**·1.5(**1,4-FIB**) is within this range.

Besides, possible lp(I)···π(C) interaction between **1,4-FIB** molecules was found (Figure 5). Although the C···I distance is around the vdW sum (3.686 (8) vs 3.68 Å), further theoretical calculations performed on experimentally determined atomic coordinates (see next section) confirmed the existence of the interaction and its noncovalent nature (estimated energy is 0.9–1.1 kcal/mol). Notably, the same interactions were found by us for **1,4-FIB** and other iodofluorobenzenes [60,79,80].

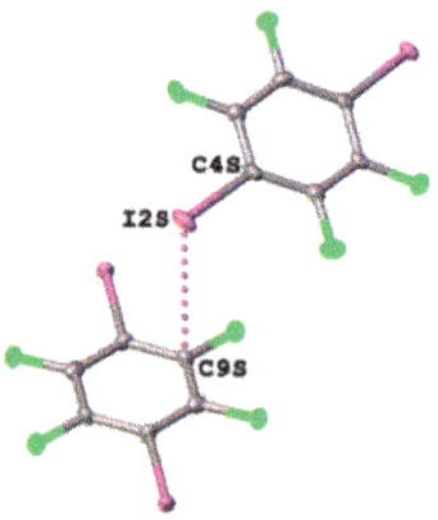

Figure 5. The lp(I)···π(C) interaction between **1,4-FIB** molecules in **ASZ**·1.5(**1,4-FIB**).

3.3. Hydrogen Bonding in ASZ·1.5(1,4-FIB)

As well as in the structure of free **ASZ**, cyano N atoms are involved in weak hydrogen bonding (theoretically estimated strength of appropriate contacts vary from 0.9 to 1.9 kcal/mol) (Figure 6 and Table 3). Apart from methyl H atoms, the hydrogen atom in the methylene group is also an HB donor, which was not observed in the **ASZ** structure previously.

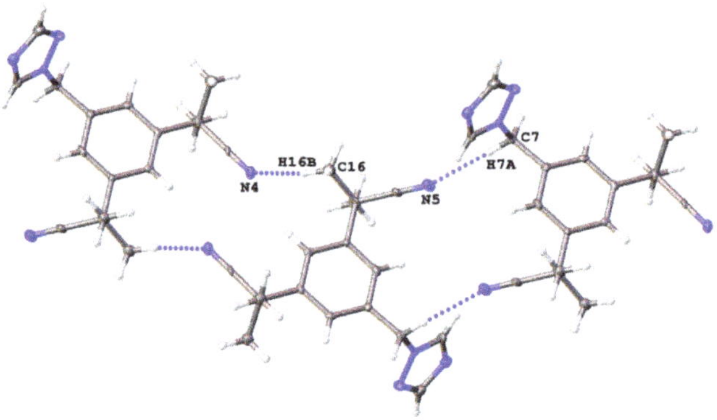

Figure 6. The C–H···N HBs in **ASZ**·1.5(**1,4-FIB**).

Table 3. Parameters of the C–H···N HBs in **ASZ**·1.5(**1,4-FIB**).

C–H···N	d(H···N), Å	R_{HN} [b]	d(C···N), Å	∠(C–I···X),°
C7–H7A···N5	2.484	0.90	3.441 (10)	168.6
C16–H16B···N4	2.733	0.99	3.62 (1)	153.9
Comparison [a]	2.75	1.00	3.25	110.0

[a] Comparison is the vdW radii sum [42] for distances and minimal HB angle. [b] $R_{HN} = d(H···N)/(R_{vdW}(H) + R_{vdW}(N))$.

3.4. Theoretical Study of Different Non-covalent Interactions in ASZ·1.5(1,4-FIB)

The supramolecular structure of **ASZ**·1.5(**1,4-FIB**) is formed by various non-covalent contacts (viz. lp-π interactions, hydrogen, and halogen bonding). We performed quantum chemical calculations and QTAIM analysis [32] to study the nature and energies of these non-covalent contacts in a model supramolecular cluster (**ASZ**)₃·(**1,4-FIB**)₄ based on the appropriate X-ray diffraction data (Supporting Information, Table S4). This approach depends very slightly on the basis set [81,82] or method [83,84] used and it was already successfully used by us previously for similar chemical systems [14,15,79,85,86] and upon studies of different non-covalent interactions (e.g., hydrogen/chalcogen/halogen bonds, stacking interactions, metallophilic interactions) in other organic and inorganic compounds [14,15,87–92]. The results of QTAIM analysis are presented in Table 4 and visualized in Figure 7.

Table 4. Values of the density of all electrons—$\rho(\mathbf{r})$, Laplacian of electron density—$\nabla^2\rho(\mathbf{r})$, energy density—H_b, potential energy density—$V(\mathbf{r})$, and Lagrangian kinetic energy—$G(\mathbf{r})$ (a.u.) at the bond critical points (3, −1), corresponding to different non-covalent interactions in $(\mathbf{ASZ})_3 \cdot (\mathbf{1,4\text{-}FIB})_4$, bond lengths—$l$ (Å), as well as energies for these contacts E_{int} (kcal/mol), defined by two approaches.*,·

Contact	$\rho(\mathbf{r})$	$\nabla^2\rho(\mathbf{r})$	Hb	$V(\mathbf{r})$	$G(\mathbf{r})$	Eint a	Eint b	l
I3S···N2	0.022	0.070	0.000	−0.017	0.017	5.3	4.6	2.913
I1S···N3	0.024	0.072	0.000	−0.019	0.018	6.0	4.8	2.883
I2S···F6S	0.006	0.026	0.001	−0.004	0.005	1.3	1.3	3.390
I2S···I3S	0.008	0.031	0.001	−0.005	0.006	1.6	1.6	3.853
C9···I1S	0.009	0.029	0.001	−0.005	0.006	1.6	1.6	3.528
C9S···I2S	0.006	0.023	0.001	−0.003	0.004	0.9	1.1	3.686
H7A···N5	0.009	0.033	0.001	−0.006	0.007	1.9	1.9	2.484
H16B···N4	0.005	0.021	0.001	−0.003	0.004	0.9	1.1	2.733

a $E_{int} = -V(\mathbf{r})/2$ [93] b $E_{int} = 0.429G(\mathbf{r})$ [94] * Note that Tsirelson et al. [95] also proposed alternative correlations developed exclusively for non-covalent interactions involving iodine atoms, viz. $E_{int} = 0.68(-V(\mathbf{r}))$ or $E_{int} = 0.67G(\mathbf{r})$.

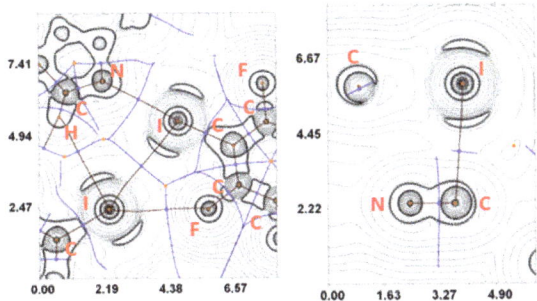

Figure 7. Contour line diagrams of the Laplacian distribution $\nabla^2\rho(\mathbf{r})$, bond paths and selected zero-flux surfaces referring to the C–I···X (X = N, F, I) halogen bonding (left) and lp(I)···π(triazole) (right) interactions in $(\mathbf{ASZ})_3 \cdot (\mathbf{1,4\text{-}FIB})_4$. Bond critical points (3, −1) are shown in blue, nuclear critical points (3, −3) in pale brown, ring critical points (3, +1) in orange, cage critical points (3, +3) in light green. Length units—Å.

The QTAIM analysis reveals the existence of bond critical points (3, −1) (BCPs) for all non-covalent interactions listed in Table 4. The properties of electron density, Laplacian of electron density and energy density in these BCPs are common for non-covalent interactions. Energies for these non-covalent contacts (vary from 0.9 to 6.0 kcal/mol) were defined according to the procedures developed by Espinosa et al. [93] and Vener et al. [94] using the equations $E_{int} = 0.5(-V(\mathbf{r}))$ or $E_{int} = 0.429G(\mathbf{r})$, respectively. The balance between the potential energy density $V(\mathbf{r})$ and Lagrangian kinetic energy $G(\mathbf{r})$ at the BCPs reveals that a covalent contribution is absent in all supramolecular contacts listed in Table 4, except I1S···N3 halogen bonding [96].

4. Conclusions

In combination with 1,2,4,5-tetrafluoro-3,6-diiodobenzene, a classical XB donor, we have identified a new halogen-bonded solid for anastrozole, an anticancer aromatase inhibitor drug. These findings continue to provide proof-of-principle for the productive employment of halogen bonds in the design and discovery of stable crystalline forms of important drug substances. Moreover, these results suggest that the range of potential XB donors for co-crystallization with basic nitrogen-rich molecular frameworks can potentially be expanded beyond the classical ones. The distinctive features of the crystal structures obtained and characterized in detail in this work are the presence of XBs with both triazole N atoms, firstly found for anastrozole. Apart from that, the adduct structure demonstrates the lp(I)···π(triazole) attractive interactions, which may also be important for the adduct formation. The findings encourage us to continue searching for yet novel opportunities to detect XBs as indispensable forces leading to the formation of a new crystal. The results of these studies will be reported in due course.

Supplementary Materials: The following are available online at http://www.mdpi.com/2073-4352/10/5/371/s1, Figure S1: Structural motifs around the C–I···N XBs including 1,2,4-triazole moiety in CCDC structures; Figure S2: Structural motifs around the lp(I)···C interactions including 1,2,4-triazole moiety in CCDC structures; Figure S3: Powder X-ray diffraction data (blue line) of mixture, obtained by mechanical grinding of 2**ASZ** + 3(**1,4-FIB**) mixture with MeOH additions; Figure S4: Powder X-ray diffraction data (blue line) of mixture, obtained by grinding of crystalline material grown from 2**ASZ** + 3(**1,4-FIB**) solution in methanol; Table S1: Parameters of the C–I···N XBs including 1,2,4-triazole moiety in CCDC structures; Table S2: Parameters of the lp(I)···C interactions including 1,2,4-triazole moiety in CCDC structures; Table S3: Crystal data and structure refinement for **ASZ**·1.5(**1,4-FIB**); Table S4: Cartesian atomic coordinates of model supramolecular cluster.

Author Contributions: Conceptualization, M.K., A.V.S., and D.M.I.; data curation, D.M.I.; formal analysis, A.S.N. and D.M.I.; funding acquisition, A.V.S.; investigation, M.A.K.; methodology, D.M.I.; project administration, D.M.I.; resources, A.V.S.; software, A.S.N.; supervision, M.K. and D.M.I.; validation, M.A.K.; visualization, A.S.N. and D.M.I.; writing—original draft, A.S.N. and D.M.I.; writing—review & editing, M.K. All authors have read and agreed to the published version of the manuscript.

Funding: This work was funded by Russian Science Foundation, grant number 17-73-20185.

Acknowledgments: Physicochemical studies were performed at the Center for X-ray Diffraction Studies belonging to Saint Petersburg State University.

Conflicts of Interest: The authors declare no conflict of interest.

References

1. Stahl, P.H.; Wermiuth, C.G.E. *Handbook of Pharmaceutical Salts Properties, Selection and Use*; Verlag Helvetica Chimica Acta: Zürich, Switzerland, 2002.
2. Trask, A.V. An overview of pharmaceutical cocrystals as intellectual property. *Mol. Pharm.* **2007**, *4*, 301–309. [CrossRef] [PubMed]
3. Trask, A.V.; Motherwell, W.D.S.; Jones, W. Pharmaceutical cocrystallization: Engineering a remedy for caffeine hydration. *Cryst. Growth Des.* **2005**, *5*, 1013–1021. [CrossRef]
4. Karki, S.; Friščić, T.; Jones, W.; Motherwell, W.D.S. Screening for pharmaceutical cocrystal hydrates via neat and liquid-assisted grinding. *Mol. Pharm.* **2007**, *4*, 347–354. [CrossRef] [PubMed]
5. Merkens, C.; Pan, F.F.; Englert, U. 3-(4-Pyridyl)-2,4-pentanedione—A bridge between coordinative, halogen, and hydrogen bonds. *CrystEngComm* **2013**, *15*, 8153–8158. [CrossRef]
6. Cinčić, D.; Friščić, T.; Jones, W. Structural Equivalence of Br and I Halogen Bonds: A Route to Isostructural Materials with Controllable Properties. *Chem. Mater.* **2008**, *20*, 6623–6626. [CrossRef]
7. Cinčić, D.; Friščić, T.; Jones, W. A cocrystallisation-based strategy to construct isostructural solids. *New J. Chem.* **2008**, *32*, 1776–1781. [CrossRef]
8. Bushuyev, O.S.; Tan, D.; Barrett, C.J.; Friščić, T. Fluorinated azobenzenes with highly strained geometries for halogen bond-driven self-assembly in the solid state. *CrystEngComm* **2015**, *17*, 73–80. [CrossRef]
9. Cinčić, D.; Friščić, T. Synthesis of an extended halogen-bonded metal-organic structure in a one-pot mechanochemical reaction that combines covalent bonding, coordination chemistry and supramolecular synthesis. *CrystEngComm* **2014**, *16*, 10169–10172. [CrossRef]
10. Troff, R.W.; Makela, T.; Topic, F.; Valkonen, A.; Raatikainen, K.; Rissanen, K. Alternative Motifs for Halogen Bonding. *Eur. J. Org. Chem.* **2013**, *2013*, 1617–1637. [CrossRef]
11. Cinčić, D.; Friščić, T.; Jones, W. A stepwise mechanism for the mechanochemical synthesis of halogen-bonded cocrystal architectures. *J. Am. Chem. Soc.* **2008**, *130*, 7524–7525. [CrossRef]
12. Carletta, A.; Spinelli, F.; d'Agostino, S.; Ventura, B.; Chierotti, M.R.; Gobetto, R.; Wouters, J.; Grepioni, F. Halogen-Bond Effects on the Thermo- and Photochromic Behaviour of Anil-Based Molecular Co-crystals. *Chem.: Eur. J.* **2017**, *23*, 5317–5329. [CrossRef] [PubMed]
13. Stilinović, V.; Horvat, G.; Hrenar, T.; Nemec, V.; Cinčić, D. Halogen and Hydrogen Bonding between (N-Halogeno)-succinimides and Pyridine Derivatives in Solution, the Solid State and In Silico. *Chem. Eur. J.* **2017**, *23*, 5244–5257. [CrossRef] [PubMed]

14. Kryukova, M.A.; Sapegin, A.V.; Novikov, A.S.; Krasavin, M.; Ivanov, D.M. New Crystal Forms for Biologically Active Compounds. Part 1: Noncovalent Interactions in Adducts of Nevirapine with XB Donors. *Crystals* **2019**, *9*, 71. [CrossRef]
15. Kryukova, M.A.; Sapegin, A.V.; Novikov, A.S.; Krasavin, M.; Ivanov, D.M. Non-covalent interactions observed in nevirapinium pentaiodide hydrate which include the rare $I_4-I^-\cdots O=C$ halogen bonding. *Z. Kristallogr. Cryst. Mater.* **2019**, *234*, 101–108. [CrossRef]
16. Wiseman, L.R.; Adkins, J.C. Anastrozole—A review of its use in the management of postmenopausal women with advanced breast cancer. *Drugs Aging* **1998**, *13*, 321–332. [CrossRef] [PubMed]
17. Augusto, T.V.; Correia-da-Silva, G.; Rodrigues, C.M.P.; Teixeira, N.; Amaral, C. Acquired resistance to aromatase inhibitors: Where we stand! *Endocr.-Relat. Cancer* **2018**, *25*, R283–R301. [CrossRef]
18. Rodgers, R.J.; Reid, G.D.; Koch, J.; Deans, R.; Ledger, W.L.; Friedlander, M.; Gilchrist, R.B.; Walters, K.A.; Abbott, J.A. The safety and efficacy of controlled ovarian hyperstimulation for fertility preservation in women with early breast cancer: A systematic review. *Hum. Reprod.* **2017**, *32*, 1033–1045. [CrossRef]
19. Arunan, E.; Desiraju, G.R.; Klein, R.A.; Sadlej, J.; Scheiner, S.; Alkorta, I.; Clary, D.C.; Crabtree, R.H.; Dannenberg, J.J.; Hobza, P.; et al. Definition of the hydrogen bond (IUPAC Recommendations 2011). *Pure Appl. Chem.* **2011**, *83*, 1637–1641. [CrossRef]
20. Tang, G.P.; Gu, J.M. 2-[3-(2-cyano-2-propyl)-5-(1,2,4-triazol-1-yl)phenyl]-2-methylpropiononitrile. *Acta Cryst. E* **2005**, *61*, O2330–O2331. [CrossRef]
21. Capucci, D.; Balestri, D.; Mazzeo, P.P.; Pelagatti, P.; Rubini, K.; Bacchi, A. Liquid Nicotine Tamed in Solid Forms by Cocrystallization. *Cryst. Growth Des.* **2017**, *17*, 4958–4964. [CrossRef]
22. Choquesillo-Lazarte, D.; Nemec, V.; Cinčić, D. Halogen bonded cocrystals of active pharmaceutical ingredients: Pyrazinamide, lidocaine and pentoxifylline in combination with haloperfluorinated compounds. *CrystEngComm* **2017**, *19*, 5293–5299. [CrossRef]
23. Sheldrick, G. SHELXT - Integrated space-group and crystal-structure determination. *Acta Cryst. A* **2015**, *71*, 3–8. [CrossRef] [PubMed]
24. Dolomanov, O.V.; Bourhis, L.J.; Gildea, R.J.; Howard, J.A.K.; Puschmann, H. OLEX2: A complete structure solution, refinement and analysis program. *J. Appl. Cryst.* **2009**, *42*, 339–341. [CrossRef]
25. Agilent Technologies Ltd. *CrysAlisPro*; Version 1.171.136.120 (release 127-106-2012); Agilent Technologies Ltd.: Santa Clara, CA, USA, 2012.
26. Chai, J.D.; Head-Gordon, M. Long-range corrected hybrid density functionals with damped atom-atom dispersion corrections. *Phys. Chem. Chem. Phys.* **2008**, *10*, 6615–6620. [CrossRef] [PubMed]
27. Frisch, M.J.; Trucks, G.W.; Schlegel, H.B.; Scuseria, G.E.; Robb, M.A.; Cheeseman, J.R.; Scalmani, G.; Barone, V.; Mennucci, B.; Petersson, G.A.; et al. *Gaussian 09, EM64L-G09RevB. 01*; Gaussian, Inc.: Wallingford, CT, USA, 2010.
28. Barros, C.L.; de Oliveira, P.J.P.; Jorge, F.E.; Canal Neto, A.; Campos, M. Gaussian basis set of double zeta quality for atoms Rb through Xe: Application in non-relativistic and relativistic calculations of atomic and molecular properties. *Mol. Phys.* **2010**, *108*, 1965–1972. [CrossRef]
29. de Berrêdo, R.C.; Jorge, F.E. All-electron double zeta basis sets for platinum: Estimating scalar relativistic effects on platinum(II) anticancer drugs. *J. Mol. Struct. THEOCHEM* **2010**, *961*, 107–112. [CrossRef]
30. Jorge, F.E.; Canal Neto, A.; Camiletti, G.G.; Machado, S.F. Contracted Gaussian basis sets for Douglas–Kroll–Hess calculations: Estimating scalar relativistic effects of some atomic and molecular properties. *J. Chem. Phys.* **2009**, *130*, 064108. [CrossRef]
31. Neto, A.C.; Jorge, F.E. All-electron double zeta basis sets for the most fifth-row atoms: Application in DFT spectroscopic constant calculations. *Chem. Phys. Lett.* **2013**, *582*, 158–162. [CrossRef]
32. Bader, R.F.W. A quantum theory of molecular structure and its applications. *Chem. Rev.* **1991**, *91*, 893–928. [CrossRef]
33. Lu, T.; Chen, F. Multiwfn: A multifunctional wavefunction analyzer. *J. Comput. Chem.* **2012**, *33*, 580–592. [CrossRef]
34. Oh, S.Y.; Nickels, C.W.; Garcia, F.; Jones, W.; Friščić, T. Switching between halogen- and hydrogen-bonding in stoichiometric variations of a cocrystal of a phosphine oxide. *CrystEngComm* **2012**, *14*, 6110–6114. [CrossRef]
35. Desiraju, G.R.; Ho, P.S.; Kloo, L.; Legon, A.C.; Marquardt, R.; Metrangolo, P.; Politzer, P.; Resnati, G.; Rissanen, K. Definition of the halogen bond (IUPAC Recommendations 2013). *Pure Appl. Chem.* **2013**, *85*, 1711–1713. [CrossRef]

36. Steiner, T. The hydrogen bond in the solid state. *Angew. Chem.-Int. Ed.* **2002**, *41*, 48–76. [CrossRef]
37. Pandiyan, B.V.; Deepa, P.; Kolandaivel, P. How do halogen bonds (S–O···I, N–O···I and C–O···I) and halogen-halogen contacts (C–I···I–C, C–F···F–C) subsist in crystal structures? A quantum chemical insight. *J. Mol. Model.* **2017**, *23*, 16. [CrossRef]
38. Li, L.L.; Liu, Z.F.; Wu, W.X.; Jin, W.J. Cocrystals with tunable luminescence colour self-assembled by a predictable method. *Acta Crystallogr. Sect. B* **2018**, *74*, 610–617. [CrossRef]
39. DeHaven, B.A.; Chen, A.L.; Shimizu, E.A.; Salpage, S.R.; Smith, M.D.; Shimizu, L.S. Synergistic effects of hydrogen and halogen bonding in co-crystals of dipyridylureas and diiodotetrafluorobenzenes. *Supramol. Chem.* **2018**, *30*, 315–327. [CrossRef]
40. Politzer, P.; Murray, J.S.; Clark, T. Halogen bonding and other s-hole interactions: A perspective. *Phys. Chem. Chem. Phys.* **2013**, *15*, 11178–11189. [CrossRef]
41. Murray, J.S.; Politzer, P. Interaction and Polarization Energy Relationships in s-Hole and p-Hole Bonding. *Crystals* **2020**, *10*, 76. [CrossRef]
42. Bondi, A. Van der Waals volumes + radii. *J. Phys. Chem.* **1964**, *68*, 441–451. [CrossRef]
43. Zhang, K.L.; Hou, C.T.; Song, J.J.; Deng, Y.; Li, L.; Ng, S.W.; Diao, G.W. Temperature and auxiliary ligand-controlled supramolecular assembly in a series of Zn(II)-organic frameworks: Syntheses, structures and properties. *CrystEngComm* **2012**, *14*, 590–600. [CrossRef]
44. Zhang, K.L.; Chang, Y.; Ng, S.W. Preparation and characterization of two supramolecular complexes with 5-amino-2,4,6-triiodoisophthalic acid under N-donor auxiliary ligand intervention. *Inorg. Chim. Acta* **2011**, *368*, 49–57. [CrossRef]
45. Wang, J.W.; Chen, C.; Li, Y.J.; Luo, Y.H.; Sun, B.W. Halogen-bonding contacts determining the crystal structure and fluorescence properties of organic salts. *New J. Chem.* **2017**, *41*, 9444–9452. [CrossRef]
46. Rode, N.D.; Sonawane, A.D.; Garud, D.R.; Joshi, R.R.; Joshi, R.A.; Likhite, A.P. First regioselective iodocyclization reaction of 3-aryl-5-(prop-2-ynylthio)-1H-1,2,4-triazoles. *Tetrahedron Lett.* **2015**, *56*, 5140–5144. [CrossRef]
47. Luo, Y.H.; Sun, Y.; Liu, Q.L.; Yang, L.J.; Wen, G.J.; Wang, M.X.; Sun, B.W. Influence of Halogen Atoms on Spin-Crossover Properties of 1,2,4-Triazole-Based 1D Iron(II) Polymers. *ChemistrySelect* **2016**, *1*, 3879–3884. [CrossRef]
48. Xiong, H.-P.; Gao, S.-H.; Li, C.-T.; Wu, Z.-J. (2RS)-2-(2,4-Difluorophenyl)-1-[(4-iodobenzyl)(methyl)amino]-3-(1H-1,2,4-triazol-1-yl)propan-2-ol. *Acta Cryst. E* **2012**, *68*, o2447–o2448. [CrossRef]
49. Li, L.; Chi, Y.; Mang, X.Y.; Zhang, G.Q.; Zhang, Y.; Zhao, T.X.; Huang, M.; Li, H.B. Synthesis, crystal structure and thermal analysis of tetraiodo-4,4'-bi-1,2,4-triazole. *Chin. Chem. Lett.* **2013**, *24*, 786–788. [CrossRef]
50. Il'inykh, E.S.; Kim, D.G.; Kodess, M.I.; Matochkina, E.G.; Slepukhin, P.A. Synthesis of novel fluorine- and iodine-containing [1,2,4]triazolo[3, 4-b][1,3]thiazines based 3-(alkenylthio)-5-(trifluoromethyl)-4H-1,2,4-triazole-3-thiols. *J. Fluorine Chem.* **2013**, *149*, 24–29. [CrossRef]
51. Song, J.; Wu, Z.H.; Wangtrakuldee, B.; Choi, S.R.; Zha, Z.H.; Ploessl, K.; Mach, R.H.; Kung, H. 4-(((4-Iodophenyl)methyl)-4H-1,2,4-triazol-4-ylamino)-benzonitrile: A Potential Imaging Agent for Aromatase. *J. Med. Chem.* **2016**, *59*, 9370–9380. [CrossRef]
52. Nagaradja, E.; Bentabed-Ababsa, G.; Scalabrini, M.; Chevallier, F.; Philippot, S.; Fontanay, S.; Duval, R.E.; Halauko, Y.S.; Ivashkevich, O.A.; Matulis, V.E.; et al. Deprotometalation-iodolysis and computed CH acidity of 1,2,3-and 1,2,4-triazoles. Application to the synthesis of resveratrol analogues. *Bioorg. Med. Chem.* **2015**, *23*, 6355–6363. [CrossRef]
53. Dong, Z.; Zhao, T.X.; Li, L.; Zhang, L.J.; Liang, D.H.; Li, H.B. Synthesis and X-Ray Crystal Structures of Tetrahalogeno-4,4'-bi-1,2,4-triazoles. *Mol. Cryst. Liq. Cryst.* **2015**, *623*, 333–342. [CrossRef]
54. Al-Salahi, R.; Al-Omar, M.; Marzouk, M.; Ng, S.W. 5-Chloro-2-methylsulfonyl-1,2,4-triazolo[1,5-a]quinazoline. *Acta Cryst. E* **2012**, *68*, o1809. [CrossRef] [PubMed]
55. Khan, I.; Panini, P.; Khan, S.U.D.; Rana, U.A.; Andleeb, H.; Chopra, D.; Hameed, S.; Simpson, J. Exploiting the Role of Molecular Electrostatic Potential, Deformation Density, Topology, and Energetics in the Characterization of S···N and Cl···N Supramolecular Motifs in Crystalline Triazolothiadiazoles. *Cryst. Growth Des.* **2016**, *16*, 1371–1386. [CrossRef]
56. Valkonen, J.; Pitkanen, I.; Pajunen, A. Molecular and crystal structure and IR spectrum of 3,5-dibromo-1,2,4-triazole. *Acta Chem. Scand.* **1985**, *39*, 711–716. [CrossRef]

57. Berski, S.; Ciunik, Z.; Drabent, K.; Latajka, Z.; Panek, J. Dominant role of C–Br···N halogen bond in molecular self-organization. Crystallographic and quantum-chemical study of Schiff-base-containing triazoles. *J. Phys. Chem. B* **2004**, *108*, 12327–12332. [CrossRef]
58. Gilandoust, M.; Harsha, K.B.; Madan Kumar, S.; Rakesh, K.S.; Lokanath, N.K.; Byrappa, K.; Rangappa, K.S. 5-Bromo-1,2,4-triazolo[1,5-a]pyrimidine. *IUCrData* **2016**, *1*, x161944. [CrossRef]
59. Eccles, K.S.; Morrison, R.E.; Sinha, A.S.; Maguire, A.R.; Lawrence, S.E. Investigating C=S···I Halogen Bonding for Cocrystallization with Primary Thioamides. *Cryst. Growth Des.* **2015**, *15*, 3442–3451. [CrossRef]
60. Eliseeva, A.A.; Ivanov, D.M.; Novikov, A.S.; Kukushkin, V.Y. Recognition of the π-hole donor ability of iodopentafluorobenzene—A conventional σ-hole donor for crystal engineering involving halogen bonding. *CrystEngComm* **2019**, *21*, 616–628. [CrossRef]
61. Mochida, T.; Miura, Y.; Shimizu, F. Assembled Structures and Cation-Anion Interactions in Crystals of Alkylimidazolium and Alkyltriazolium Iodides with Ferrocenyl Substituents. *Cryst. Growth Des.* **2011**, *11*, 262–268. [CrossRef]
62. Guino-o, M.A.; Talbot, M.O.; Snits, M.M.; Pham, T.N.; Audi, M.C.; Janzen, D.E. Crystal structures of five 1-alkyl-4-aryl-1,2,4-triazol-1-ium halide salts. *Acta Cryst. E* **2015**, *71*, 628–635. [CrossRef]
63. Zhang, W.Y.; Yuan, J.Y. Poly(1-Vinyl-1,2,4-triazolium) Poly(Ionic Liquid)s: Synthesis and the Unique Behavior in Loading Metal Ions. *Macromol. Rapid Commun.* **2016**, *37*, 1124–1129. [CrossRef]
64. Gao, Y.; Twamley, B.; Shreeve, J.M. The first (ferrocenylmethyl)imidazolium and (ferrocenylmethyl)triazolium room temperature ionic liquids. *Inorg. Chem.* **2004**, *43*, 3406–3412. [CrossRef]
65. Darwich, C.; Karaghiosoff, K.; Klapotke, T.M.; Sabate, C.M. Synthesis and characterization of 3,4,5-Triamino-1,2,4-triazolium and 1-Methyl-3,4,5-triamino-1,2,4-triazolium iodides. *Z. Anorg. Allg. Chem.* **2008**, *634*, 61–68. [CrossRef]
66. McCrary, P.D.; Chatel, G.; Alaniz, S.A.; Cojocaru, O.A.; Beasley, P.A.; Flores, L.A.; Kelley, S.P.; Barber, P.S.; Rogers, R.D. Evaluating Ionic Liquids as Hypergolic Fuels: Exploring Reactivity from Molecular Structure. *Energy Fuels* **2014**, *28*, 3460–3473. [CrossRef]
67. Elnajjar, F.O.; Binder, J.F.; Kosnik, S.C.; Macdonald, C.L.B. 1,2,4-Triazol-5-ylidenes versus Imidazol-2-ylidenes for the Stabilization of Phosphorus(I) Cations. *Z. Anorg. Allg. Chem.* **2016**, *642*, 1251–1258. [CrossRef]
68. Talbot, M.O.; Pham, T.N.; Guino-o, M.A.; Guzei, I.A.; Vinokur, A.I.; Young, V.G. Investigation of ligand steric effect on the hydrogen gas produced via a nickel-catalyzed dehydrogenation of ammonia-borane utilizing unsymmetrical triazolylidene ligands. *Polyhedron* **2016**, *114*, 415–421. [CrossRef]
69. Ghazal, B.; Machacek, M.; Shalaby, M.A.; Novakova, V.; Zimcik, P.; Makhseed, S. Phthalocyanines and Tetrapyrazinoporphyrazines with Two Cationic Donuts: High Photodynamic Activity as a Result of Rigid Spatial Arrangement of Peripheral Substituents. *J. Med. Chem.* **2017**, *60*, 6060–6076. [CrossRef]
70. Zhang, H.; Wang, Z.Q.; Ghiviriga, I.; Pillai, G.G.; Jabeen, F.; Arami, J.A.; Zhou, W.F.; Steel, P.J.; Hall, C.D.; Katritzky, A.R. Synthesis, characterization and energetic properties of novel 1-methyl-1,2,4-triazolium N-aryl/N-pyridinyl ylids. *Tetrahedron Lett.* **2017**, *58*, 1079–1085. [CrossRef]
71. Yan, H.R.; Wang, J.; Yu, Y.H.; Hou, G.F.; Zhang, H.X.; Gao, J.S. Two cationic $[(Cu_xI_y)^{x-y}]_n$ motif based coordination polymers and their photocatalytic properties. *RSC Adv.* **2016**, *6*, 71206–71213. [CrossRef]
72. Jiang, Y.L.; Wang, Y.L.; Lin, J.X.; Liu, Q.Y.; Lu, Z.H.; Zhang, N.; Jia Jia, W.; Li, L.Q. Syntheses, structures and properties of coordination polymers of cadmium(II) with 4-methyl-1,2,4-triazole-3-thiol ligand. *CrystEngComm* **2011**, *13*, 1697–1706. [CrossRef]
73. Li, B.Y.; Peng, Y.; Li, G.H.; Hua, J.; Yu, Y.; Jin, D.; Shi, Z.; Feng, S.H. Design and Construction of Coordination Polymers by 4-Amino-3,5-bis(n-pyridyl)-1,2,4-triazole (n = 2, 3, 4) Isomers in a Copper(I) Halide System: Diverse Structures Tuned by Isomeric and Anion Effects. *Cryst. Growth Des.* **2010**, *10*, 2192–2201. [CrossRef]
74. Kuttatheyil, A.V.; Handke, M.; Bergmann, J.; Lassig, D.; Lincke, J.; Haase, J.; Bertmer, M.; Krautscheid, H. ^{113}Cd Solid-State NMR for Probing the Coordination Sphere in Metal-Organic Frameworks. *Chem. Eur. J.* **2015**, *21*, 1118–1124. [CrossRef]
75. Wang, X.; Guo, W.; Guo, Y.M. Controllable assemblies of Cd(II) supramolecular coordination complexes based on a versatile tripyridyltriazole ligand and halide/pseduohalide anions. *J. Mol. Struct.* **2015**, *1096*, 136–141. [CrossRef]
76. Yan, J.Z.; Lu, L.P. Syntheses, Crystal Structures and Luminescence Properties of Two Cu_4I_4 Coordination Polymers Based on 3,5-Dialkyl-1,2,4-triazole. *Chinese J. Inorg. Chem.* **2017**, *33*, 1697–1704. [CrossRef]

77. Tan, T.T.Y.; Schick, S.; Hahn, F.E. Synthesis and Reactivity of Ir^{III} Complexes Bearing C-Metalated Pyrazolato Ligands. *Organometallics* **2019**, *38*, 567–574. [CrossRef]
78. Libnow, S.; Wille, S.; Christiansen, A.; Hein, M.; Reinke, H.; Kockerling, M.; Miethchen, R. Synthesis and reactivity of halogenated 1,2,4-triazole nucleoside analogues with high potential for chemical modifications. *Synth.-Stuttg.* **2006**, *2006*, 496–508. [CrossRef]
79. Novikov, A.S.; Ivanov, D.M.; Bikbaeva, Z.M.; Bokach, N.A.; Kukushkin, V.Y. Noncovalent Interactions Involving Iodofluorobenzenes: The Interplay of Halogen Bonding and Weak Ip(O)···π-Hole$_{(arene)}$ Interactions. *Cryst. Growth Des.* **2018**, *18*, 7641–7654. [CrossRef]
80. Bikbaeva, Z.M.; Ivanov, D.M.; Novikov, A.S.; Ananyev, I.V.; Bokach, N.A.; Kukushkin, V.Y. Electrophilic-Nucleophilic Dualism of Nickel(II) toward Ni···I Noncovalent Interactions: Semicoordination of Iodine Centers via Electron Belt and Halogen Bonding via σ-Hole. *Inorg. Chem.* **2017**, *56*, 13562–13578. [CrossRef]
81. Bikbaeva, Z.M.; Novikov, A.S.; Suslonov, V.V.; Bokach, N.A.; Kukushkin, V.Y. Metal-mediated reactions between dialkylcyanamides and acetamidoxime generate unusual (nitrosoguanidinate)nickel(II) complexes. *Dalton Trans.* **2017**, *46*, 10090–10101. [CrossRef]
82. Andrusenko, E.V.; Kabin, E.V.; Novikov, A.S.; Bokach, N.A.; Starova, G.L.; Kukushkin, V.Y. Metal-mediated generation of triazapentadienate-terminated di- and trinuclear μ^2-pyrazolate Ni^{II} species and control of their nuclearity. *New J. Chem.* **2017**, *41*, 316–325. [CrossRef]
83. Mikherdov, A.S.; Novikov, A.S.; Kinzhalov, M.A.; Boyarskiy, V.P.; Starova, G.L.; Ivanov, A.Y.; Kukushkin, V.Y. Halides Held by Bifurcated Chalcogen–Hydrogen Bonds. Effect of μ$_{(S,N-H)}$Cl Contacts on Dimerization of Cl(carbene)Pd^{II} Species. *Inorg. Chem.* **2018**, *57*, 3420–3433. [CrossRef]
84. Mikherdov, A.S.; Kinzhalov, M.A.; Novikov, A.S.; Boyarskiy, V.P.; Boyarskaya, I.A.; Avdontceva, M.S.; Kukushkin, V.Y. Ligation-Enhanced π-Hole···π Interactions Involving Isocyanides: Effect of π-Hole···π Noncovalent Bonding on Conformational Stabilization of Acyclic Diaminocarbene Ligands. *Inorg. Chem.* **2018**, *57*, 6722–6733. [CrossRef] [PubMed]
85. Adonin, S.A.; Bondarenko, M.A.; Novikov, A.S.; Abramov, P.A.; Sokolov, M.; Fedin, V.P. Halogen bonding in the structures of pentaiodobenzoic acid and its salts. *CrystEngComm* **2019**, *21*, 6666–6670. [CrossRef]
86. Afanasenko, A.M.; Novikov, A.S.; Chulkova, T.G.; Grigoriev, Y.M.; Kolesnikov, I.E.; Selivanov, S.I.; Starova, G.L.; Zolotarev, A.A.; Vereshchagin, A.N.; Elinson, M.N. Intermolecular interactions-photophysical properties relationships in phenanthrene-9,10-dicarbonitrile assemblies. *J. Mol. Struct.* **2020**, *1199*, 126789. [CrossRef]
87. Yandanova, E.S.; Ivanov, D.M.; Kuznetsov, M.L.; Starikov, A.G.; Starova, G.L.; Kukushkin, V.Y. Recognition of S···Cl Chalcogen Bonding in Metal-Bound Alkylthiocyanates. *Cryst. Growth Des.* **2016**, *16*, 2979–2987. [CrossRef]
88. Bulatova, M.; Melekhova, A.A.; Novikov, A.S.; Ivanov, D.M.; Bokach, N.A. Redox reactive (RNC)Cu^{II} species stabilized in the solid state via halogen bond with I$_2$. *Z. Kristallogr. Cryst. Mater.* **2018**, *233*, 371–377. [CrossRef]
89. Rozhkov, A.V.; Novikov, A.S.; Ivanov, D.M.; Bolotin, D.S.; Bokach, N.A.; Kukushkin, V.Y. Structure-Directing Weak Interactions with 1,4-Diiodotetrafluorobenzene Convert One-Dimensional Arrays of [M^{II}(acac)$_2$] Species into Three-Dimensional Networks. *Cryst. Growth Des.* **2018**, *18*, 3626–3636. [CrossRef]
90. Kinzhalov, M.A.; Kashina, M.V.; Mikherdov, A.S.; Mozheeva, E.A.; Novikov, A.S.; Smirnov, A.S.; Ivanov, D.M.; Kryukova, M.A.; Ivanov, A.Y.; Smirnov, S.N.; et al. Dramatically Enhanced Solubility of Halide-Containing Organometallic Species in Diiodomethane: The Role of Solvent···Complex Halogen Bonding. *Angew. Chem. Int. Ed.* **2018**, *57*, 12785–12789. [CrossRef]
91. Zelenkov, L.E.; Ivanov, D.M.; Avdontceva, M.S.; Novikov, A.S.; Bokach, N.A. Tetrachloromethane as halogen bond donor toward metal-bound halides. *Z. Kristallogr. Cryst. Mater.* **2019**, *234*, 9–17. [CrossRef]
92. Baykov, S.V.; Dabranskaya, U.; Ivanov, D.M.; Novikov, A.S.; Boyarskiy, V.P. Pt/Pd and I/Br Isostructural Exchange Provides Formation of C–I···Pd, C–Br···Pt, and C–Br···Pd Metal-Involving Halogen Bonding. *Cryst. Growth Des.* **2018**, *18*, 5973–5980. [CrossRef]
93. Espinosa, E.; Molins, E.; Lecomte, C. Hydrogen bond strengths revealed by topological analyses of experimentally observed electron densities. *Chem. Phys. Lett.* **1998**, *285*, 170–173. [CrossRef]

94. Vener, M.V.; Egorova, A.N.; Churakov, A.V.; Tsirelson, V.G. Intermolecular hydrogen bond energies in crystals evaluated using electron density properties: DFT computations with periodic boundary conditions. *J. Comput. Chem.* **2012**, *33*, 2303–2309. [CrossRef] [PubMed]
95. Bartashevich, E.V.; Tsirelson, V.G. Interplay between non-covalent interactions in complexes and crystals with halogen bonds. *Russ. Chem. Rev.* **2014**, *83*, 1181–1203. [CrossRef]
96. Espinosa, E.; Alkorta, I.; Elguero, J.; Molins, E. From weak to strong interactions: A comprehensive analysis of the topological and energetic properties of the electron density distribution involving X–H···F–Y systems. *J. Chem. Phys.* **2002**, *117*, 5529–5542. [CrossRef]

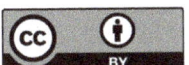

© 2020 by the authors. Licensee MDPI, Basel, Switzerland. This article is an open access article distributed under the terms and conditions of the Creative Commons Attribution (CC BY) license (http://creativecommons.org/licenses/by/4.0/).

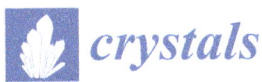

Article

Pharmaceutical Salts of Enrofloxacin with Organic Acids

Hong Pang [1], Yu-Bin Sun [1], Jun-Wen Zhou [1], Meng-Juan Xie [1], Hao Lin [1], Yan Yong [2], Liang-Zhu Chen [2] and Bing-Hu Fang [1,2,*]

[1] National Laboratory of Safety Evaluation (Environmental Assessment) of Veterinary Drugs, South China Agricultural University, Guangzhou 510000, China; pang_h163@163.com (H.P.); 18826231020@163.com (Y.-B.S.); zhou_j_wen@163.com (J.-W.Z.); xie_mjuan@163.com (M.-J.X.); 18319772187@163.com (H.L.)

[2] Guangdong Dahuanong Animal Health Products Co. Ltd., Yunfu 527400, China; xiaoyner@126.com (Y.Y.); che_lizh@163.com (L.-Z.C.)

* Correspondence: fangbh@scau.edu.cn

Received: 1 July 2020; Accepted: 24 July 2020; Published: 27 July 2020

Abstract: Enrofloxacin is a poorly soluble antibacterial drug of the fluoroquinolones class used in veterinary medicine. The main purpose of this work was to investigate the structural and pharmaceutical properties of new enrofloxacin salts. Enrofloxacin anhydrate and its organic salts with tartaric acid, nicotinic acid and suberic acid formed as pure crystalline anhydrous solids. All the crystals were grown from a mixed solution by slow evaporation at room temperature. These products were then characterized by field-emission scanning electron microscopy, powder X-ray diffraction, Fourier transform infrared spectroscopy and differential scanning calorimetry. Further, X-ray single crystal diffraction analysis was used to study the crystal structure. The intermolecular interactions and packing arrangements in the crystal structures were studied, and the solubility of these salts in water was determined using high-performance liquid chromatography. The results show that the new salts of enrofloxacin developed in this study exhibited excellent water solubility.

Keywords: enrofloxacin; salts; crystal structure; organic acids; solubility

1. Introduction

Crystal engineering through multicomponent crystals has attracted substantial attention in the pharmaceutical field in recent years [1,2] because of the possibility of improved solubility and bioavailability of newly designed drug compounds (polymorphs, salt and cocrystals) [3,4]. The formation of the salt/cocrystal is based on the crystal engineering concepts [5]. The salt/cocrystal formation provides an enormous scope for the manipulation and modification of crucial pharmaceutical physical properties such as the dissolution rate, solubility, thermodynamic stability and bioavailability [6,7]. Proton transfer is a decisive factor that distinguishes salts from cocrystals: In salt formation, proton transfer and ionization occur, while these do not occur in the formation of cocrystals [8]. Salts and cocrystals have been employed in the pharmaceutical industry because of their excellent solubility [9]. Although cocrystallization has many exciting advantages, salt formation still represents a widely accepted method to obtain higher solubility of the drug [10].

Most of the active pharmaceutical ingredients (APIs) available in the current market cause formulation difficulties because of poor water solubility, which may lead to poor oral bioavailability [11,12]. Hence, improving the solubility and bioavailability of APIs without changing their stability and other characteristics has become a challenging task. Notably, every crystal structure is the result of mutual balance between numerous noncovalent interactions, but the hydrogen bond remains an important factor in supramolecular assembly [13]. The design of supramolecular heterosynthons derived from organic salts was hypothesized on the basis of the supramolecular synthon strategy in the context of crystal engineering [14,15]. Recently, this strategy has been effectively adopted in the field of pharmaceutical crystallization [16].

Enrofloxacin (1-cyclopropyl-7-(4-ethylpiperazin-1-yl)-6-fluoro-4-oxo-1,4-dihydroquinoline-3-carboxylate) shows a wide spectrum of antibacterial activity, and it belongs to the class of fluoroquinolone antibiotics [17]. As an important synthetic bacteriostatic drug, it has been widely used in stock raising. In good clinical trials, its effectiveness in treating uncomplicated and complicated urinary tract infections, urethral and cervical gonococcal infections, respiratory tract infections, and skin and tissue infections has been proven [18]. It exhibits concentration-dependent antibacterial activity [19]. Enrofloxacin exists in a zwitterionic form within a neutral aqueous solution due to the acid/base interaction between the basic nitrogen of the piperazine and the carboxylic acid group [20,21]. Therefore, in water at pH ≈ 7, enrofloxacin exhibits a low solubility (0.45 mg/mL) [21]. In addition, low solubility of enrofloxacin is one of the unfavourable properties in formulation [22]. Therefore, a method to improve its solubility without compromising performance has been sought. A weak organic acid can be used as an organic counterionic component for salt formation [23,24]. These acids can potentially present the formation of salts with multiple stoichiometries due to the containment of carboxylic group. This approach is widely used in pharmaceutical industries to enhance solubility, bioavailability and controlled release of drugs [25]. Therefore, we adopted crystal engineering concepts to select pharmaceutically acceptable organic counterions to form salts with enrofloxacin.

In this study, we prepared enrofloxacin anhydrate and salt trihydrate with tartaric acid and salt solvate with nicotinic acid and suberic acid, and we analysed the crystal structures of these compounds. The obtained crystal compounds were characterized by field-emission scanning electron microscopy (FESEM), Fourier transform infrared spectroscopy (FT-IR), powder X-ray diffraction (PXRD) and differential scanning calorimetry (DSC). All the crystal structure data were successfully resolved by single-crystal X-ray diffraction (SCXRD), and the crystal conformations and packing arrangements were studied in detail. Finally, the solubility of the new phases in water was also determined by high-performance liquid chromatography (HPLC). The new salts were found to exhibit significantly improved solubility and were therefore suitable for use in drug formulation.

2. Experimental

2.1. Materials

Enrofloxacin ($C_{19}H_{22}FN_3O_3$, 98%) was obtained from Nanjing Kangmanlin Biomedical Technology Co. Ltd. (Nanjing, China). These organic acids (tartaric acid ($C_4H_6O_6$, 99.5%), nicotinic acid ($C_6H_5NO_2$, 99.5%), suberic acid ($C_6H_{10}O_4$, 99%)) were purchased from Shanghai Macklin Biochemical Co., Ltd. (Shanghai, China). The chromatography grade organic solvents (methanol (MeOH), acetonitrile (ACN), triethylamine (TEA), phosphate) were purchased from Tianjin Kemio Chemical Reagent Co., Ltd. (Tianjin, China). All of the analytical-grade organic solvents (ethanol (EtOH), dichloromethane (DCM), N,N-Dimethylformamide (DMF)) were obtained from Tianjin Damao Chemical Reagent Factory (Tianjin, China) and these were used without further purification. Purified water was prepared using the Millipore Milli-Q system.

2.2. Crystallization of Enrofloxacin Anhydrate

Enrofloxacin Anhydrate (**1**): Enrofloxacin (230 mg, 0.64 mmol) was added to 4 mL of an ethanol/dichloromethane mixed solvent (1:1 *v/v*) for crystallization. The **1** crystals in the suspension were then filtered and dried in air (yield: 77%).

2.3. Preparation of Salts and Crystallization

Enrofloxacin and various acids in equal molar ratios were dissolved in a mixed solvent in a 50-mL conical flask, and this mixture was stirred at 50 °C until a completely clear solution was obtained.

The solution was then allowed to slowly evaporate at room temperature to obtain single crystals of the products. Diffraction-quality crystals were obtained within 1–5 days. Each sample was scaled up 20 times for the solubility determination.

Enrofloxacin Tartrate Trihydrate (**2**): A 1:1 mixture of enrofloxacin (460 mg, 1.28 mmol) and tartaric acid (180 mg, 1.28 mmol) was added to 12 mL of a water/ethanol/dichloromethane mixed solvent (4:7:3 *v/v/v*) for crystallization. Then, **2** was obtained by filtration and drying in air (yield: 76%).

Enrofloxacin Nicotinat-EtOH Salt Solvate (**3**): A 1:1 mixture of enrofloxacin (230 mg, 0.64 mmol) and nicotinic acid (83.7 mg, 0.64 mmol) was added to 5 mL of an ethanol/dichloromethane mixed solvent (3:2 *v/v*) for crystallization. The resulting **3** crystals were filtered and dried in air (yield: 86%).

Enrofloxacin Suberate-2EtOH Salt Solvate (**4**): A 1:1 mixture of enrofloxacin (230 mg, 0.64 mmol) and suberic acid (110 mg, 0.64 mmol) was added to 4 mL of an ethanol/dichloromethane mixed solvent (1:1 *v/v*) for crystallization. Crystals were then obtained by filtration and drying (yield: 77%).

2.4. Field-Emission Scanning Electron Microscopy (FESEM)

The surface morphology of the samples was investigated by FESEM (Heidelberg, Germany) using a Zeiss Sigma 300.

2.5. Powder X-ray Diffraction (PXRD)

PXRD measurements of the new compounds were carried out on a Rigaku-Ultima IV X-ray powder diffractometer (Tokyo, Japan) using Cu Kα radiation (λ = 1.54178 Å) at 40 kV and 40 mA. Samples were analysed in the 2θ range from 5° to 80° with a scanning rate of 8°/min. These data were collected at room temperature and analysed using Jade 6.0 software (Livermore, CA, USA).

2.6. Fourier Transform Infrared (FT-IR)

FT–IR spectra were collected using a Bruker Vertex 70 spectrometer and measured in the range of 4000–400 cm^{-1} with an RT-DLaTGS detector (Ettlingen, Germany). The KBr diffuse-reflectance mode was used (sample concentration: 1 mg in 100 mg of KBr) for recording the IR spectra of these samples. Data were analysed using the OPUS software (San Francisco, CA, USA).

2.7. Single Crystal X-ray Diffraction (SCXRD)

X-ray diffraction data were collected using a Rigaku Oxford Diffraction SuperNova diffractometer (Oxford, UK) equipped with a monochromator mirror for Cu Kα (λ = 1.54184 Å) radiation at 150 K. Data reduction was carried out using the CrysAlisPro software, and absorption correction was implemented in the SCALE3 ABSPACK scaling algorithm. The structure was solved (direct methods) and refined (using least squares minimization) with Olex2 [26] using SHELX [27] structure solution programs. All the non-H atoms were refined anisotropically. In addition, all the figures, including the packing and molecular structure diagrams, were drawn using Olex2 and PLATON [28]. Table 1 gives the pertinent crystal lographic data, and Table 2 gives the hydrogen-bond parameters.

Table 1. Crystallographic Data for Compounds 1–4.

Crystal Parameters	1	2	3	4
Empirical formula	$C_{19}H_{22}FN_3O_3$	$C_{23}H_{31}FN_3O_{10.5}$	$C_{27}H_{33}FN_4O_6$	$C_{29}H_{42}FN_3O_8$
Formula weight	359.39	536.51	528.57	579.65
Temperature/K	150.03(12)	150.00(10)	150.00(10)	150.00(10)
Crystal system	monoclinic	triclinic	triclinic	triclinic
Space group	$P2_1/n$	$P\bar{1}$	$P\bar{1}$	$P\bar{1}$
a/Å	13.9309(2)	7.4444(4)	8.4841(4)	6.9755(2)
b/Å	6.87600(10)	11.2932(6)	12.1821(6)	9.3315(4)
c/Å	18.5133(3)	15.5835(9)	13.6436(6)	23.4431(9)
α/°	90	86.475(4)	115.392(4)	99.065(3)
β/°	100.9240(10)	77.366(4)	93.462(4)	95.004(3)
γ/°	90	74.427(5)	92.054(4)	104.306(3)
Volume/Å³	1741.23(5)	1231.46(12)	1268.59(11)	1447.42(10)
Z	4	2	2	2
ϱ_{calc} g/cm³	1.371	1.447	1.384	1.330
μ/mm^{-1}	0.839	1.023	0.861	0.841
F(000)	760.0	566.0	560.0	620.0
Crystal size/mm³	0.7 × 0.4 × 0.4	0.2 × 0.02 × 0.01	0.4 × 0.3 × 0.25	0.25 × 0.15 × 0.03
Radiation	CuKα (λ = 1.54184)	CuKα (λ = 1.54184)	CuKα (λ = 1.54184)	CuKα (λ = 1.54178)
2θ range for data collection/°	7.314 to 146.554	8.128 to 148.07	7.198 to 134.982	7.704 to 137.998
Index ranges	−13 ≤ h ≤ 17, −8 ≤ k ≤ 5, −22 ≤ l ≤ 20	−9 ≤ h ≤ 9, −14 ≤ k ≤ 11, −19 ≤ l ≤ 19	−10 ≤ h ≤ 9, −14 ≤ k ≤ 14, −16 ≤ l ≤ 14	−7 ≤ h ≤ 8, −11 ≤ k ≤ 11, −28 ≤ l ≤ 27
Reflections collected	5229	8302	6853	10,171
Independent reflections	3299 [R_{int} = 0.0297, R_{sigma} = 0.0325]	4827 [R_{int} = 0.0317, R_{sigma} = 0.0427]	4494 [R_{int} = 0.0339, R_{sigma} = 0.0366]	5318 [R_{int} = 0.0262, R_{sigma} = 0.0340]
Data/restraints/parameters	3299/0/238	4827/0/369	4494/0/348	5318/72/462
Goodness-of-fit on F²	1.062	1.030	1.054	1.018
Final R indexes [I>=2σ (I)]	R_1 = 0.0509, wR_2 = 0.1325	R_1 = 0.0483, wR_2 = 0.1236	R_1 = 0.0532, wR_2 = 0.1475	R_1 = 0.0695, wR_2 = 0.1736
Final R indexes [all data]	R_1 = 0.0528, wR_2 = 0.1355	R_1 = 0.0580, wR_2 = 0.1307	R_1 = 0.0585, wR_2 = 0.1531	R_1 = 0.0792, wR_2 = 0.1838
Largest diff. peak/hole/e Å^{-3}	0.25/−0.40	0.36/−0.42	0.76/−0.56	0.45/−0.49
CCDC	2000796	2000797	2000798	2000799

Table 2. Hydrogen Bond Geometry Parameters in Compounds 1–4.

D–H⋯A	D⋯A (Å)	H⋯A (Å)	D–H⋯A (Deg)
			Compound 1
O1–H1⋯O3	2.5460(14)	1.78	154
C2–H2⋯O2	2.7950(16)	2.46	101
C8–H8A⋯O1	3.4690(16)	2.56	157
C8–H8B⋯O3	3.2816(16)	2.33	167
C9–H9⋯O3	3.2232(15)	2.45	135
C15–H15B⋯F1	2.8895(15)	2.24	123
			Compound 2
O1–H1⋯O3	2.5182(19)	1.76	153
N3–H3⋯O7	3.022(2)	2.21	139
N3–H3⋯O9	2.835(2)	1.99	142
O6–H6⋯O4	2.624(3)	2.15	117
O6–H6⋯O11	3.051(12)	2.37	141

Table 2. Cont.

D–H···A	D···A (Å)	H···A (Å)	D–H···A (Deg)
O6–H6···O12	3.097(13)	2.37	148
O7–H7···O5	2.610(2)	1.80	171
O8–H8···O4	2.439(3)	1.29(5)	174(4)
O10–H10A···O6	2.684(4)	1.90	154
O10–H10B···O2	2.805(3)	2.00	158
O11–H11A···O6	3.051(12)	2.47	126
O11–H11A···O7	3.367(12)	2.54	165
O11–H11B···O4	2.870(11)	2.40	116
O11–H11B···O9	2.909(12)	2.12	153
O12–H12A···O11	2.823(15)	2.00	164
O12–H12A···O12	2.715(16)	1.90	160
O12–H12B···O4	2.985(10)	2.50	117
O12–H12B···O9	3.057(13)	2.25	158
C2–H2···O2	2.836(2)	2.53	100
C7–H7B···O2	3.567(3)	2.60	175
C9–H9···O3	3.306(3)	2.38	157
C10–H10···O3	3.411(3)	2.51	163
C14–H14A···O8	3.325(2)	2.39	162
C15–H15A···F1	2.872(2)	2.22	123
C17–H17A···O1	3.165(2)	2.25	156
C18–H18B···O6	3.015(3)	2.55	109
C19–H19A···O7	3.343(3)	2.56	139
C19–H19A···O11	3.194(13)	2.46	133
C21–H21···O8	2.884(3)	2.51	102
Compound 3			
O1–H1···O3	2.536(2)	1.77	154
N3–H3···O4	2.618(2)	1.64	172
O6–H6···O5	2.761(3)	1.94	178
C2–H2···O2	2.799(3)	2.48	101
C8–H8B···O3	3.363(3)	2.45	157
C14–H14B···O6	3.460(3)	2.54	158
C15–H15A···F1	2.861(3)	2.22	123
C16–H16A···O4	3.241(2)	2.48	135
C17–H17A···O3	3.349(2)	2.52	144
C18–H18B···O2	3.224(3)	2.44	138
C23–H23···O4	2.792(3)	2.46	101
Compound 4			
O1–H1···O3	2.740(12)	1.95	162
N3–H3···O6	2.667(3)	1.74	155
O5–H5···O6	2.567(3)	1.75	174
O8–H8···O7	2.731(6)	1.94	162
C2–H2···O2	2.723(9)	2.27	109
C7–H7A···F1	3.430(8)	2.46	174
C8–H8A···O8	3.040(8)	2.59	108
C9–H9···O3	3.347(7)	2.57	137
C15–H15A···F1	2.882(3)	2.26	121
C16–H16B···O1	3.358(10)	2.44	158
C16–H16B···O1A	3.435(8)	2.49	166
C17–H17B···O4	3.320(3)	2.39	161
C29–H29B···O1A	3.203(10)	2.53	127

2.8. Differential Scanning Calorimetry (DSC)

Thermal analyses of these samples were performed on a DSC (Q200 V24.10 Build 122) instrument (New Castle, DE, USA): 2–3 mg of the crystals was placed in standard aluminium pans and scanned at 20 °C/min in the range 25–280 °C under a nitrogen gas flow of 50 mL/min. Data were analysed using the Universal Analysis 2000 software (New Castle, DE, USA).

2.9. Solubility Analyses

The solubility of these products was determined according to the shake-flask method [29]. Excess amounts (100 mg) of the crystals were added to the screw-capped glass vials containing

2.5 mL of ultrapure water, and the resulting suspensions was shaken at room temperature. After 24 h, the suspensions were filtered through 0.22-µm polycarbonate filters, and the compounds' concentrations were determined using the Agilent 1260 Infinity II HPLC system (Palo Alto, CA, USA) equipped with a 1260 Multi λ Fluorescence detector with the wavelength of the excited and emitted spectra of crystals being 280 nm and 450 nm, respectively. The C18 HPLC column (Poroshell 120 EC-C18, 4.6 mm × 100 mm, 2.7 µm) was employed, and acetonitrile, methanol and triethylamine phosphate (pH = 2.5) were used as the mobile phase (1:24:75, $v:v::v$) with a flow rate of 1 mL/min. Each solubility test was performed in triplicate.

3. Results and Discussion

3.1. Field-Emission Scanning Electron Microscopy (FESEM)

The FESEM (Heidelberg, Germany) images provide information about the crystal morphology of several new crystals (Figure 1). Needle-shaped or long rod-shaped forms are seen for the products **1** and **2**, whereas **3** and **4** displayed rectangular blocks and fragmentary crystals.

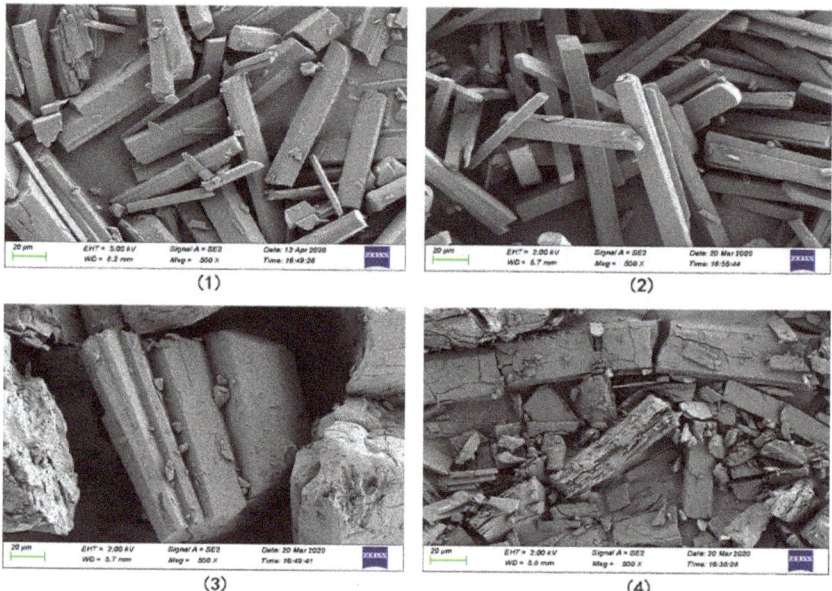

Figure 1. Field-emission scanning electron microscopy (FESEM) photos of compounds **1–4**.

3.2. PXRD Analysis

PXRD enables the study and characterization of novel crystalline materials [30]. PXRD patterns of the four crystal samples are shown in Figure 2. The patterns for **1** were different from those of the starting material and from the previously published PXRD patterns for the polymorphic form [31]. The purity of all products was confirmed by comparing the PXRD patterns with the simulated patterns obtained from the single crystal data (see the Supplementary Materials, Figures S1–S4). No apparent peaks corresponding to impurities were observed, so the obtained powder compounds were considered to be of high chemical purity. Further, these PXRD patterns of enrofloxacin compounds **2–4** differ significantly from the patterns of individual APIs, proving the formation of the new crystalline phases.

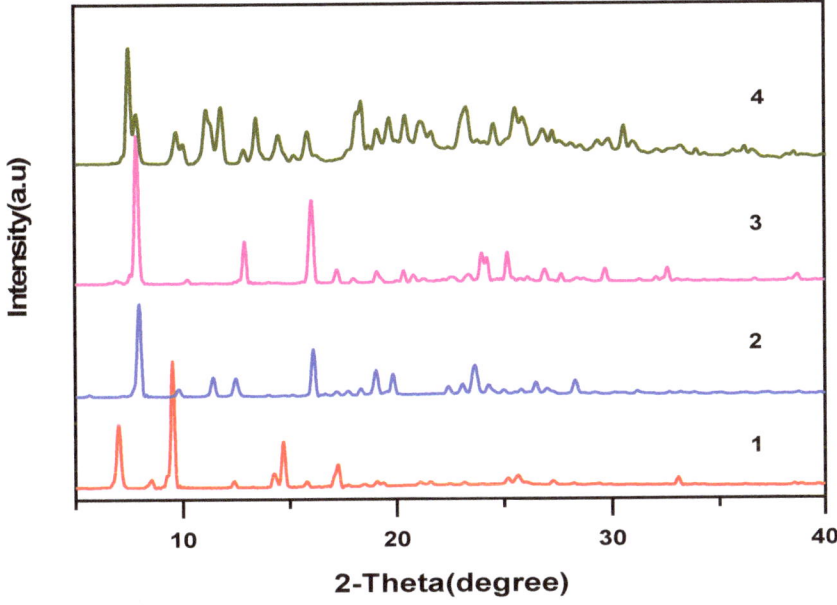

Figure 2. Powder X-ray diffraction (PXRD) patterns of compounds **1–4**.

3.3. Spectroscopic Characterization

The FTIR analysis results for the products are given in Figure 3. The absorption band of crystalline enrofloxacin was located at 1737 cm^{-1} because of the carbonyl stretching of its unionized carboxylic acid C=O group [31]. The C=O band in **1** was at 1736.4 cm^{-1}, which indicates that the enrofloxacin exists as a neutral molecule. Slight peak shifts were also seen in compounds **2–4**, in particular, for the carboxylic acid C=O stretching, which shifted to 1728.8 cm^{-1}, 1728.5 cm^{-1} and 1729.3 cm^{-1}, respectively. This can be attributed to intermolecular interactions such as the formation of hydrogen bonds [32]. The terminal amino group of the piperazine ring was protonated in the process of crystallization, and this is proved by the presence of broad bands from 2600 cm^{-1} to 3000 cm^{-1}. However, confirming this is difficult because the broad IR absorption bands possibly overlap with others, e.g., in the case of the C–H stretching [33]. However, Karanam et al. reported FTIR analysis results that showed that enrofloxacin salts were protonated in the process of crystallization [34]. The medium-intensity broad band in the region of 3300–3500 cm^{-1} is attributed to the O–H stretching of the water molecule **2** and ethanol molecule **3–4**. The existence of enrofloxacin as a neutral molecular and in the ionic state in the crystal structures was confirmed by SCXRD analysis.

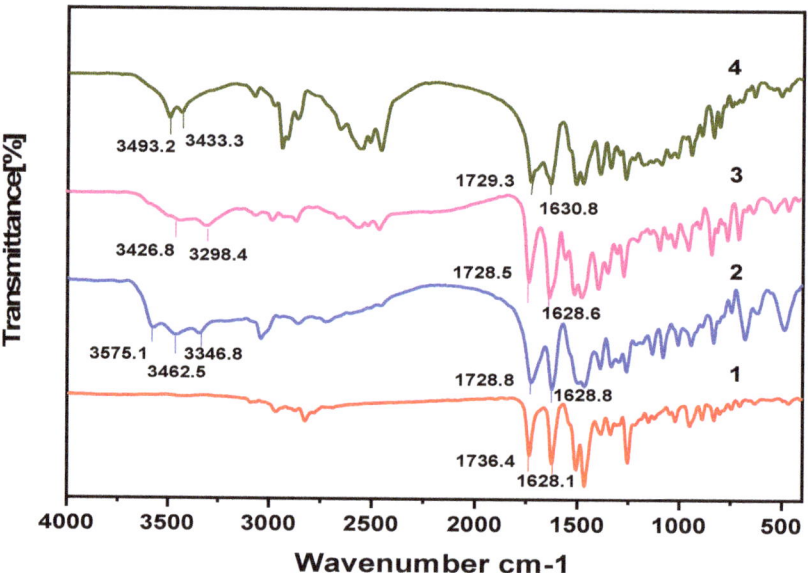

Figure 3. Fourier transform infrared (FTIR) spectrum of compounds 1–4.

3.4. Crystal Structure Analysis

3.4.1. Crystallization of Enrofloxacin Anhydrate (1)

Single crystals suitable for X-ray diffraction were obtained to determine the structures of the anhydrous form with a neutral molecule (no proton transfer from carboxylic acid to piperazinyl N atom; Figure 4a). The enrofloxacin anhydrate crystallized in the monoclinic $P2_1/n$ space group with one molecule in the asymmetric unit. In addition, the piperazine ring in enrofloxacin usually exhibits a stable chair conformation with a torsion angle of C12–N2–C15–C16 = 158.25°. It has the same crystal structure compared with the previous published [34]. The carboxylic acid group participated in intramolecular O–H···O hydrogen bonding with the carbonyl oxygen atom of the quinolone moiety. The crystal structure was stacked with $\pi\cdots\pi$ (3.598 Å) interactions and was further stabilized by weak C–H···O and C–H···F hydrogen bonds Table 2 in enrofloxacin (Figure 4b).

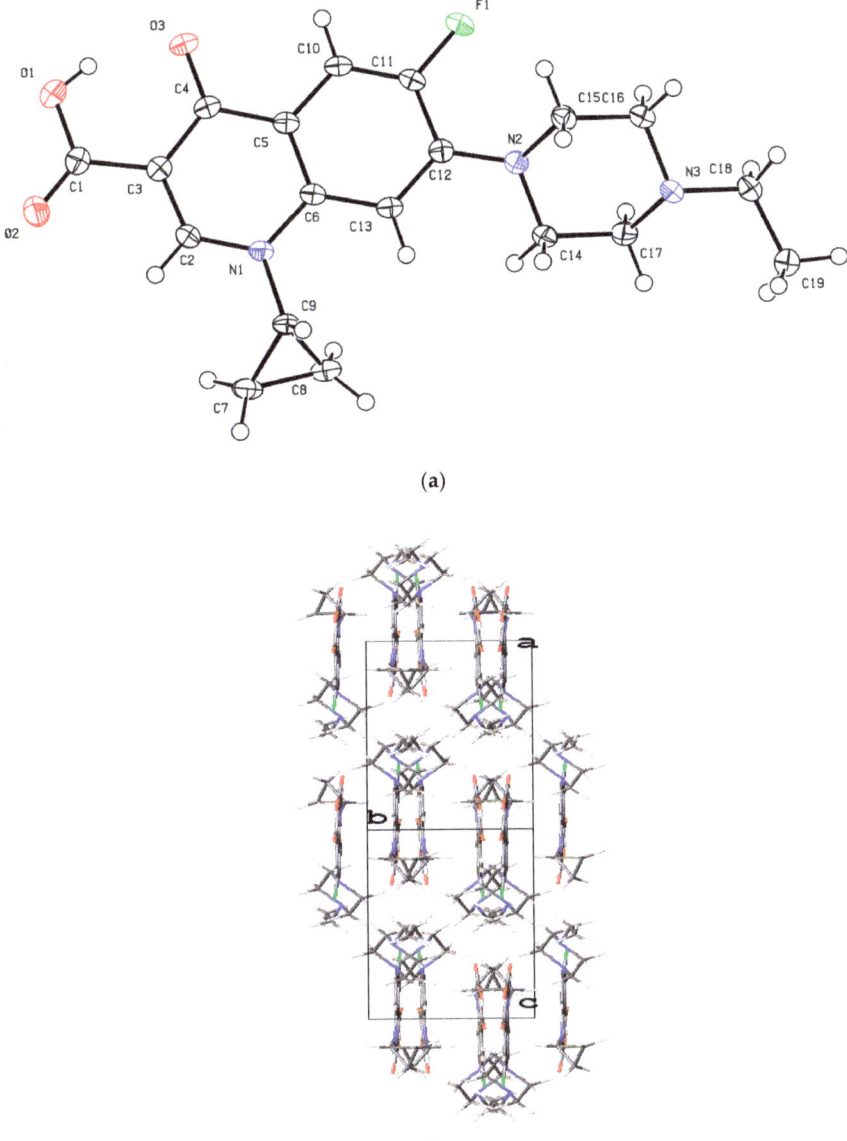

Figure 4. (**a**) The molecular structure diagram of the product **1** (ellipsoids were drawn at the 50% probability level). (**b**) Molecular packing projections for product **1** along the [101] direction.

3.4.2. Enrofloxacin Tartrate Trihydrate (2)

The novel enrofloxacin salt trihydrate **2** crystallized in the triclinic $P\bar{1}$ space group. The 1:1 salt structure of enrofloxacin tartrate trihydrate contains an enrofloxacin cation, a tartrate anion and three H_2O molecules in the asymmetric unit (Figure 5a). One of the carboxylic acid groups of tartaric acid transferred one proton to the piperazinyl-ring N atom of the enrofloxacin molecule, resulting in a tartrate anion and enrofloxacin cation in the crystal structure (Figure 5b). The carboxylic acid group of enrofloxacin was involved in intramolecular O−H···O hydrogen bonding with the quinolone oxygen atom. The product 2 displayed a unique hydrogen-bonding pattern with the formation of multicomponent crystals. The enrofloxacin cation interacted with the tartrate ion via N$^+$–H···O interactions to form the crystal structure, rather than forming hydrogen bonds with ionized oxygen atoms. Further, one of the water molecules connected the enrofloxacin cation and tartrate anion via O–H···O interactions (Figure 5c).

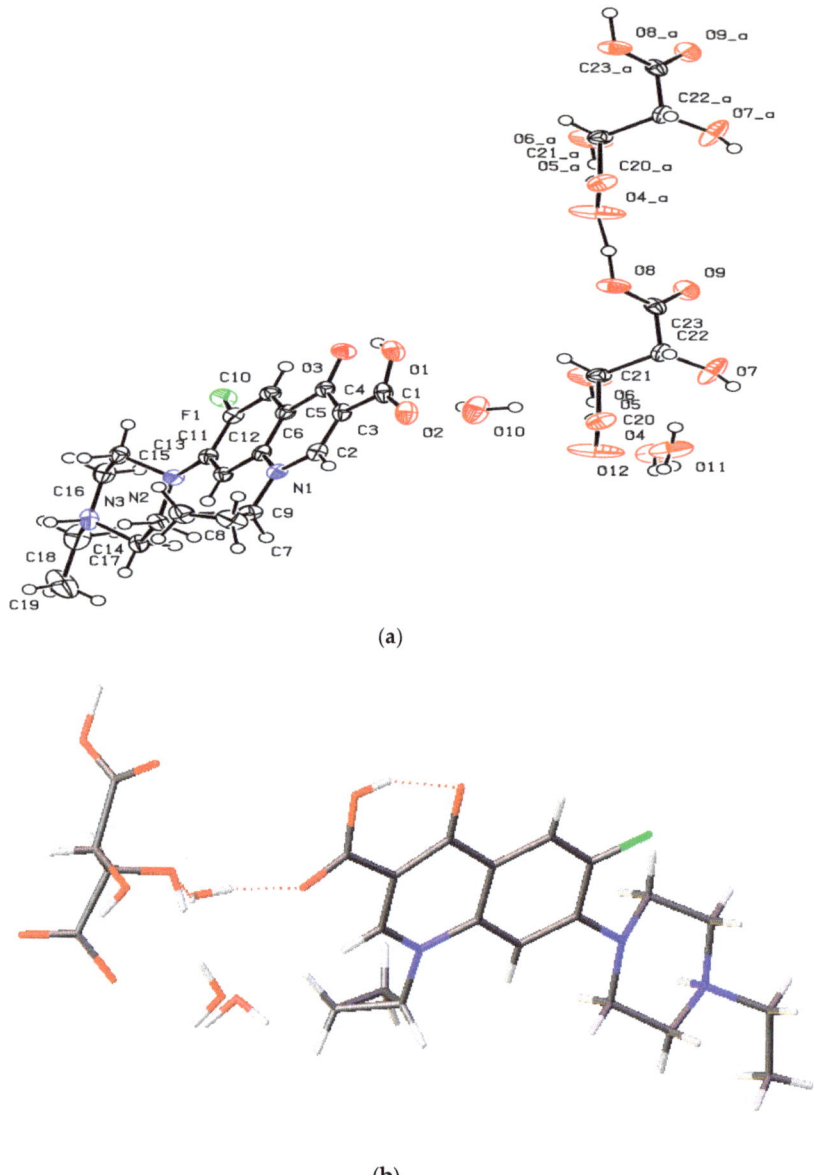

(a)

(b)

Figure 5. *Cont.*

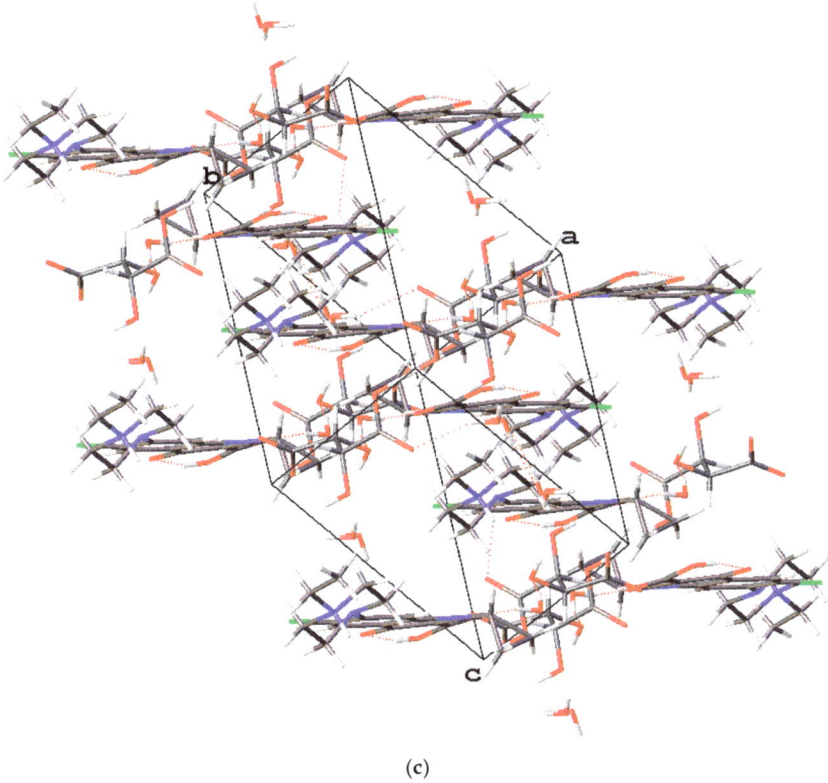

(c)

Figure 5. (**a**) The molecular structure diagram of the salt trihydrate **2** (ellipsoids were drawn at the 50% probability level). (**b**) Interaction between enrofloxacin and tartaric acid molecules in the crystal via O–H···O hydrogen bonds. (**c**) Molecular packing projections for salt trihydrate **2** along the [111] direction.

3.4.3. Enrofloxacin Nicotinate-EtOH Salt Solvate (3)

The novel enrofloxacin salt solvate **3** had a triclinic system and space group $P\bar{1}$. Its crystal contained an enrofloxacin cation, a nicotinate anion and an EtOH molecule in the asymmetric unit (Figure 6a). The carboxylic acid group of **3** was involved in intramolecular O–H···O hydrogen bonding with the quinolone oxygen atom. The nicotinic acid was ionized by proton transfer to the enrofloxacin molecule to form N^+–H···O^-, while the EtOH molecule formed the O–H···O hydrogen bond with the carboxylic acid C=O group of nicotinate (Figure 6b). The quinolone moieties of the enrofloxacin molecules stacked via π···π (3.538 Å) interactions (Figure 6c).

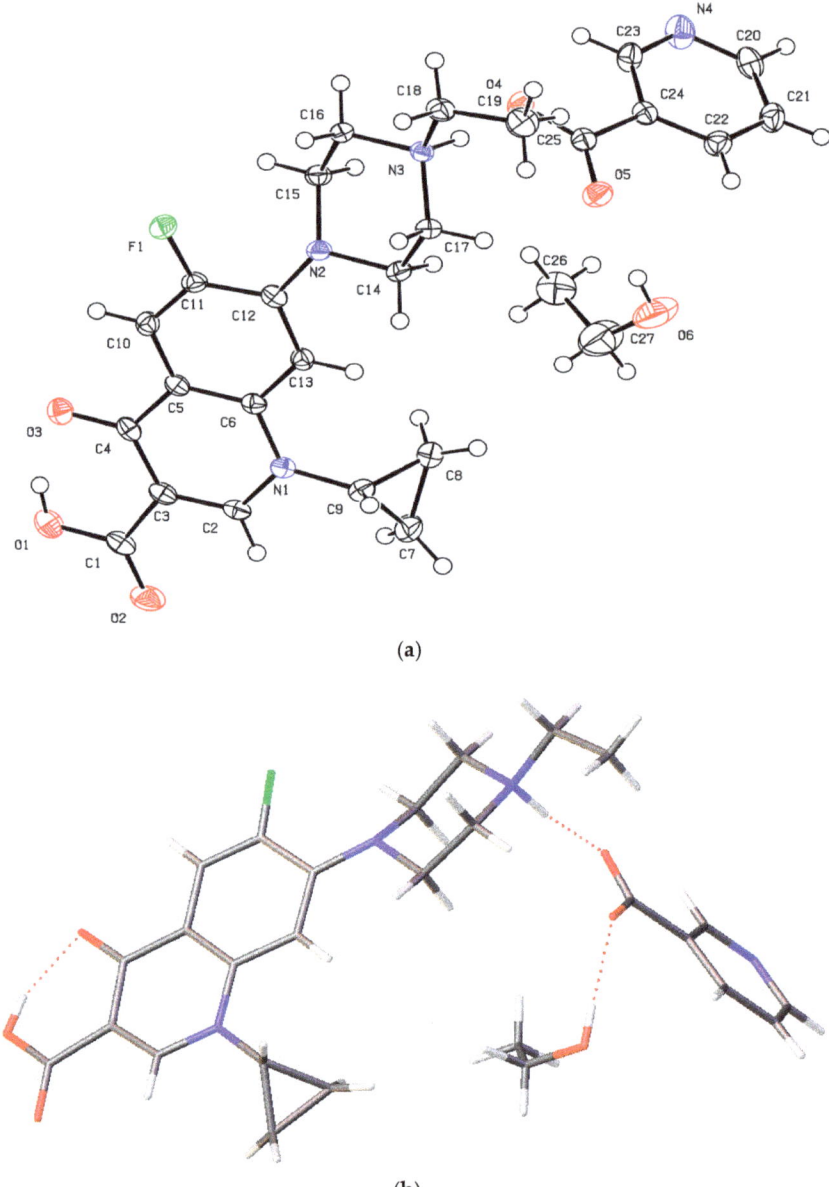

(a)

(b)

Figure 6. *Cont.*

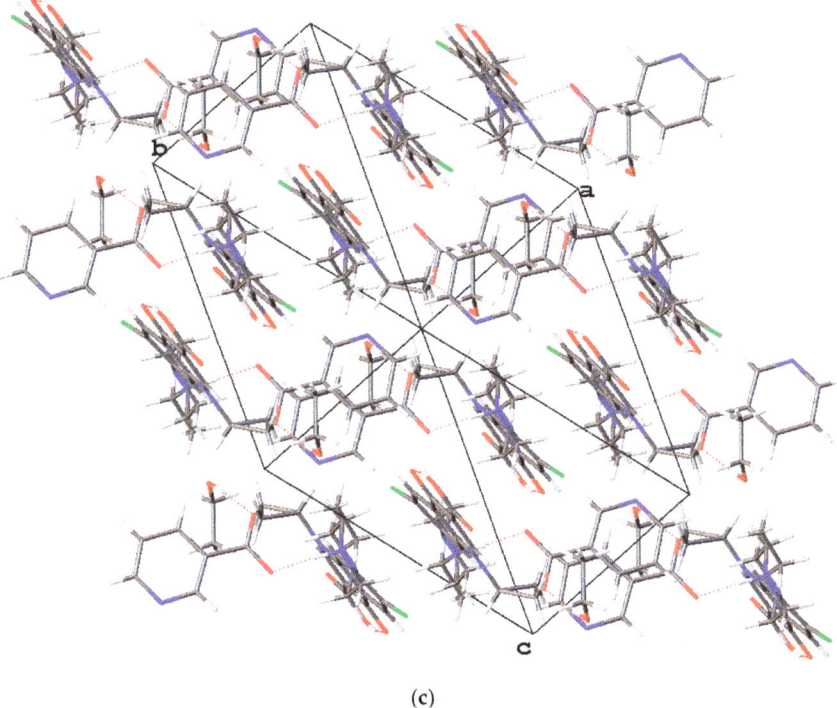

(c)

Figure 6. (a) The molecular structure diagram of the salt solvate **3** (ellipsoids were drawn at the 50% probability level). (b) Interaction between enrofloxacin and nicotinic acid molecules in the crystal via $N^+-H\cdots O^-$ and $O-H\cdots O$ hydrogen bonds. (c) Molecular packing projections for salt solvate **3** along the [111] direction.

3.4.4. Enrofloxacin Suberate-2EtOH Salt Solvate (4)

The novel enrofloxacin salt solvate **4** had a triclinic system and space group $P\bar{1}$ with an enrofloxacin cation, a suberate anion and two EtOH molecules in the asymmetric unit. The carboxylic acid and cyclopropyl groups of the enrofloxacin molecule were observed to exhibit disorder in this crystal structure (Figure 7a). One of the carboxylic acid groups of the suberic acid transferred one proton to the piperazinyl-ring N atom of the enrofloxacin molecule, thereby forming a suberate anion and enrofloxacin cations in the crystal structure (Figure 7b). The carboxylic acid group of **4** was involved in intramolecular $O-H\cdots O$ hydrogen bonding with the quinolone oxygen atom. Enrofloxacin interactsedwith the suberate ion via $N^+-H\cdots O^-$ interactions in the crystal structure, while the EtOH molecule formed the $O-H\cdots O$ hydrogen bond with the carboxylic acid C=O group of the suberate ion. The quinolone moieties of the enrofloxacin molecule stacked via $\pi\cdots\pi$ (3.872 Å) interactions (Figure 7c).

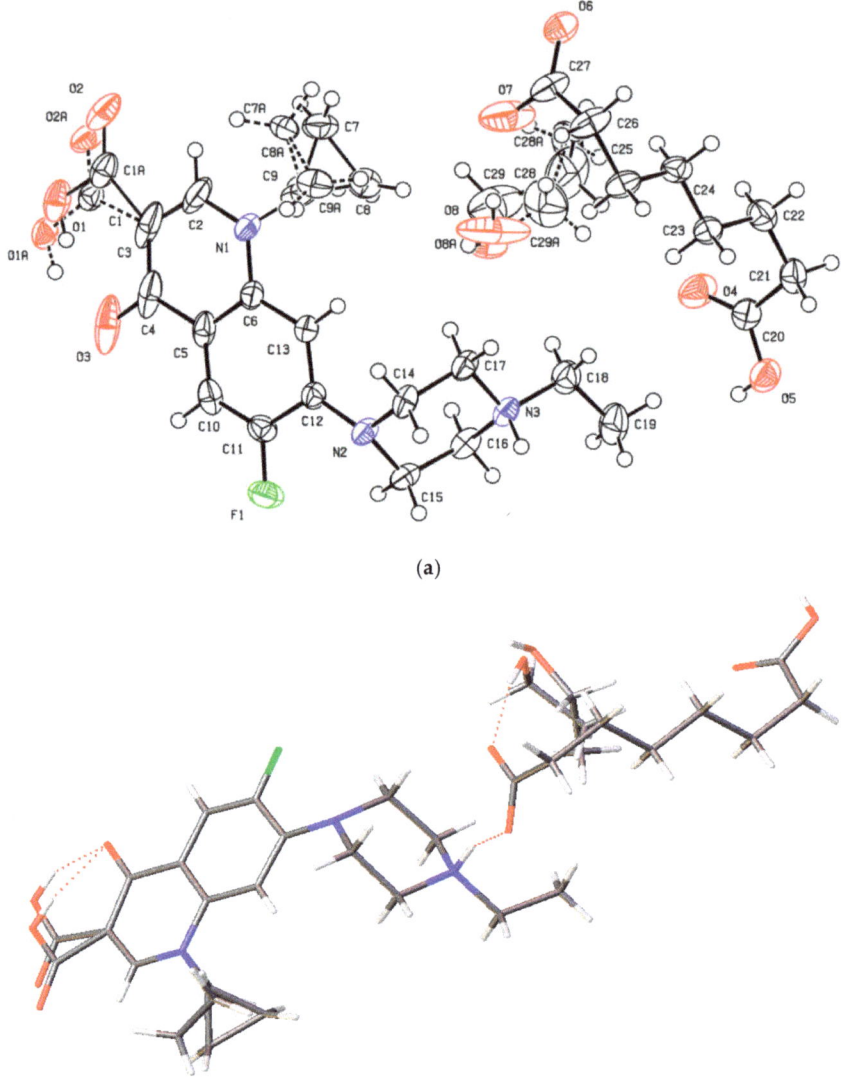

(a)

(b)

Figure 7. *Cont.*

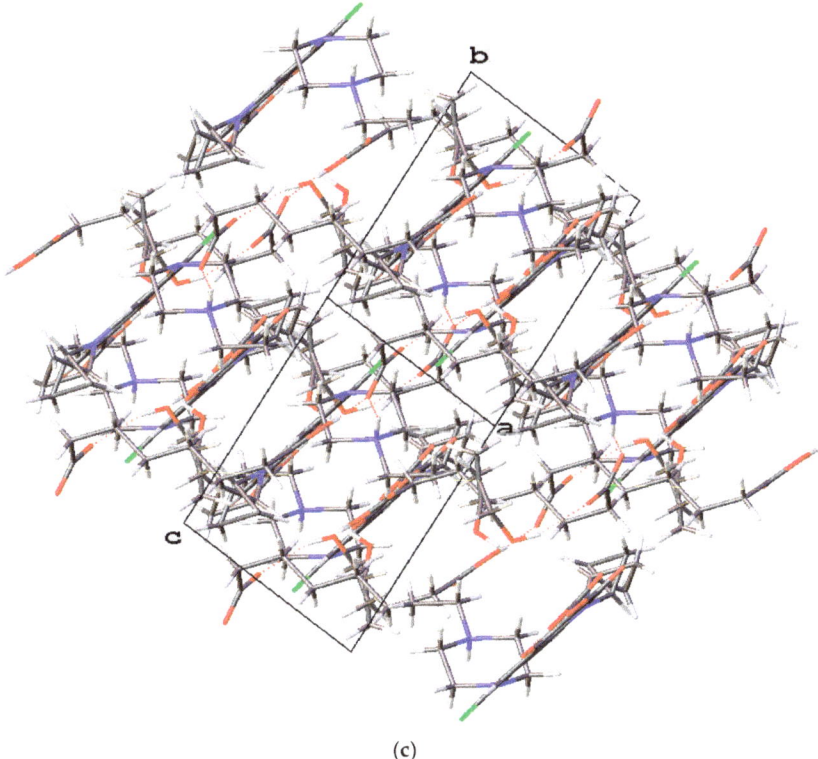

(c)

Figure 7. (a) The molecular structure diagram of the salt solvate **4** (ellipsoids were drawn at the 50% probability level). (b) Interaction between enrofloxacin and suberic acid molecules in the crystal by N^+–H···O^- and O–H···O hydrogen bonds. (c) Molecular packing projections for salt solvate **4** along the [011] direction.

3.5. Thermal Analysis

DSC curves showing the thermal behaviour of the products **1**–**4** are shown in Figure 8. The endothermic peak for melting of **1** was found at 228 °C. In the case of **2**, the endothermic melting peak was at 228 °C, and this was followed by a phase transition. The endothermic transitions between 75 °C and 125 °C in the DSC thermograms for **2** showed the loss of water molecules from the crystal structure. In the DSC thermogram for **3**, several steps of small endothermic transitions at about 120–180 °C due to solvent loss were observed, followed by a four-step endothermic melting transition of the salt solvate Further, **4** was found to melt at 112 °C.

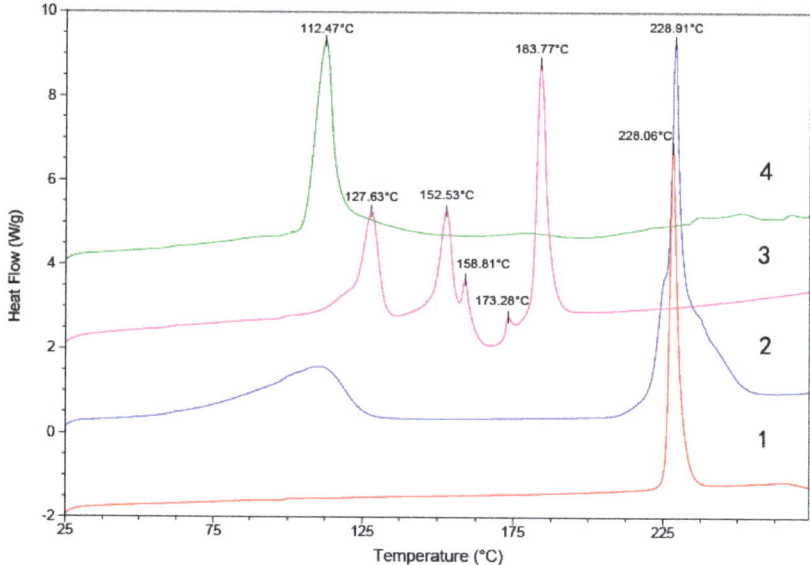

Figure 8. Differential scanning calorimetry (DSC) diagrams of compounds **1–4**.

3.6. Results for Solubility Study

The solubility data are presented in Table 3. The solubility of commercially available enrofloxacin in water was 0.14 mg/mL, which is similar to the previously reported values [21]. The solubilities of **1** and the commercially available enrofloxacin are similar. As expected, the enrofloxacin salts showed a considerable improvement in solubility: **2–4** were found to be 57- to 406-times more soluble than pure enrofloxacin. Correlating the solubility with crystal structures is difficult because the limited experimental/calculated data on crystal packing, etc. However, it can be speculated that the solubility enhancement in the case of the salts was a result of greater ionization.

Table 3. Solubility Data for Compounds **1–4**.

Compound	Saturation Solubility [a] in Water (mg/mL)
enrofloxacin [b]	0.14
1	0.14
2	8.53
3	56.83
4	8.04

[a] Solubility measured after 24 h of equilibration. [b] Solubility of commercially available enrofloxacin.

4. Discussion

Enrofloxacin anhydrate was crystallized, and the crystal structure was determined. Further, new salts formed using tartaric acid, nicotinic acid and suberic acid have been reported for the first time. The novel salts were prepared efficiently via evaporation using a mixed solvent has been found to be highly rewarding. These compounds formed a layered structure, and these layers were stacked via hydrogen bonds and π⋯π interactions. In the structure of salts, the piperazinyl moieties of enrofloxacin interacted with the carboxylate ions. These carboxylate ions connected the H_2O and EtOH molecules formed a stacking structure. The enrofloxacin salts prepared in this study showed a 57- to 406-fold higher solubility than the starting material.

Supplementary Materials: The following are available online at http://www.mdpi.com/2073-4352/10/8/646/s1. The PXRD patterns with the simulated patterns obtained from the single crystal data.CIF files giving crystal data can be obtained free of charge from the Cambridge Crystallographic Data Centre via the Internet www.ccdc.cam.ac.uk/data_request/cif.

Author Contributions: Writing–original draft, H.P.; Conceptualization, Y.-B.S.; Formal analysis, Y.Y., and L.-Z.C.; Funding acquisition, B.-H.F.; Investigation, J.-W.Z.; Methodology, M.-J.X.; Software, H.L. All authors have read and agreed to the published version of the manuscript.

Funding: This research was funded by the Natural Science Foundation of China (No. 31872522).

Conflicts of Interest: There are no conflict to declare.

References

1. Vishweshwar, P.; McMahon, J.A.; Peterson, M.L.; Hickey, M.B.; Shattock, T.R.; Zaworotko, M.J. Crystal engineering of pharmaceutical co-crystals from polymorphic active pharmaceutical ingredients. *Chem. Commun.* **2005**, *36*, 4601. [CrossRef] [PubMed]
2. Maeno, Y.; Fukami, T.; Kawahata, M.; Yamaguchi, K.; Tagami, T.; Ozeki, T.; Suzuki, T.; Tomono, K. Novel pharmaceutical cocrystal consisting of paracetamol and trimethylglycine, a new promising cocrystal former. *Int. J. Pharmaceut.* **2014**, *473*, 179–186. [CrossRef]
3. Blagden, N.; de Matas, M.; Gavan, P.T.; York, P. Crystal engineering of active pharmaceutical ingredients to improve solubility and dissolution rates. *Adv. Drug Deliv. Rev.* **2007**, *59*, 617–630. [CrossRef] [PubMed]
4. McNamara, D.P.; Childs, S.L.; Giordano, J.; Iarriccio, A.; Cassidy, J.; Shet, M.S.; Mannion, R.; O'Donnell, E.; Park, A. Use of a Glutaric Acid Cocrystal to Improve Oral Bioavailability of a Low Solubility API. *Pharm. Res. Dordr.* **2006**, *23*, 1888–1897. [CrossRef]
5. Jones, W.; Motherwell, W.D.S.; Trask, A.V. Pharmaceutical Cocrystals: An Emerging Approach to Physical Property Enhancement. *MRS Bull.* **2006**, *11*, 875–879. [CrossRef]
6. Thakuria, R.; Delori, A.; Jones, W.; Lipert, M.P.; Roy, L.; Rodríguez-Hornedo, N. Pharmaceutical cocrystals and poorly soluble drugs. *Int. J. Pharm.* **2013**, *453*, 101–125. [CrossRef] [PubMed]
7. Darwish, S.; Zeglinski, J.; Krishna, G.R.; Shaikh, R.; Khraisheh, M.; Walker, G.M.; Croker, D.M. A New 1:1 Drug-Drug Cocrystal of Theophylline and Aspirin: Discovery, Characterization, and Construction of Ternary Phase Diagrams. *Cryst. Growth Des.* **2018**, *18*, 7526–7532. [CrossRef]
8. Aakeröy, C.B.; Fasulo, M.E.; Desper, J. Cocrystal or Salt: Does It Really Matter? *Mol. Pharm.* **2007**, *4*, 317–322. [CrossRef]
9. Basavoju, S.; Boström, D.; Velaga, S.P. Pharmaceutical Cocrystal and Salts of Norfloxacin. *Cryst. Growth Des.* **2006**, *6*, 2699–2708. [CrossRef]
10. Berge, S.M.; Bighley, L.D.; Monkhouse, D.C. Pharmaceutical salts. *J. Pharm. Sci.* **1977**, *66*, 1–19. [CrossRef]
11. Datta, S.; Grant, D.J.W. Crystal structures of drugs: Advances in determination, prediction and engineering. *Nat. Rev. Drug Discov.* **2004**, *3*, 42–57. [CrossRef] [PubMed]
12. Meyer, M.C. Drug Product Selection—Part 2: Scientific basis of bioavailability and bioequivalence testing. *Am. Pharm.* **1991**, *NS31*, 47–52. [CrossRef]
13. Fleischman, S.G.; Kuduva, S.S.; McMahon, J.A.; Moulton, B.; Bailey Walsh, R.D.; Rodríguez-Hornedo, N.; Zaworotko, M.J. Crystal Engineering of the Composition of Pharmaceutical Phases: Multiple-Component Crystalline Solids Involving Carbamazepine. *Cryst. Growth Des.* **2003**, *3*, 909–919. [CrossRef]
14. Childs, S.L.; Chyall, L.J.; Dunlap, J.T.; Smolenskaya, V.N.; Stahly, B.C.; Stahly, G.P. Crystal Engineering Approach to Forming Cocrystals of Amine Hydrochlorides with Organic Acids. Molecular Complexes of Fluoxetine Hydrochloride with Benzoic, Succinic, and Fumaric Acids. *J. Am. Chem. Soc.* **2004**, *126*, 13335–13342. [CrossRef]
15. Bis, J.A.; Zaworotko, M.J. The 2-Aminopyridinium-carboxylate Supramolecular Heterosynthon: A Robust Motif for Generation of Multiple-Component Crystals. *Cryst. Growth Des.* **2005**, *5*, 1169–1179. [CrossRef]
16. Douroumis, D.; Ross, S.A.; Nokhodchi, A. Advanced methodologies for cocrystal synthesis. *Adv. Drug Deliv. Rev.* **2017**, *117*, 178–195. [CrossRef]
17. Efthimiadou, E.K.; Katsaros, N.; Karaliota, A.; Psomas, G. Synthesis, characterization, antibacterial activity, and interaction with DNA of the vanadyl-enrofloxacin complex. *Bioorg. Med. Chem. Lett.* **2007**, *17*, 1238–1242. [CrossRef]

18. Fan, J.; Sun, D.; Yu, H.; Kerwin, S.M.; Hurley, L.H. Self-Assembly of a Quinobenzoxazine-Mg2+ Complex on DNA: A New Paradigm for the Structure of a Drug-DNA Complex and Implications for the Structure of the Quinolone Bacterial Gyrase-DNA Complex. *J. Med. Chem.* **1995**, *38*, 408–424. [CrossRef]
19. TerHune, T.N.; Skogerboe, T.L.; Shostrom, V.K.; Weigel, D.J. Comparison of pharmacokinetics of danofloxacin and enrofloxacin in calves challenged with Mannheimia haemolytica. *Am. J. Vet. Res.* **2005**, *66*, 342–349. [CrossRef]
20. Barrón, D.; Irles, A.; Barbosa, J. Prediction of electrophoretic mobilities in non-aqueous capillary electrophoresis: Optimal separation of quinolones in acetonitrile–water media. *J. Chromatogr. A* **2000**, *871*, 367–380. [CrossRef]
21. Lizondo, M.; Pons, M.; Gallardo, M.; Estelrich, J. Physicochemical properties of enrofloxacin. *J. Pharm. Biomed.* **1997**, *15*, 1845–1849. [CrossRef]
22. Romañuk, C.B.; Manzo, R.H.; Linck, Y.G.; Chattah, A.K.; Monti, G.A.; Olivera, M.E. Characterization of the Solubility and Solid-State Properties of Saccharin Salts of Fluoroquinolones. *J. Pharm. Sci.* **2009**, *10*, 3788–3801. [CrossRef] [PubMed]
23. Xu, Y.; Jiang, L.; Mei, X. Supramolecular structures and physicochemical properties of norfloxacin salts. *Acta Crystallogr. Sect. B Struct. Sci. Cryst. Eng. Mater.* **2014**, *70*, 750–760. [CrossRef] [PubMed]
24. Surov, A.O.; Manin, A.N.; Voronin, A.P.; Drozd, K.V.; Simagina, A.A.; Churakov, A.V.; Perlovich, G.L. Pharmaceutical salts of ciprofloxacin with dicarboxylic acids. *Eur. J. Pharm. Sci.* **2015**, *77*, 112–121. [CrossRef]
25. Banerjee, R.; Bhatt, P.M.; Ravindra, N.V.; Desiraju, G.R. Saccharin Salts of Active Pharmaceutical Ingredients, Their Crystal Structures, and Increased Water Solubilities. *Cryst. Growth Des.* **2005**, *5*, 2299–2309. [CrossRef]
26. Dolomanov, O.V.; Bourhis, L.J.; Gildea, R.J.; Howard, J.A.K.; Puschmann, H. OLEX2: A complete structure solution, refinement and analysis program. *J. Appl. Crystallogr.* **2009**, *42*, 339–341. [CrossRef]
27. Sheldrick, G.M. SHELXT-Integrated space-group and crystal-structure determination. *Acta Crystallogr. Sect. A Found. Adv.* **2015**, *71*, 3–8. [CrossRef]
28. Spek, A.L. Structure validation in chemical crystallography. *Acta Cryst.* **2009**, *D65*, 148–155.
29. Glomme, A.; März, J.; Dressman, J.B. Comparison of a Miniaturized Shake-Flask Solubility Method with Automated Potentiometric Acid/Base Titrations and Calculated Solubilities. *J. Pharm. Sci.* **2005**, *94*, 1–16. [CrossRef]
30. Shaibat, M.A.; Casabianca, L.B.; Wickramasinghe, N.P.; Guggenheim, S.; de Dios, A.C.; Ishii, Y. Characterization of Polymorphs and Solid-State Reactions for Paramagnetic Systems by13 C Solid-State NMR and ab Initio Calculations. *J. Am. Chem. Soc.* **2007**, *129*, 10968–10969. [CrossRef]
31. Mesallati, H.; Umerska, A.; Tajber, L. Fluoroquinolone Amorphous Polymeric Salts and Dispersions for Veterinary Uses. *Pharmaceutics* **2019**, *11*, 268. [CrossRef] [PubMed]
32. Löbmann, K.; Laitinen, R.; Grohganz, H.; Strachan, C.; Rades, T.; Gordon, K.C. A theoretical and spectroscopic study of co-amorphous naproxen and indomethacin. *Int. J. Pharm.* **2013**, *453*, 80–87. [CrossRef] [PubMed]
33. Gunasekaran, S.; Anita, B. Spectral investigation and normal coordinate analysis of piperazine. *Indian J. Pure Appl. Phys.* **2008**, *46*, 833–838.
34. Karanam, M.; Choudhury, A.R. Structural Landscape of Pure Enrofloxacin and Its Novel Salts: Enhanced Solubility for Better Pharmaceutical Applicability. *Cryst. Growth Des.* **2013**, *13*, 1626–1637. [CrossRef]

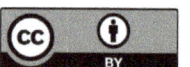

© 2020 by the authors. Licensee MDPI, Basel, Switzerland. This article is an open access article distributed under the terms and conditions of the Creative Commons Attribution (CC BY) license (http://creativecommons.org/licenses/by/4.0/).

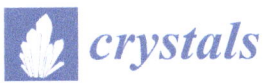

Article

Single Crystal X-Ray Structure for the Disordered Two Independent Molecules of Novel Isoflavone: Synthesis, Hirshfeld Surface Analysis, Inhibition and Docking Studies on IKKβ of 3-(2,3-dihydrobenzo [b][1,4]dioxin-6-yl)-6,7-dimethoxy-4H-chromen-4-one

Soon Young Shin [1], Young Han Lee [1], Yoongho Lim [2], Ha Jin Lee [3], Ji Hye Lee [4], Miri Yoo [4], Seunghyun Ahn [4,*] and Dongsoo Koh [4,*]

[1] Department of Biological Chemistry, Konkuk University, Seoul 05029, Korea; shinsy@konkuk.ac.kr (S.Y.S.); yhlee58@gmail.com (Y.H.L.)
[2] Division of Bioscience and Biotechnology, BMIC, Konkuk University, Seoul 05029, Korea; yoongho@konkuk.ac.kr
[3] Western Seoul Center, Korea Basic Science Institute, Seoul 03759, Korea; hajinlee@kbsi.re.kr
[4] Department of Applied Chemistry, Dongduk Women's University, Seoul 02748, Korea; dwg1993@naver.com (J.H.L.); mil2425@naver.com (M.Y.)
* Correspondence: mistahn321@naver.com (S.A.); dskoh@dongduk.ac.kr (D.K.)

Received: 14 September 2020; Accepted: 6 October 2020; Published: 9 October 2020

Abstract: The structure of the isoflavone compound, 3-(2,3-dihydrobenzo[b][1,4] dioxin-6-yl)-6,7-dimethoxy-4H-chromen-4-one (**5**), was elucidated by 2D-NMR spectra, mass spectrum and single crystal X-ray crystallography. Compound **5**, $C_{19}H_{16}O_6$, was crystallized in the monoclinic space group $P2_1/c$ with the cell parameters; a = 12.0654(5) Å, b = 11.0666(5) Å, c = 23.9550(11) Å, β = 101.3757(16)°, V = 3135.7(2) Å^3, and Z = 8. The asymmetric unit of compound **5** consists of two independent molecules **5I** and **5II**. Both molecules exhibit the disorder of each methylene group present in their 1,4-dioxane rings with relative occupancies of 0.599(10) (**5I**) and 0.812(9) (**5II**) for the major component **A**, and 0.401(10) (**5I**) and 0.188(9) (**5II**) for the minor component **B**, respectively. Each independent molecule revealed remarkable discrepancies in bond lengths, bond angles and dihedral angles in the disordered regions of 1,4-dioxane rings. The common feature of the molecules **5I** and **5II** are a chromone ring and a benzodioxin ring, which are more tilted towards each other in **5I** than in **5II**. An additional difference between the molecules is seen in the relative disposition of two methoxy substituents. In the crystal, the molecule **5II** forms inversion dimers which are linked into chains along an *a*-axis direction by intermolecular C–H···O interactions. Additional C–H···O hydrogen bonds connected the molecules **5I** and **5II** each other to form a three-dimensional network. Hirshfeld surface analysis evaluated the relative intermolecular interactions which contribute to each crystal structure **5I** and **5II**. Western blot analysis demonstrated that compound **5** inhibited the TNFα-induced phosphorylation of IKKα/β, resulting in attenuating further downstream NF-κB signaling. A molecular docking study predicted the possible binding of compound **5** to the active site of IKKβ. Compound **5** showed an inhibitory effect on the clonogenicity of HCT116 human colon cancer cells. These results suggest that compound **5** can be used as a platform for the development of an anti-cancer agent targeting IKKα/β.

Keywords: disordered crystal structure; hydrogen bonding; in silico docking; Hirshfeld surface; NF-κB signaling; IKKβ inhibitor

1. Introduction

The NF-κB family of transcription factors plays crucial roles in cellular proliferation, survival, and immune responses. These consist of five members, including c-Rel, p65/RelA, RelB, p50/NF-κB1, and p52/NF-κB2 [1]. The most abundant form is a p65/RelA and p50/NF-κB1. In resting cells, NF-κB dimers remain in an inactive form in the cytoplasm during their association with an inhibitor of κB (IκB) [2]. Upon cellular activation by extracellular stimuli, the upstream IκB kinase (IKK) complex consisting of IKKα, IKKβ, and IKKγ phosphorylates IκB to degrade IκB, allowing the activation of NF-κB [3]. The activated NF-κB complex immediately translocates to the nucleus, thereby regulating the expression of many genes involved in cell survival, cell cycle progression, angiogenesis, invasion, and metastasis [4]. Tumor necrosis factor α (TNFα) is a potent pro-inflammatory cytokine that promotes tumor progression in most types of malignant tumors [5]. It stimulates NF-κB through the activation of IKK [6]. Structure-based drug design (SBDD) and ligand-based drug design (LBDD) are the main streams of computer-aided drug design. Integrated drug design methods have been new trends in this area by combining information from both the ligand and the proteins [7,8]. For the integrated computer-aided studies, three-dimensional molecular structures of proteins and small molecules are prerequisites. Since the three-dimensional x ray structures of the IKKβ protein were revealed [9,10], the development of various inhibitors has been investigated and many inhibitors are commercially available [11–21]. However, it is uncommon for flavonoid compounds to be studied as IKKβ inhibitors [22,23]. Since flavonoids are second metabolites with phytoalexin properties and present in excess amount in plants, many studies and developments have been achieved as dietary supplements [24,25]. Flavonoids have also been reported to exhibit a variety of physiological activities and have been used in the development of a wide range of pharmaceuticals [26–28]. Chalcones, flavones, flavonols and isoflavones are diverse forms of flavonoids. In light of our research results, each form of flavonoid has been found to represent unique biological activities [29–33]. In this study, it was intended to investigate the anticancer activity through the IKKβ inhibitory effect after synthesizing the isoflavone compound **5** and revealing its solid-state structure by single crystal x-ray diffraction.

2. Materials and Methods

2.1. General

NMR experiments were carried out on a Bruker Avance 400 spectrometer Q (Bruker, Karlsruhe, Germany). The detailed procedures and parameters for the NMR experiments followed to the methods reported previously [34]. Other general experimental methods were followed by the methods reported previously [35].

2.2. Crystal Structure Determination

Single crystals were obtained by the slow evaporation of the ethanol solution of the isoflavone **5** at ambient temperature. A single crystal of the dimensions 0.393 × 0.305 × 0.134 mm^3 was selected and x-ray data were collected at 223 K on a Bruker D8 Venture equipped (Bruker, Madison, EI, USA) with IμS micro-focus sealed tube Mo Kα (λ = 0.71073 Å) and a PHOTON 100 CMOS detector. Bruker SAINT was utilized for the cell refinement and data reduction [36]. The structure was solved by direct methods and refined by full-matrix least-squares on F^2 using SHELXTL [37]. Detailed refining methods followed previously reported methods [35], and the outcomes of the crystallographic data collection, structural determination and refinement are summarized in Table 1 (CCDC deposition number 2027508). All relevant information which include bond distances, angles, fractional coordinates, and the equivalent isotropic displacement parameters can be obtained free of charge from the CCDC (Cambridge Crystallographic Data Centre), 12 Union Road, Cambridge CB2 1EZ, UK; Fax: +44 1223 336033; E-mail: deposit@ccdc.cam.ac.uk.

Table 1. Crystal data and structure refinement for compound 5.

CCDC deposit number	2027508
Empirical formula	$C_{19}H_{16}O_6$
Formula weight	340.32
Temperature	223(2) K
Wavelength	0.71073 Å
Crystal system	Monoclinic
Space group	$P2_1/c$
Unit cell dimensions	a = 12.0654(5) Å b = 11.0666(5) Å c = 123.9550(11) Å β = 101.3757(16)°.
Volume	3135.7(2) Å^3
Z	8
Density (calculated)	1.442 Mg/m^3
Absorption coefficient	0.108 mm^{-1}
F(000)	1424
Crystal size	0.393 × 0.305 × 0.134 mm^3
Theta range for data collection	1.722 to 28.347°
Index ranges	$-16 \leq h \leq 16, -14 \leq k \leq 14, -31 \leq l \leq 31$
Reflections collected	102751
Independent reflections	7798 [R(int) = 0.0604]
Completeness to theta = 25.242°	99.7 %
Max. and min. transmission	0.7457 and 0.6970
Refinement method	Full-matrix least-squares on F^2
Data/restraints/parameters	7798/12/492
Goodness-of-fit on F^2	1.063
Final R indices [I>2sigma(I)]	R1 = 0.0430, wR2 = 0.1004
R indices (all data)	R1 = 0.0666, wR2 = 0.1179
Largest diff. peak and hole	0.226 and -0.206 e.Å^{-3}

2.3. Hirshfeld Surfaces

The Hirshfeld surface analyses were carried out using the program CrystalExplorer 17.5 (University of Western Australia, Perth, Australia) [38,39]. The normalized contact distances (dnorm) were mapped into the Hirshfeld surface, which enabled the visualization of intermolecular interactions by using different colors. In the color scale, the red color denotes closest contact because it indicates the sum of di (the distance from the surface to the nearest nucleus internal to the surface) and d_e (the distance from the surface to the nearest nucleus external to the surface) and de is shorter than the sum of the relevant van der Waals radii. On the other hand, the white and blue color represent the weak and negligible intermolecular interactions, respectively. The Hirshfeld surfaces and their associated two-dimensional fingerprint plots were used to quantify the various intermolecular interactions in the title compound.

2.4. In Silico Docking with IκB Kinaseβ (IKKβ)

In silico dockings to elucidate the molecular binding mode between isoflavone 5 and IκB kinaseβ (IKKβ) were performed on an Intel Core 2 Quad Q6600 (2.4 GHz) Linux PC with Sybyl 7.3 (Tripos,

St. Louis, MO, USA). The three-dimensional structure of IκB kinaseβ (IKKβ) was adopted from a protein data bank deposited as 4KIK.pdb [40]. The detailed experimental procedures followed to the methods previously reported [41].

2.5. Cells and Cell Culture

HCT116 human colon cancer cells were obtained from the American Type Culture Collection (ATCC, Rockville, MD). The cells were grown in Dulbecco's modified Eagle medium (DMEM) supplemented with 10% (v/v) heat-inactivated fetal bovine serum (HyClone, Logan, UT, USA).

2.6. Western Blot Analysis

HCT116 cells treated with or without 10 ng/mL TNFα (Calbiochem, San Diego, CA, USA) in the presence or absence of compound **5** were lysed in a cell lysis buffer containing 20 mM HEPES (pH 7.2), 1% (v/v) Triton X-100, 10% (v/v) glycerol, 150 mM NaCl, 10 μg/mL leupeptin, and 1 mM phenylmethylsulfonyl fluoride (PMSF). Protein extracts (20 μg per sample) were separated via 10% (w/v) SDS-polyacrylamide gel electrophoresis, transferred to nitrocellulose membranes and incubated with the appropriate primary and secondary antibodies. Primary antibodies against phospho (p)-IKKα/β (Ser176/180), p-IκBα (Ser32), p-p65/RelA (Ser536) were obtained from Cell Signaling Technology (Beverly, MA, USA), and an antibody against glyceraldehyde phosphate dehydrogenase (GAPDH) was from Santa Cruz Biotechnology (Santa Cruz, CA, USA). All the primary antibodies were diluted to 1:1000 concentration in 50 mM Tris-buffered saline (pH 7.6) containing 5% nonfat dry milk solution and 0.05% Tween-20. The antibody-bound blots were developed using an enhanced chemiluminescence detection system (GE Healthcare, Piscataway, NJ, USA).

2.7. Clonogenic Assay

To measure the long-term growth inhibitory effect of compound **5** against cancer cells, the clonogenic survival assay was performed as reported previously with a minor modification [42]. Briefly, HCT116 human colon cancer cells were plated at a density of 4×10^3 cells per well in 24-well culture plates (BD Falcon™; Becton Dickson Immunocytometry System). After attachment, the cells were incubated in the presence or absence of compound **5** at different concentrations (0, 1, 5, and 10 μM) for 7 days, and fixed with 6% glutaraldehyde, followed by staining with 0.1% crystal violet. Its half-maximal clonogenic growth inhibitory concentration (GI_{50}) was determined using the SigmaPlot software (SYSTAT, Chicago, IL, USA) [43].

3. Results and Discussion

3.1. Synthesis

The title compound **5** was synthesized as shown in Scheme 1 by literature methods [34,44,45]. The final compound **5** was obtained by palladium-catalyzed Suzuki reaction between boronic acid (**4**) derivative and 3-iodoflavone (**3**) in three steps from the commercially available starting material.

3.1.1. Synthesis of (E)-3-(dimethylamino)-1-(2-hydroxy-4,5-dimethoxyphenyl)prop-2-en-1-one (2)

The previously reported literature procedures were used, but starting with 2-hydroxy-4,5-dimethoxyacetophenone (**1**) [34,44]. ^{1}H NMR (400 MHz, DMSO) δ 14.76 (s, 1H), 7.83 (d, J = 12.0 Hz, 1H), 7.31 (s, 1H), 6.41 (s, 1H), 5.85 (d, J = 12.0 Hz, 1H), 3.78 (s, 3H), 3.75 (s, 3H), 3.17 (s, 3H), 2.99 (s, 3H). ^{13}C NMR (100 MHz, DMSO) δ 189.35, 159.65, 154.95, 154.74, 141.13, 111.98, 111.41, 100.78, 89.38, 56.95, 55.71, 44.96, 37.54.

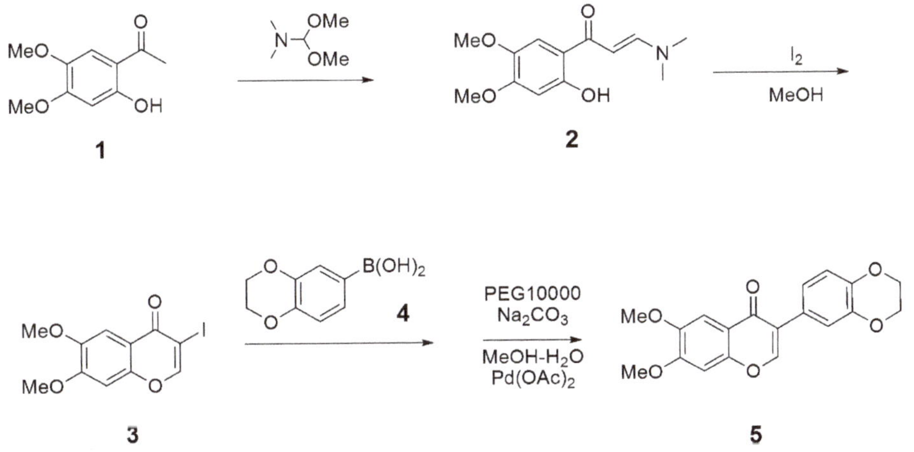

Scheme 1. Synthetic procedures for the title compound 5.

3.1.2. Synthesis of 3-iodo-6,7-dimethoxy-4H-chromen-4-one (3)

The slightly modified literature procedures were used, but starting with previously obtained enamine **2** [34,44]. After the completion of the reaction, the precipitate was formed. The resulting solid was filtered and was washed with cold methanol. The solid compound of iodoflavone (**3**) was pure and used for the next reaction without further purifications. ^{1}H NMR (400 MHz, DMSO) δ 8.73 (s, 1H), 7.37 (s, 1H), 7.31 (s, 1H), 3.90 (s, 3H), 3.85 (s, 3H). ^{13}C NMR (101 MHz, DMSO) δ 171.82, 158.31, 154.69, 152.04, 147.91, 114.46, 104.22, 100.44, 86.58, 56.62, 56.00.

3.1.3. Synthesis of 3-(2,3-dihydrobenzo[b][1,4]dioxin-6-yl)-6,7-dimethoxy-4H-chromen-4-one (5)

The previously reported literature procedures were used but starting with the 3-iodo flavone compound (**3**) [34,45]. For the complete assignment for the proton atoms and carbon atoms, additional two-dimensional NMR such as HMBC (heteronuclear multiple bond correlation), HMQC (heteronuclear multiple-quantum correlation) and TOCSY (total correlation spectroscopy) were performed (Supplementary Materials). ^{1}H NMR (400 MHz, DMSO-d_6) δ 8.34 (s, 1H, H-2), 7.47 (s, 1H, H-5), 7.16 (s, 1H, H-8), 7.15 (d, 1H, H-2′, J = 2.1 Hz), 7.06 (dd, 1H, H-6′, J = 8.4, 2.1 Hz), 6.88 (d, 1H, H-5′, J = 8.4 Hz), 4.27 (s, 4H, 3′, 4′-CH$_2$), 3.93 (s, 3H, 7-OCH$_3$), 3.88 (s, 3H, 6-OCH$_3$); ^{13}C NMR (400 MHz, DMSO-d_6) δ 173.9 (C-4), 154.2 (C-7), 152.8 (C-2), 151.5 (C-9), 147.4 (C-6), 143.0 (C-4′), 142.8 (C-3′), 124.9 (C-1′), 122.4 (C-3), 121.5 (C-6′), 117.3 (C-2′), 117.0 (C-10), 116.4 (C-5′), 104.4 (C-5), 100.1 (C-8), 63.90 (C-3′), 63.86 (C-4′), 56.1 (7-OCH$_3$), 55.7 (6-OCH$_3$). HR/MS (m/z): Calcd. for (M+H)$^+$: 341.0980; Found: 341.1032.

3.2. Crystal Structure of Isoflavone Compound 5

The asymmetric unit of compound **5** consists of two independent molecules **5I** (C1–C19) and **5II** (C20–C38). In each independent molecules, two methylene groups C18–C19 (**5I**) and C37–C38 (**5II**) in corresponding 1, 4-dioxane rings are disordered over two positions with relative occupancies of 0.599(10) (**5I**) and 0.812(9) (**5II**) for the major component **A**, and 0.401(10) (**5I**) and 0.188(9) (**5II**) for the minor component **B**, respectively (Figure 1A). From a macroscopic point of view, two independent molecules **5I** and **5II** are roughly superimposed over each other as shown in Figure 1B.

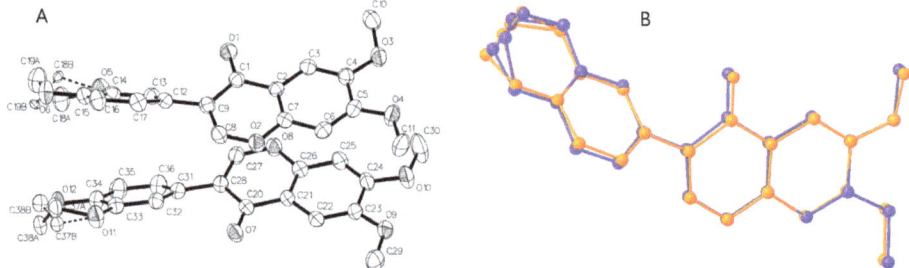

Figure 1. (**A**) Molecular structure of the title compound **5** with atomic labelling. The asymmetric part of the unit cell incorporates two independent molecules **5I** (C1–C19) and **5II** (C20–C38). Displacement ellipsoids are drawn at the 30% probability level. The minor component of the disordered moiety is drawn with open bonds. (**B**) An overlay diagram of two independent crystals **5I** (orange color) and **5II** (blue color) of title compound **5**. H atoms are omitted for clarity.

There are relative differences in the corresponding bond distances, bond angles, and torsional angles among the conformers **5IA–5IIB**. In the C1–C19 molecule (**5I**), the two dioxane rings at major component **5IA** and minor component **5IB** are both in the half-chair conformations. The atom C18A shows maximum deviation from the dioxane ring of C14–C15–O6–C19A–C18A–O5 (r.m.s. deviation = 0.212 Å) by 0.351 Å in the major component **5IA**. The atom C19B shows maximum deviation from the ring of C14–C15–O6–C19B–C18B–O5 (rmsd = 0.201 Å) by 0.338 Å in the minor component **5IB**. The dihedral angle formed between plane of the dimethoxy-substituted benzene ring (C2–C7; rmsd = 0.004 Å) and a plane of dioxane-attached benzene ring (C12–C17; rmsd = 0.003 Å) is 47.45(4)°. The methoxy groups are slightly twisted from the benzene ring by torsion angle of C3–C4–O3–C10 = 10.6(2)° at C4 and C6–C5–O4–C11 = −5.5(2)° at C5, respectively, in the molecule **5I** (Figure 2).

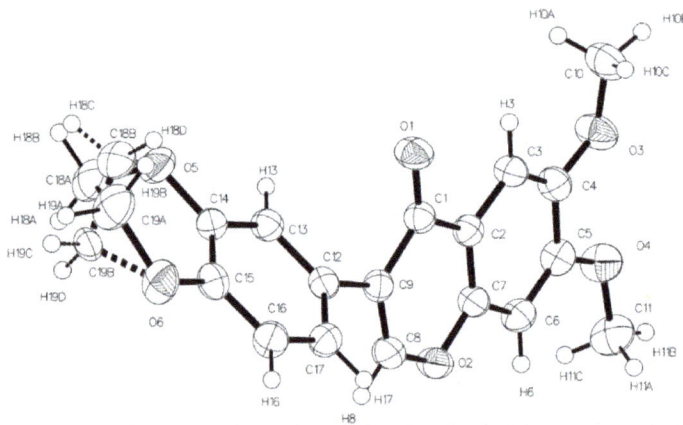

Figure 2. View of the molecular structure of the independent molecule **5I** with the atom label including all hydrogens. It shows a disordered structure in the 1, 4-dioxane rings. Displacement ellipsoids are drawn at the 30% probability level.

Both the dioxane ring (C33–C34–O11–C38A–C37A–O12 (rmsd 0.204 Å)) of the major component and the dioxane ring (C33–C34–O11–C38B–C37B–O12 (rmsd 0.226 Å)) of a minor component lie in the half-chair conformations in molecule **5II** as well. The maximum deviations from each dioxane ring are 0.332 Å at C37A, and 0.383 Å at C38B, respectively. For the independent molecule **5II** (C20–C38), the dihedral angle formed between the corresponding two benzene rings of (C21–C26; rmsd = 0.004 Å) and (C31–C36; rmsd = 0.003Å) is 34.82(2)°, which is slightly less twisted compared to molecule **5I**. In addition, the methoxy groups are almost coplanar with the benzene ring by the torsion angle of C25–C24–O10–C30 = −1.5(3)° at C23 and C22–C23–O9–C29 = 2.6(2)° at C24, respectively (Figure 3).

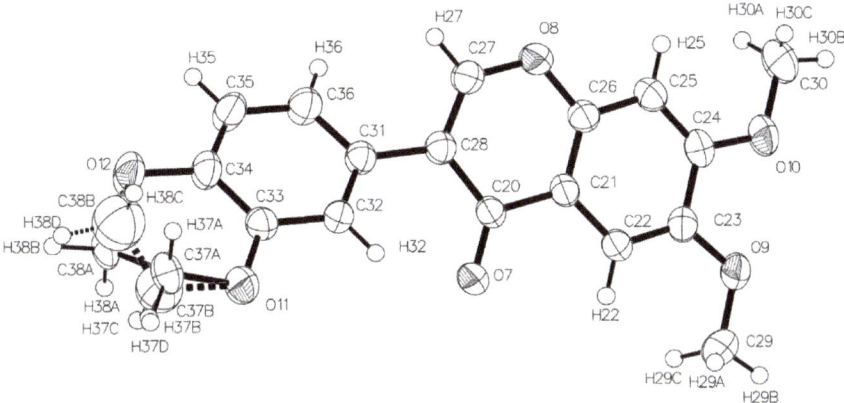

Figure 3. View of the molecular structure of independent molecule **5II** with the atom label including all hydrogens. It shows disordered structure in 1, 4-dioxane rings. Displacement ellipsoids are drawn at the 30% probability level.

There are distinctive discrepancies in the bond lengths and bond angles in the distorted regions of molecules **5IA**, **5IB**, **5IIA** and **5IIB**. Comparing the bond lengths between two conformers (**A** and **B**) of each independent molecule (**5I**, **5II**), the molecule **5I** revealed significant difference in bond lengths around the disordered area. For the major conformer **5IA**, the bond lengths were O(5)–C(18A) = 1.412(4) Å, C(18A)–C(19A) = 1.506(8) Å, C(19A)–O(6) =1.495(4) Å, respectively, and for the minor conformers **5IB**, those are O(5)–C(18B) = 1.513(7) Å, C(18B)–C(19B) = 1.458(13) Å, C(19B)–O(6) =1.402(6) Å, respectively. When they are compared in an inter-molecular manner, the bond lengths of O(5)–C(18B) and C(18B)–C(19B) in crystal **5I** are longer than those of the corresponding O(11)–C(37B) and C(37B)–C(38B) in crystal **5II**. Bond angles C(38B)–C(37B)–O(11) = 110.9(15)° and C(37B)–C(38B)–O(12) = 105.2(16)° in molecule **5IIB** are smaller than the corresponding bond angles O(5)–C(18B)–C(19B) = 113.2(7)° and O(6)–C(19B)–C(18B) = 106.5(8)° in molecule **5IB** (Table 2).

Table 2. Selected bond lengths (Å) and bond angles (°) in the distorted regions of crystal **5IA**, **5IB**, **5IIA** and **5IIB**, which show distinctive discrepancy. Torsional angles (°) were shown for the difference in the methoxy group substitutions.

I		II	
O(5)–C(18A)	1.412(4)	O(11)–C(37A)	1.447(3)
O(5)–C(18B)	1.513(7)	O(11)–C(37B)	1.422(14)
C(18A)–C(19A)	1.506(8)	C(37A)–C(38A)	1.507(6)
C(18B)–C(19B)	1.458(13)	C(37B)–C(38B)	1.45(3)
C(19A)–O(6)	1.495(4)	C(38A)–O(12)	1.452(3)
C(19B)–O(6)	1.402(6)	C(38B)–O(12)	1.449(15)
O(5)–C(18A)–C(19A)	107.5(4)	O(11)–C(37A)–C(38A)	109.2(3)
C(18A)–C(19A)–O(6)	109.5(4)	O(12)–C(38A)–C(37A)	108.8(3)
O(5)–C(18B)–C(19B)	113.2(7)	C(38B)–C(37B)–O(11)	110.9(15)
O(6)–C(19B)–C(18B)	106.5(8)	C(37B)–C(38B)–O(12)	105.2(16)
C(15)–O(6)–C(19A)	111.59(18)	C(34)–O(12)–C(38A)	113.50(15)
C(15)–O(6)–C(19B)	113.9(3)	C(34)–O(12)–C(38B)	108.9(5)
C(3)–C(4)–O(3)–C(10)	10.6(3)	C(22)–C(23)–O(9)–C(29)	2.6(2)
C(6)–C(5)–O(4)–C(11)	−5.5(2)	C(25)–C(24)–O(10)–C(30)	−1.5(3)

In the crystal, the pairs of the intermolecular C37–H37B···O11 hydrogen bonds form inversion dimers with $R^2_2(6)$ graph-set motifs. The dimers are linked into chains along the a axis direction by pairs of the C38–H38B···O9 hydrogen bonds in the molecule **II** (Figure 4, Table 3).

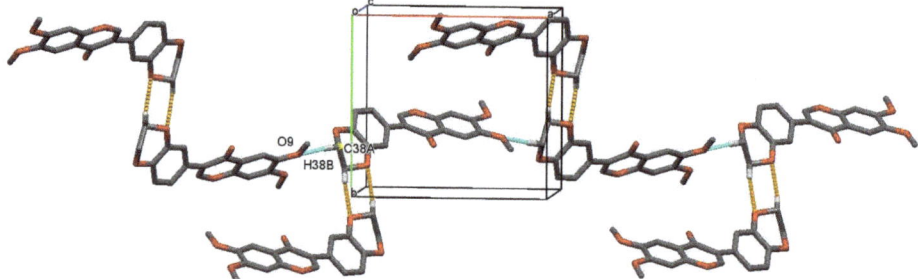

Figure 4. Pairs of hydrogen bonds form an inversion dimer (orange dashed line) which are linked into chains along the *a*-axis.

Table 3. Intermolecular hydrogen bonds involved in the crystal packing of compound **5** (Å and °).

D–H ... A	d(D–H)	d(H ... A)	d(D ... A)	<(DHA)
C(29)–H(29B) ... O(1)#1	0.97	2.43	3.396(2)	172.2
C(38A)–H(38B) ... O(9)#2	0.98	2.46	3.396(3)	157.8
C(10)–H(10B) ... O(7)#3	0.97	2.48	3.424(2)	165.6
C(37A)–H(37B) ... O(11)#4	0.98	2.59	3.071(4)	110.7

Symmetry transformations used to generate equivalent atoms: #1 x+1, y, z; #2 x−1, -y+3/2, z−1/2; #3 x, −y+3/2, z+1/2; #4 −x, −y+1, −z.

The two molecules **5I** and **5II** are connected to each other by intermolecular hydrogen bonds C11–H11B···O12 and C29–H29B···O1 to form an ac-plane from two-dimensional supramolecules (Figure 5, Table 3).

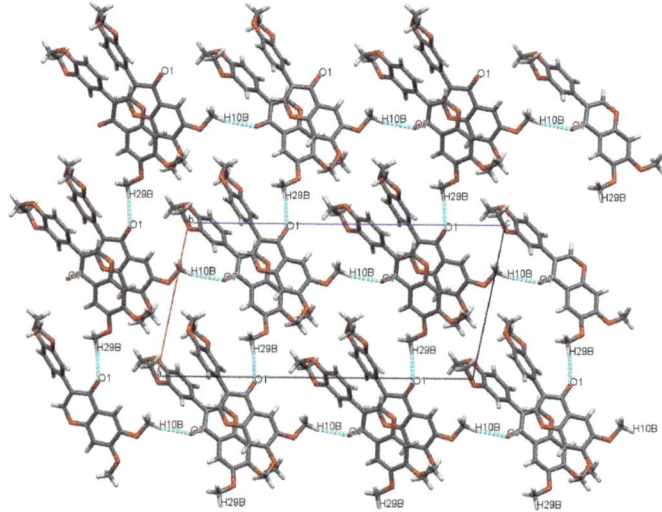

Figure 5. A view along the b axis of the crystal packing of compound **5**. The molecule **I** and **II** are linked via intermolecular hydrogen bonds C11–H11B···O12 and C29–H29B···O1. For clarity, the hydrogen atoms not involved in H bonds are omitted.

3.3. Hirshfeld Surface analysis of Compound 5

In order to quantify the intermolecular interactions in the crystals of the titled compound **5**, a Hirshfeld surface (HS) analysis was carried out. Based on the Hirshfeld analysis on all conformers, two independent molecules (**5I** and **5II**) showed different dnorm, shape index (SI) and curvedness, however, each set of conformers **A** and **B** revealed the same Hirshfeld analysis results [46]. The 3D Hirshfeld surfaces of two independent molecules (**5I** and **5II**) were illustrated in Figure 6A,B, which maps dnorm, shape index and curvedness. The deep red spots on the dnorm Hirshfeld surfaces of each molecule represent the close contact interactions, which are mainly responsible for the significant intermolecular C–H···O interactions. Shape index and curvedness can also be used to identify the characteristic packing modes. The shape indexes of **5I** and **5II** show red concave regions on the surface around the acceptor atoms and blue regions around the donor H atoms. The maps of curvedness for **5I** and **5II** show no flat surface patches representing that there are no stacking interactions between the molecules [47].

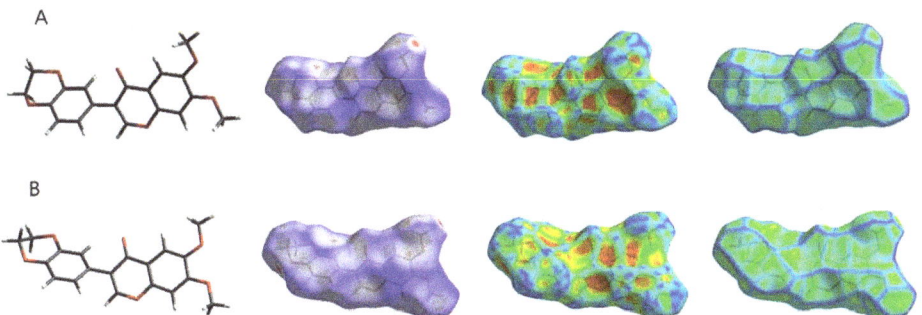

Figure 6. (**A**) Hirshfeld surfaces of molecule **5I** mapped with d_{norm}, shape index and curvedness. (**B**) Hirshfeld surfaces of molecule **5II** mapped with d_{norm}, shape index and curvedness.

According to two-dimensional fingerprint plots analysis, the dominant interaction in each molecule **5I** and **5II** originates from H···H contacts, which are the major contributors of 43.5% and 42.5% to the total Hirshfeld surface, respectively. The contribution from the O···H/H···O contacts of 25.1% and 29.1% of each molecule **5I** and **5II** is represented by a pair of sharp spikes that are characteristic of hydrogen-bonding interactions. Other meaningful interactions include C···H/H···C with contributions of 17.8% and 16.7% from **5I** and **5II**, respectively (Figure 7A–H).

The overall contribution to the total Hirshfeld surface is illustrated in Figure 8.

3.4. In Silico Docking with IKKβ

The docking calculations were carried out using the protein structure of IKKβ (The Protein Data Bank code; 4KIK.pdb). Using the Sybyl program, the apo-protein of IKKβ was obtained by removing the original ligand **K252a** contained in 4KIK.pdb. The original ligand K252a was again docked to the apo-protein, to confirm that the flexible docking procedure worked well. Through a flexible docking procedure repeated 30 times, 30 complexes between apo-protein and **K252a** were obtained. Their binding energy ranged from −28.44 to −10.24 kcal/mol and their binding poses were good to be comparable with 4KIK.pdb.The binding pocket of IKKβ was determined using the LigPlot software as previously reported [48]. They are composed of 16 residues; 14 residues, namely Leu21, Gly22, Thr23, Val25, Ala42, Lys44, Glu61, Val74, Met96, Tyr98, Glu149, Asn150, Ile165, and Asp166 are involved in hydrophobic interactions, and two residues, Glu97 and Cys99 are involved in hydrogen bonds. Using the three-dimensional structure of compound **5** obtained in this study, docking with apo-protein was performed in the same way as the original ligand. The binding energy generated by the 30 iterations ranged from −15.92 to −13.09 kcal/mol. The interactions between IKKβ and compound **5** were analyzed using the LigPlot progam. Six residues including Thr23, Val29, Glu61, Met65, Met96, and Ile165 showed the hydrophobic interactions with the ligand and three residues including Gly27, Lys44, and Asp166 formed hydrogen bonds (H bonds) with the ligand (Figure 9A). The binding pocket of compound **5** resided in IKKβ was visualized using the PyMOL program (PyMOL Molecular Graphics System, version 1.0r1, Schrödinger, LLC, Portland, OR, USA). Isoflavone compound **5** in IKKβ exhibited a slightly different binding pattern from those of the original ligand **K252a**. However, both isoflavone **5** and original ligand **K252a** have been shown to bind well at the active site of the IKKβ protein (Figure 9B).

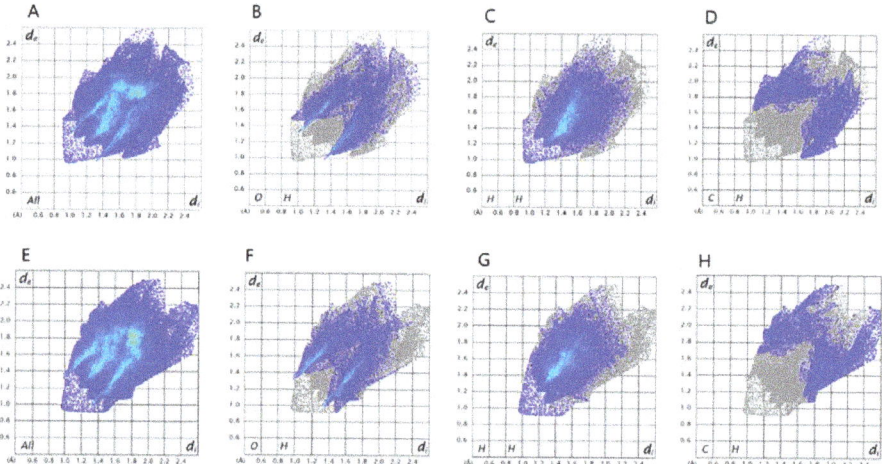

Figure 7. Two-dimensional fingerprint plots of the most important intermolecular contacts in each molecule **I** and **II**. For **I**: full (**A**) and resolved into O···H (**B**), H···H (**C**), C···H (**D**). For **II**: full (**E**) and resolved into O···H (**F**), H···H (**G**), C···H (**H**).

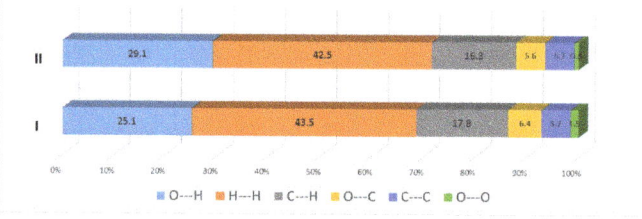

Figure 8. Summary of the overall detailed intermolecular interactions and their contribution to each crystal structure **I** and **II**. For **I**; H···H; 43.5%, O···H; 25.1%, O···C; 6.4%, C···H; 17.8%, C···C; 5.7%, O···O; 1.5%, For **II**; H···H; 42.5%, O···H; 29.1%, O···C; 5.6%, C···H; 16.3%, C···C; 5.7%, O···O; 0.8%.

3.5. Effect of Compound 5 on the Inhibition of IKK Pathway

To validate the in silico docking prediction that IKKβ is a target for compound **5**, we tested the effect of compound **5** on the inhibition of the IKK signaling pathway using a cell-based kinase assay. We confirmed that the phosphorylation of IKKα/β and its downstream targets IκB and p65/RelA was rapidly induced within 10 min and then gradually decreased upon 10 ng/mL TNFα stimulation (Figure 10A). Under this experimental condition, we determined whether compound **5** inhibited the TNFα-induced IKK activity. HCT116 cells were pre-treated with different concentrations of compound **5** (0, 50, 100 μM) for 30 min and then stimulated with 10 ng/mL TNFα for 10 min. We observed that pre-treatment with compound **5** dose-dependently reduced phosphorylation of IKKα/β and its downstream target IκB and p65/RelA, induced by TNFα (Figure 10B). These data suggest that compound **5** inhibits TNFα-induced NF-κB activation through the targeting of IKK.

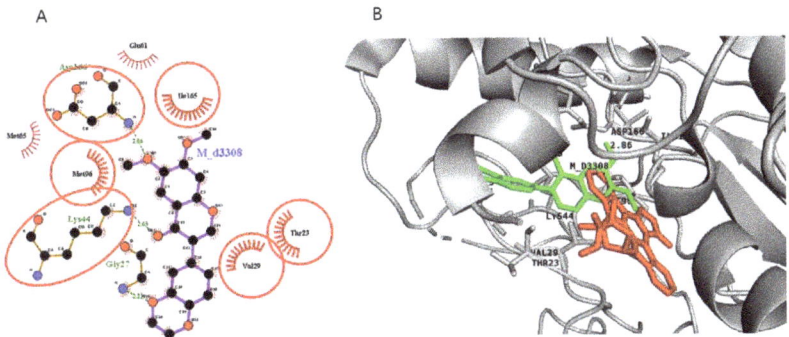

Figure 9. (**A**) The residues participating in the binding sites of the compound **5**-IKKβ complex analyzed by using the LigPlot program. (**B**) Three-dimensional image of the IKKβ and compound **5** complex, where compound **5** is colored in green and the original ligand **K252a** contained in IKKβ is colored in red.

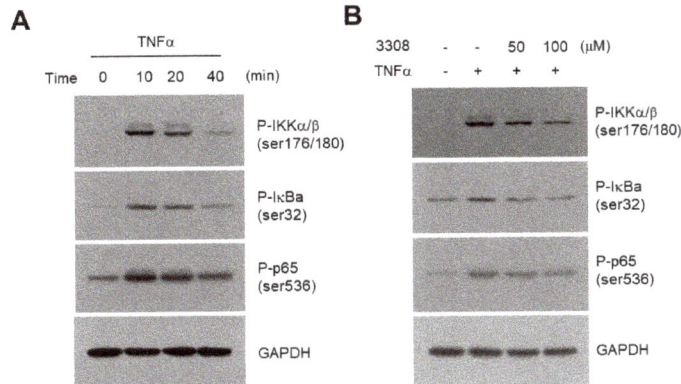

Figure 10. Effect of compound **5** on the inhibition of the IKK signaling pathway in HCT116 colon cancer cells. (**A**) HCT116 cells were starved with 0.5% fetal bovine serum for 24 h, followed by stimulation with 10 ng/mL TNFα for the indicated times. Whole-cell lysates were prepared, and Western blotting was performed using the phospho-specific antibody against IKKα/β (Ser176/180), IκBα (Ser32), and p65/RelA NF-κB (Ser536). Glyceraldehyde phosphate dehydrogenase (GAPDH) was used as an internal control. (**B**) HCT116 cells were starved with 0.5% FBS for 24 h, followed by pre-treatment with compound **5** (5 or 20 μM) 30 min before stimulation with 10 ng/mL TNFα. After 10 min, whole-cell lysates were prepared, and Western blotting was performed using the phospho-specific antibody against IKKα/β (Ser176/180), IκBα (Ser32), and p65/RelA NF-κB (Ser536). GAPDH was used as an internal control.

3.6. Effect of Compound 5 on the Inhibition of Clonogenicity of HCT116 Cells

To support the idea that NF-κB inhibition through IKK targeting by compound **5** exerts an antiproliferation effect, we tested the inhibitory activity of compound **5** on the clonogenicity of HCT116 human colon cancer cells. Clonogenic assay is an in vitro non-destructive method known to reflect the in vivo evaluation of anticancer drugs. Treatment with compound **5** for 7 days resulted in a dose-dependent loss of clonogenicity of HCT116 cells (Figure 11). Its GI_{50} value was determined to be

17.2 µM. These data suggest that IKK targeting by compound **5** reduced the individual cell ability to proliferate into viable colonies.

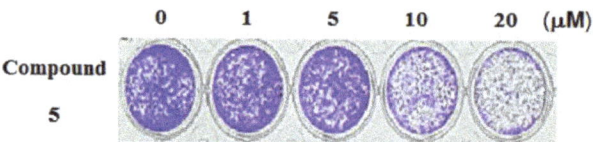

Figure 11. Effect of compound **5** on the inhibition of clonogenicity of HCT116 colon cancer cells.

NF-κB is constitutively activated in most cancer cells. The inhibition of NF-κB in cancer cells causes the induction of the cell cycle arrest and apoptosis. Therefore, pharmacological NF-κB inhibitors have been widely used for cancer prevention and therapy. The full activation of p65/RelA NF-κB is necessary for the release of the NF-κB complex from IκB. IKK phosphorylates IκB on Serine-32, triggering the proteasome-dependent proteolysis of IκB and releasing NF-κB from IκB. IKK also phosphorylates and degrades the Forkhead transcription factor FOXO3a that is involved in cell cycle arrest and apoptosis [49] and activates insulin receptor substrate (IRS) to impair insulin signaling [50], suggesting that IKK inhibition can exhibit multiple anticancer activities in addition to inhibiting NF-κB. Previous study has demonstrated that the most effective and selective approach for NF-κB inhibition might be offered by the IKK inhibitor [51], suggesting that the selective targeting of IKK is a promising therapeutic strategy for anticancer drug development. In this study, we identified compound **5** that inhibits the NF-κB signaling pathway through targeting the upstream kinase IKKβ.

4. Conclusions

The title compound **5**, $C_{19}H_{16}O_6$, was crystallized in the monoclinic space group $P2_1/c$ and consists of two independent molecules **5I** and **5II**. Both molecules exhibit the disorder of each methylene groups present in the 1,4-dioxane ring with occupancies 0.6289 (17) and 0.3711 (17), respectively. Based on the Hirshfeld analysis, two independent crystals (**5I** and **5II**) showed differences in the dnorm, shape index (SI), curvedness and the overall contribution to the total Hirshfeld surface. In the crystal, the molecule **5II** forms inversion dimers which are linked into chains along the a axis direction by intermolecular C–H···O interactions. Western blot analysis demonstrated that compound **5** inhibited the TNFα-induced phosphorylation of IKKα/β. A molecular docking study predicted the possible binding of compound **5** to the active site of IKKβ. We found that isoflavone derivative **5** inhibited the TNFα-induced phosphorylation of IKKα/β and its downstream IκB and p65/RelA NF-κB, which suggest that compound **5** can be used as a platform for the development of anti-cancer agent targeting IKKα/β.

Supplementary Materials: The following are available online at http://www.mdpi.com/2073-4352/10/10/911/s1, CIF file and NMR spectra for reaction intermediates compounds **2**, **3**, and final product compound **5**: Figure S1: 1H NMR spectrum of compound **2**; Figure S2: 13C-NMR spectrum of compound **2**; Figure S3: 1H-NMR spectrum of compound **3**.; Figure S4: 13C-NMR spectrum of compound **3**; Figure S5: 1H-NMR spectrum of compound **5**; Figure S6: 13C-NMR spectrum of compound **5**; Figure S7: 2D-HMBC spectrum of compound **5**; Figure S8: 2D-HMQC spectrum of compound **5**; Figure S9: 2D-TOSCY spectrum of compound **5**.

Author Contributions: Conceptualization, D.K. and S.Y.S.; investigation, S.A., J.H.L. and M.Y.; validation, Y.H.L., H.J.L. and Y.L.; writing—original draft, S.A., D.K. writing—review and editing, S.Y.S. All authors have read and agreed to the published version of the manuscript.

Funding: The authors acknowledge financial support from the Basic Science Research Program (award No. NRF-2019R1F1A1058747). S.Y. Shin was supported by the KU Research Professor Program of Konkuk University.

Conflicts of Interest: The authors declare no conflict of interest.

References

1. Luo, J.-L.; Kamata, H.; Karin, M. IKK/NF-κB signaling: Balancing life and death—A new approach to cancer therapy. *J. Clin. Investig.* **2005**, *115*, 2625–2632. [CrossRef] [PubMed]
2. Tang, E.D.; Inohara, N.; Wang, C.-Y.; Nuñez, G.; Guan, K.-L. Roles for homotypic interactions and transautophosphorylation in IκB kinase beta (IKKβ) activation. *J. Biol. Chem.* **2003**, *278*, 38566–38570. [CrossRef] [PubMed]
3. Chen, A.; Koehler, A.N. Transcription Factor Inhibition: Lessons Learned and Emerging Targets. *Trends Mol. Med.* **2020**, *26*, 508–518. [CrossRef]
4. Karin, M.; Cao, Y.; Greten, F.R.; Li, Z.W. NF-kappaB in cancer: From innocent bystander to major culprit. *Nat. Rev. Cancer* **2002**, *2*, 301–310. [CrossRef]
5. Balkwill, F. Tumour necrosis factor and cancer. *Nat. Rev. Cancer* **2009**, *9*, 361–371. [CrossRef]
6. Gaur, U.; Aggarwal, B.B. Regulation of proliferation, survival and apoptosis by members of the TNF superfamily. *Biochem. Pharmacol.* **2003**, *66*, 1403–1408. [CrossRef]
7. Wilson, G.L.; Lill, M.A. Integrating structure-based and ligand-based approaches for computational drug design. *Future Med. Chem.* **2011**, *3*, 735–750. [CrossRef]
8. Batool, M.; Ahmad, B.; Choi, S. A Structure-Based Drug Discovery Paradigm. *Int. J. Mol. Sci.* **2019**, *20*, 2783. [CrossRef]
9. Rushe, M.; Silvian, L.; Bixler, S.; Chen, L.L.; Cheung, A.; Bowes, S.; Cuervo, H.; Berkowitz, S.; Zheng, T.; Guckian, K.; et al. Structure of a NEMO/IKK—Associating Domain Reveals Architecture of the Interaction Site. *Structure* **2008**, *16*, 798–808. [CrossRef]
10. Xu, G.; Lo, Y.-C.; Li, Q.; Napolitano, G.; Wu, X.; Jiang, X.; Dreano, M.; Karin, M.; Wu, H. Crystal structure of inhibitor of κB kinase β. *Nat. Cell Biol.* **2011**, *472*, 325–330. [CrossRef]
11. Dong, T.; Li, C.; Wang, X.; Dian, L.; Zhang, X.; Li, L.; Chen, S.; Cao, R.; Li, L.; Huang, N.; et al. Ainsliadimer A selectively inhibits IKKα/β by covalently binding a conserved cysteine. *Nat. Commun.* **2015**, *6*, 6522. [CrossRef] [PubMed]
12. Elkamhawy, A.; Kim, N.Y.; Hassan, A.H.; Park, J.-E.; Paik, S.; Yang, J.-E.; Oh, K.-S.; Lee, B.H.; Lee, M.Y.; Shin, K.J.; et al. Thiazolidine-2,4-dione-based irreversible allosteric IKK-β kinase inhibitors: Optimization into in vivo active anti-inflammatory agents. *Eur. J. Med. Chem.* **2020**, *188*, 111955. [CrossRef] [PubMed]
13. Heyninck, K.; Lahtela-Kakkonen, M.; Van der Veken, P.; Haegeman, G.; Vanden Berghe, W. Withaferin a inhibits NK-κB activation by targeting cysteine 179 in IKKβ. *Biochem. Pharmacol.* **2014**, *91*, 501–509. [CrossRef] [PubMed]
14. Sordi, R.; Chiazza, F.; Johnson, F.L.; Patel, N.S.A.; Brohi, K.; Collino, M.; Thiemermann, C. Inhibition of IκB Kinase Attenuates the Organ Injury and Dysfunction Associated with Hemorrhagic Shock. *Mol. Med.* **2015**, *21*, 563–575. [CrossRef] [PubMed]
15. Uota, S.; Dewan, Z.; Saitoh, Y.; Muto, S.; Itai, A.; Utsunomiya, A.; Watanabe, T.; Yamamoto, N.; Yamaoka, S. An IκB kinase 2 inhibitor IMD-0354 suppresses the survival of adult T-cell leukemia cells. *Cancer Sci.* **2011**, *103*, 100–106. [CrossRef]
16. Choi, S.I.; Lee, S.Y.; Jung, W.J.; Lee, S.H.; Lee, E.J.; Min, K.H.; Hur, G.Y.; Lee, S.H.; Lee, S.Y.; Kim, J.H.; et al. The effect of an IκB-kinase-beta (IKKβ) inhibitor on tobacco smoke-induced pulmonary inflammation. *Exp. Lung Res.* **2016**, *42*, 182–189. [CrossRef]
17. Bassères, D.S.; Ebbs, A.; Cogswell, P.C.; Baldwin, A.S. IKK is a therapeutic target in KRSA-induced lung cancer with disrupted p53 activity. *Genes Cancer* **2014**, *5*, 41–55. [CrossRef]
18. Nan, J.; Du, Y.; Chen, X.; Bai, Q.; Wang, Y.; Zhang, X.; Zhu, N.; Zhang, J.; Hou, J.; Wang, Q.; et al. TPCA-1 is a direct dual inhibitor of STAT3 and NK-κB and regresses mutant EGFR-associated human non-small cell lung cancers. *Mol. Cancer Ther.* **2014**, *13*, 617–629. [CrossRef]
19. Liu, Q.; Wu, H.; Chim, S.M.; Zhou, L.; Zhao, J.; Feng, H.; Wei, Q.; Wang, Q.; Zheng, M.H.; Tan, R.X.; et al. SC-514, a selective inhibitor of IKKβ attenuates RANKL-induced osteoclastogenesis and NK-κB activation. *Biochem. Pharmacol.* **2013**, *86*, 1775–1783. [CrossRef]
20. Deng, C.; Lipstein, M.; Rodriguez, R.; Serrano, X.O.; McIntosh, C.; Tsai, W.Y.; Wasmuth, A.S.; Jaken, S.; O'Connor, O.A. The novel IKK2 inhibitor LY2409881 potently synergizes with histone deacetylase inhibitors in preclinical models of lymphoma through the downregulation of NK-κB. *Clin. Cancer Res.* **2015**, *21*, 134–145. [CrossRef]

21. Ping, H.; Yang, F.; Wang, M.; Niu, Y.; Xing, N. IKK inhibitor suppresses epithelial-mesenchymal transition and induces cell death in prostate cancer. *Oncol. Rep.* **2016**, *36*, 1658–1664. [CrossRef] [PubMed]
22. Yan, F.; Yang, F.; Wang, R.; Yao, X.J.; Bai, L.; Zeng, X.; Huang, J.; Wong, V.K.W.; Lam, C.W.K.; Zhou, H.; et al. Isoliquiritigenin suppresses human T Lymphocyte activation via covalently binding cysteine 46 of IκB kinase. *Oncotarget* **2016**, *8*, 34223–34235. [CrossRef] [PubMed]
23. Shin, S.Y.; Woo, Y.; Hyun, J.; Yong, Y.; Koh, D.; Lee, Y.H.; Lim, Y. Relationship between the structures of flavonoids and their NF-κB-dependent transcriptional activities. *Bioorg. Med. Chem. Lett.* **2011**, *21*, 6036–6041. [CrossRef] [PubMed]
24. Jeandet, P. Phytolexins: Current progress and future prospects. *Molecules* **2015**, *20*, 2770–2774. [CrossRef]
25. Guven, H.; Arici, A.; Simsek, O. Flavonoids in Our Foods: A Short Review. *J. Basic Clin. Health Sci.* **2019**, *3*, 96–106. [CrossRef]
26. Zhao, L.; Yuan, X.; Wang, J.; Feng, Y.; Ji, F.; Li, Z.; Bian, J. A review on flavones targeting serine/threonine protein kinases for potential anticancer drugs. *Bioorg. Med. Chem.* **2019**, *27*, 677–685. [CrossRef]
27. Zhuang, C.; Zhang, W.; Sheng, C.; Zhang, W.; Xing, C.; Miao, Z. Chalcone: A Privileged Structure in Medicinal Chemistry. *Chem. Rev.* **2017**, *117*, 7762–7810. [CrossRef]
28. Singh, M.; Kaur, M.; Silakari, O. Flavones: An important scaffold for medicinal chemistry. *Eur. J. Med. Chem.* **2014**, *84*, 206–239. [CrossRef]
29. Seo, G.; Hyun, C.; Koh, D.; Park, S.; Lim, Y.; Kim, Y.M.; Cho, M. A Novel Synthetic Material, BMM, Accelerates Wound Repair by Stimulating Re-Epithelialization and Fibroblast Activation. *Int. J. Mol. Sci.* **2018**, *19*, 1164. [CrossRef]
30. Sophors, P.; Kim, Y.M.; Seo, G.; Huh, J.-S.; Lim, Y.; Koh, D.S.; Cho, M. A synthetic isoflavone, DCMF, promotes human keratinocyte migration by activating Src/FAK signaling pathway. *Biochem. Biophys. Res. Commun.* **2016**, *472*, 332–338. [CrossRef]
31. Shin, S.Y.; Lee, J.M.; Lee, M.S.; Koh, D.; Jung, H.; Lim, Y.; Lee, Y.H. Targeting Cancer Cells via the Reactive Oxygen Species-Mediated Unfolded Protein Response with a Novel Synthetic Polyphenol Conjugate. *Clin. Cancer Res.* **2014**, *20*, 4302–4313. [CrossRef]
32. Shin, S.; Yoon, H.; Ahn, S.; Kim, D.-W.; Bae, D.-H.; Koh, D.; Lee, Y.H.; Lim, Y. Structural Properties of Polyphenols Causing Cell Cycle Arrest at G1 Phase in HCT116 Human Colorectal Cancer Cell Lines. *Int. J. Mol. Sci.* **2013**, *14*, 16970–16985. [CrossRef]
33. Jo, G.; Ahn, S.; Kim, B.-G.; Park, H.R.; Kim, Y.H.; Choo, H.A.; Koh, D.; Chong, Y.; Ahn, J.-H.; Lim, Y. Chromenylchalcones with inhibitory effects on monoamine oxidase B. *Bioorg. Med. Chem.* **2013**, *21*, 7890–7897. [CrossRef]
34. Ahn, S.; Sung, J.; Lee, J.H.; Yoo, M.; Lim, Y.; Shin, S.Y.; Koh, D. Synthesis, Single Crystal X-Ray Structure, Hirshfeld Surface Analysis, DFT Computations, Docking Studies on Aurora Kinases and an Anticancer Property of 3-(2,3-Dihydrobenzo[b][1,4]dioxin-6-yl)-6-methoxy-4H-chromen-4-one. *Crystals* **2020**, *10*, 413. [CrossRef]
35. Hwang, D.; Hyun, J.; Jo, G.; Koh, D.; Lim, Y. Synthesis and complete assignment of NMR data of 20 chalcones. *Magn. Reson. Chem.* **2010**, *49*, 41–45. [CrossRef]
36. Bruker. *APEX2, SAINT and SADABS*; Bruker AXS Inc.: Madison, WI, USA, 2012.
37. Sheldrick, G.M. Crystal structure refinement with SHELXL. *Acta Crystallogr. Sect. C Struct. Chem.* **2015**, *71*, 3–8. [CrossRef]
38. Turner, M.J.; McKinnon, J.J.; Wolff, S.K.; Grimwood, D.J.; Spackman, P.R.; Jayatilaka, D.; Spackman, M.A. *CrystalExplorer17*; University of Western Australia: Crawley, Australia, 2017.
39. McKinnon, J.J.; Jayatilaka, D.; Spackman, M.A. Towards quantitative analysis of intermolecular interactions with Hirshfeld surfaces. *Chem. Commun.* **2007**, *37*, 3814–3816. [CrossRef]
40. Liu, S.; Misquitta, Y.R.; Olland, A.; Johnson, M.A.; Kelleher, K.S.; Kriz, R.; Lin, L.L.; Stahl, M.; Mosyak, L. Crystal Structure of a Human IκB Kinase β Asymmetric Dimer. *J. Biol. Chem.* **2013**, *288*, 22758–22767. [CrossRef]
41. Shin, S.Y.; Lee, Y.; Kim, B.S.; Lee, J.; Ahn, S.; Koh, D.; Lim, Y.; Lee, Y.H. Inhibitory Effect of Synthetic Flavone Derivatives on Pan-Aurora Kinases: Induction of G2/M Cell-Cycle Arrest and Apoptosis in HCT116 Human Colon Cancer Cells. *Int. J. Mol. Sci.* **2018**, *19*, 4086. [CrossRef]
42. Franken, N.A.P.; Rodermond, H.M.; Stap, J.; Haveman, J.; Van Bree, C. Clonogenic assay of cells in vitro. *Nat. Protoc.* **2006**, *1*, 2315–2319. [CrossRef]

43. Kim, B.S.; Shin, S.Y.; Ahn, S.; Koh, D.; Lee, Y.H.; Lim, Y. Biological evaluation of 2-pyrazolinyl-1-carbothioamide derivatives against HCT116 human colorectal cancer cell lines and elucidation on QSAR and molecular binding modes. *Bioorg. Med. Chem.* **2017**, *25*, 5423–5432. [CrossRef] [PubMed]
44. Biegasiewicz, K.F.; Gordon, J.S.; Rodriguez, D.A.; Priefer, R. Development of a general approach to the synthesis of a library of isoflavonoid derivatives. *Tetrahedron Lett.* **2014**, *55*, 5210–5212. [CrossRef]
45. Liu, L.; Zhang, Y.; Wang, Y. Phosphine-free palladium acetate catalyzed Suzuki reaction in water. *J. Org. Chem.* **2005**, *70*, 6122–6125. [CrossRef] [PubMed]
46. Bisseyou, Y.B.M.; Ouattara, M.; Soro, P.A.; Kakou-Yao, R.; Tenon, A.J. Crystal structure, Hirshfeld surface analysis and contact enrichment ratios of 1-(2,7-dimethylimidazo[1,2-a]pyridin-3-yl)-2-(1,3-dithiolan-2-ylidene)ethanone monohydrate. *Acta Crystallogr. Sect. E Crystallogr. Commun.* **2019**, *75*, 1934–1939. [CrossRef] [PubMed]
47. Spackman, M.A.; Jayatilaka, D. Hirshfeld surface analysis. *CrystEngComm* **2009**, *11*, 19–32. [CrossRef]
48. Cardoso, M.V.D.O.; Moreira, D.R.M.; Filho, G.B.O.; Cavalcanti, S.M.T.; Coelho, L.C.D.; Espíndola, J.W.P.; Gonzalez, L.R.; Rabello, M.M.; Hernandes, M.Z.; Ferreira, P.M.P.; et al. Design, synthesis and structure–activity relationship of phthalimides endowed with dual antiproliferative and immunomodulatory activities. *Eur. J. Med. Chem.* **2015**, *96*, 491–503. [CrossRef]
49. Hu, M.C.-T.; Lee, D.-F.; Xia, W.; Golfman, L.S.; Ou-Yang, F.; Yang, J.-Y.; Zou, Y.; Bao, S.; Hanada, N.; Saso, H.; et al. IκB Kinase Promotes Tumorigenesis through Inhibition of Forkhead FOXO3a. *Cell* **2004**, *117*, 225–237. [CrossRef]
50. Gao, Z.; Hwang, D.; Bataille, F.; Lefevre, M.; York, D.; Quon, M.J.; Ye, J. Serine Phosphorylation of Insulin Receptor Substrate 1 by Inhibitor κB Kinase Complex. *J. Biol. Chem.* **2002**, *277*, 48115–48121. [CrossRef]
51. Karin, M.; Yamamoto, Y.; Wang, Q.M. The IKK NF-κB system: A treasure trove for drug development. *Nat. Rev. Drug Discov.* **2004**, *3*, 17–26. [CrossRef]

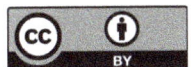

© 2020 by the authors. Licensee MDPI, Basel, Switzerland. This article is an open access article distributed under the terms and conditions of the Creative Commons Attribution (CC BY) license (http://creativecommons.org/licenses/by/4.0/).

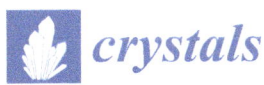

Article

Crystal Structure and Solid-State Conformational Analysis of Active Pharmaceutical Ingredient Venetoclax

Franc Perdih [1], Nina Žigart [2,3] and Zdenko Časar [2,3,*]

[1] Faculty of Chemistry and Chemical Technology, University of Ljubljana, Večna pot 113, SI-1001 Ljubljana, Slovenia; franc.perdih@fkkt.uni-lj.si
[2] Sandoz Development Center Slovenia, Lek Pharmaceuticals d.d, SI-1526 Ljubljana, Slovenia; nina.zigart@novartis.com
[3] Faculty of Pharmacy, University of Ljubljana, Aškerčeva cesta 7, SI-1000 Ljubljana, Slovenia
* Correspondence: zdenko.casar@sandoz.com or zdenko.casar@ffa.uni-lj.si; Tel.: +386-1580-2079

Abstract: Venetoclax is an orally bioavailable, B-cell lymphoma-2 selective inhibitor used for the treatment of chronic lymphocytic leukemia, small lymphocytic lymphoma, and acute myeloid leukemia. Venetoclax's crystal structure was until now determined only when it was bound to a B-cell lymphoma-2 (BCL-2) protein, while the crystal structure of this active pharmaceutical ingredient alone has not been reported yet. Herein, we present the first successful crystallization, which provided crystals of venetoclax suitable for X-ray diffraction analysis. The crystal structure of venetoclax hydrate was successfully determined. The asymmetric unit is composed of two crystallographically independent molecules of venetoclax and two molecules of interstitial water. Intramolecular N–H···O hydrogen bonding is present in both molecules, and a molecular overlay shows differences in their molecular conformations, which is also observed in respect to venetoclax molecules from known crystal structures of BCL-2:venetoclax complexes. A supramolecular structure is achieved through various N–H···N, O–H···O, C–H···O, C–H···π, C–Cl···π, ONO···π, and π···π interactions. The obtained crystals were additionally characterized with spectroscopic techniques, such as IR and Raman, as well as with thermal analysis.

Keywords: venetoclax; crystals; crystal structure; hydrate; conformation; X-ray diffraction

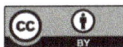

1. Introduction

The B-cell lymphoma-2 (BCL-2) family of proteins, consisting of three distinctive protein groups (anti-apoptotic proteins, pro-apoptotic effectors, and pro-apoptotic initiators/sensitizers), regulate cell death through their direct binding interactions triggering a mitochondrial apoptotic pathway that results in caspase activation and apoptosis [1–16]. BCL-2 anti-apoptotic family members play a key role in cancer cell survival as well as in drug resistance [17–22]. Therefore, they are primary inhibition targets for the treatment of several cancers as their inhibition restores the apoptotic ability of malignant cells [23–27]. Venetoclax (Figure 1) is an orally bioavailable, B-cell lymphoma-2 (BCL-2) selective inhibitor and the first-in-class oral BCL-2 inhibitor for the treatment of lymphoid malignancies [28–35]. Venetoclax was first approved by the FDA in 2016 for the treatment of patients with chronic lymphocytic leukemia (CLL) and later for small lymphocytic lymphoma (SLL) and for the treatment of newly diagnosed acute myeloid leukemia (AML) in combination with azacitidine, decitabine, or low-dose cytarabine [36–39]. According to the IMS Health data, the market value of venetoclax accounted for nearly USD 735 M in 2019. Moreover, there are many ongoing clinical trials involving venetoclax in various combination therapies [40], which puts venetoclax on the list of highly valuable drugs.

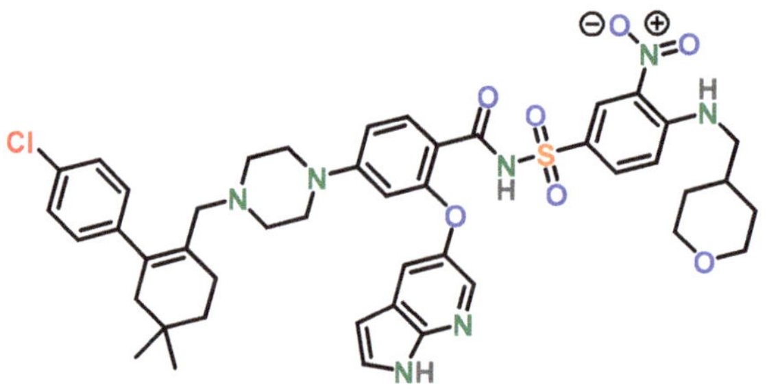

Venetoclax (VEN)

Figure 1. Structure of venetoclax.

Recently, crystal structures of BCL-2 and a BCL-2 mutants bound to venetoclax were reported in the literature [41], which provided the first insights into conformational preferences of venetoclax within the target protein. Surprisingly, although there are several patent literature reports on the salts, polymorphs, hydrates, and solvates of venetoclax [42–44], the crystal structure of active pharmaceutical ingredient venetoclax has not been described in the literature yet. This could be attributed to the well-known challenges related to the growth of single crystals of sufficient size and quality suitable for single crystal X-ray diffraction analysis [45–47]. Since venetoclax (Figure 1) contains several rotatable bonds, it is reasonable to expect that venetoclax could adopt several conformation states with overall rich conformational space. Therefore, the crystal structure of venetoclax could provide new information on the conformations found in a small molecule crystal structure, which could be compared to that of the molecule bound to BCL-2. Such comparison is of high relevance because it could establish if the small molecule crystal conformations are comparable to the protein-bound conformations of venetoclax and therefore relevant to structure-based drug design in this group of compounds. In addition, increasing our knowledge of the conformations adopted by venetoclax could provide a better understanding and exploitation of lesser-known interactions, which could provide more efficient drug design efforts in the future [48–54]. In this report, we provide details on the successful preparation of crystals of venetoclax suitable for single crystal X-ray diffraction analysis, the first crystal structure of venetoclax's hydrate form, and conformational analysis of its small molecule crystal structure in comparison with the venetoclax bound to BCL-2.

2. Materials and Methods

2.1. Materials

For the purpose of this study, venetoclax was obtained from MSN Laboratories (Hyderabad, India). Acetonitrile (ACN) was purchased from J. T. Baker, now part of Avantor® (Radnor, PA, USA). FTIR grade potassium bromide (KBr) and analytical grade ammonium bicarbonate were purchased from Merck KGaA (Darmstadt, Germany).

2.2. Characterization Methods

2.2.1. Attenuated Total Reflection Fourier Transform Infrared (ATR-FTIR) Measurements

ATR-FTIR spectra were collected with a Nicolet iS50FT-IR spectrometer (Thermo Fisher Scientific, Waltham, MA, USA), using a single reflection diamond ATR cell.

2.2.2. Raman Measurements

Raman spectra were collected with a Nicolet iS50FT-IR spectrometer (Thermo Fisher Scientific, Waltham, MA, USA), equipped with the iS50 Raman accessory.

2.2.3. Differential Scanning Calorimetry (DSC) Measurements

DSC thermograms were acquired using the differential scanning calorimeter DSC 3+ Star^e System instrument (Mettler Toledo, Polaris Parkway Columbus, OH, USA) operating at 10 °C/min.

2.2.4. Thermogravimetric Analysis (TGA) Measurements

TGA data were acquired using the TGA/DSC 1 Star^e System (Mettler Toledo, Polaris Parkway Columbus, OH, USA) operating at 10 °C/min.

2.2.5. X-ray Single Crystal Analysis

Single crystal X-ray diffraction data of **VEN·H$_2$O** were collected on an Agilent Technologies SuperNova Dual diffractometer (Agilent, UK) with an Atlas detector using monochromated Cu-Kα radiation (λ = 1.54184 Å) at 150 K. The data were processed using *CrysAlis Pro* [55]. The structure was solved by the SHELXT program [56] and refined by a full-matrix least-squares procedure based on F^2 with SHELXL [57] using the Olex2 program suite [58]. All non-hydrogen atoms were refined anisotropically. Water atom O16 was refined to be disordered over two positions in a ratio of 0.879(5):0.121(5). Hydrogen atoms were readily located in different Fourier maps, except for the atoms on water oxygen atom O16 which were not included in the refinement. Hydrogen atoms bonded to carbon atoms were subsequently treated as riding atoms in geometrically idealized positions with U_{iso}(H) = kU_{eq}(C), where k = 1.5 for methyl groups, which were permitted to rotate but not to tilt, and 1.2 for all other H atoms. Hydrogen atoms bonded to nitrogen and oxygen atoms were refined, fixing the bond lengths and isotropic temperature factors as U_{iso}(H) = kU_{eq}(N,O), where k = 1.2 in case of N atoms and 1.5 in case of O atoms. The hydrogen atom H15B on water molecule O15 had to be treated, fixing the coordinates. The crystallographic data are listed in Table 1.

Table 1. Crystallographic data of venetoclax (**VEN·H$_2$O**).

Parameter	VEN·H$_2$O
CCDC number	2063224
Formula	C$_{45}$H$_{50}$ClN$_7$O$_7$S·H$_2$O
M_r	886.44
T (K)	150.00(10)
Crystal system	triclinic
Space group	P–1
a (Å)	12.6058(3)
b (Å)	13.6947(3)
c (Å)	26.0490(6)
α (°)	83.7790(18)
β (°)	87.6244(18)
γ (°)	81.3877(18)
Volume (Å^3)	4418.55(17)
Z	4
D_c (g/cm^3)	1.333
μ (mm^{-1})	1.714
F(000)	1872.0
Reflections collected	34794
R_{int}	0.0305
Data/restraints/parameters	16756/8/1152
R, wR_2 [$I > 2\sigma(I)$] [a]	0.0463, 0.1239
R, wR_2 (all data) [a]	0.0619, 0.1323
GOF, S [b]	1.039
Largest diff. peak/hole / e Å^{-3}	1.00/−0.50

[a] $R = \sum ||F_o| - |F_c||/\sum |F_o|$, $wR_2 = \{\sum[w(F_o^2 - F_c^2)^2]/\sum[w(F_o^2)^2]\}^{1/2}$. [b] $S = \{\sum[(F_o^2 - F_c^2)^2]/(n - p)\}^{1/2}$, where n is the number of reflections and p is the total number of refined parameters.

2.2.6. Powder X-ray Diffraction Analysis

Powder X-ray diffraction pattern (p-XRD) of prepared **VEN·H$_2$O** was obtained with an X'Pert PRO diffractometer (PANalytical, Almelo, Netherlands) equipped with a Ge(111) Johannson type monochromator in reflection mode using CuKα1 radiation (λ = 1.54060 Å) and the full range of the 128 channel linear RTMS detector. The diffractogram was recorded at a tube voltage of 45 kV, tube current of 40 mA, and applying a step size of 0.034° 2θ with an exposure time of 100 s per step in the angular range of 3° to 50° 2θ under ambient conditions. Since no characteristic reflections were visible above 40° 2θ, the diffractogram is shown in the range of 3–40° 2θ.

2.3. Synthesis and Characterization of Venetoclax Hydrate

Venetoclax (100 mg) was placed into an Erlenmeyer flask and 100 mL of ACN–NH$_4$HCO$_3$ (10 mM solution) = 8:2 solvent mixture was added. The obtained suspension was sonicated in an ultrasonic bath for 5 minutes. The obtained turbid solution was left to stand at ambient temperature for 2 hours and then filtered through a polytetrafluoroethylene (PTFE) filter. The obtained yellow solution was placed into a glass laboratory bottle and left to stand unclosed at ambient temperature for 60 days. During this time, the solvent evaporated affording agglomerated crystals on the bottom of the bottle and needle-shaped crystals that were deposited on the walls of the glass bottle. The agglomerated crystals on the bottom of the glass bottle were discarded while the needle-like crystals suitable for the single crystal X-ray analysis obtained from the walls of the glass bottle were collected for further analysis. DSC (10 °K/min): 49 °C onset, 64 °C peak (endothermic transition) and 168 °C onset, 182 °C peak (endothermic transition); ATR-FTIR: 565, 663, 734, 760, 816, 831, 865, 902, 985, 1098, 1125, 1141, 1171, 1231, 1244, 1255, 1346, 1410, 1434, 1521, 1569, 1578, 1607, 1677, 2842, 2917, 3303, 3364 cm^{-1}; Raman: 796, 838, 1068, 1142, 1161, 1172, 1232, 1272, 1363, 1427, 1496, 1607, 1678, 2847, 2892, 2919, 2941, 2961, 3065, 3083 cm^{-1}; p-XRD (Cu-Kα): 6.5, 7.0, 7.7, 9.8, 10.8, 11.4, 11.7, 12.6, 13.1, 14.3, 15.6, 16.7, 16.8, 17.3, 17.7, 18.2, 18.5, 19.9, 20.0, 20.5, 21.4, 21.9, 22.5, 23.0, 23.4, 24.3, 24.9, 26.1, 26.4, 28.7, 29.2, 29.5° 2θ.

3. Results and Discussion

3.1. Preparation of Venetoclax Hydrate

In our previous studies on the stability and liquid chromatography analytical method development for venetoclax, we observed that venetoclax formed crystals after a few days from some of the solvents used for the dissolution of venetoclax [59,60]. Therefore, we performed a targeted crystallization experiment from the most promising solvent system identified in our previous study [60]. For this purpose, venetoclax was dissolved in an ACN–NH$_4$HCO$_3$ (10 mM solution) = 8:2 solvent mixture, and the solution was left to stand for 60 days at ambient temperature in a laboratory glass bottle. The yellow needle-shaped crystals that were formed on the walls of the glass bottle after evaporation of the solvent were collected and used for further analysis. This proved that the obtained crystalline venetoclax was suitable for single crystal X-ray diffraction. Thermal analysis and X-ray data indicated that the obtained crystals represented a venetoclax hydrate form that was previously reported in the patent literature, although it was obtained by desolvation of the venetoclax ethyl acetate solvate at ambient conditions and characterized only with a p-XRD [42].

3.2. Characterization of Venetoclax Hydrate

3.2.1. Infrared Spectral Analysis

In the IR spectrum of venetoclax hydrate (Figure 2) the most diagnostic bands are associated with the shoulder of an OH band of water in the 3700–3400 cm^{-1} region, N–H stretching vibrations (3364 and 3303 cm^{-1}), C–H stretching vibrations of the benzene rings (3141 and 3105 cm^{-1}), C–H stretching vibrations of CH$_2$ and CH$_3$ groups (2917 and 2842 cm^{-1}), C=O stretching vibration of an amide bond (1677 cm^{-1}), and stretching vibrations that are probably associated with C=C aromatic rings, the –NO$_2$ group, and the –SO$_2$ group (1607, 1569, 1521, 1362, 1346 and 1141 cm^{-1}).

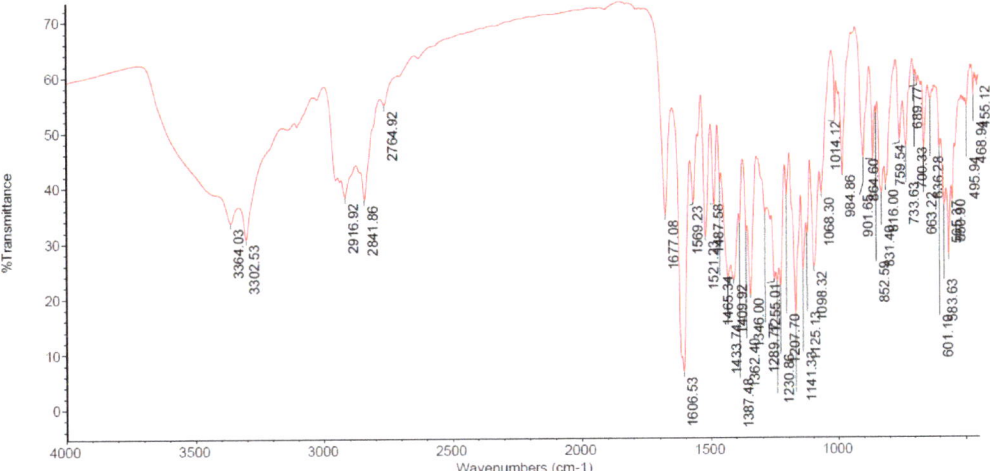

Figure 2. IR spectrum of VEN·H$_2$O.

3.2.2. Raman Spectral Analysis

The Raman spectrum of venetoclax hydrate (Figure 3) displays CH stretching of unsaturated carbons in the region above 3000 cm^{-1}, while CH stretching of saturated carbons populates the region from 3000 to 2840 cm^{-1}. The most diagnostic bands in the Raman spectrum are located at 1678 cm^{-1} (C=O stretch of an amide bond) and a very strong aryl C=C stretch 1607 cm^{-1}.

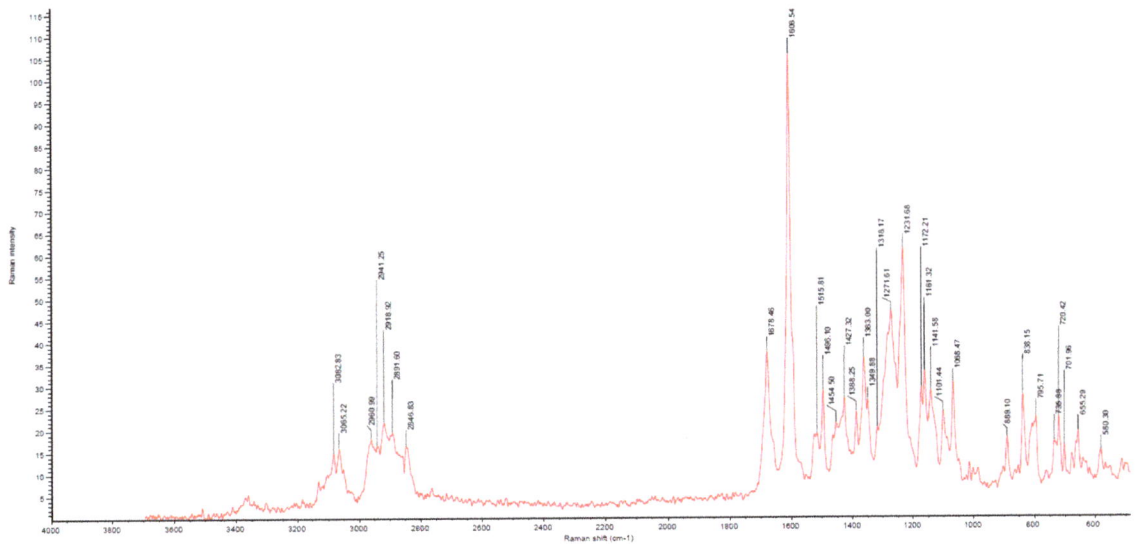

Figure 3. Raman spectrum of VEN·H$_2$O.

3.2.3. Thermal Analyses

The thermal behavior of the obtained crystalline venetoclax is shown in Figure 4. In the DSC thermogram (Figure 4, top), two endothermic transitions were observed: the first transition at 49 °C (onset) and 64 °C (peak), which is probably associated with partial dehydration, and the second transition at 168 °C (onset) and 182 °C (peak), which is probably associated with the melting of the form obtained after dehydration. After both endothermic phenomena, an exothermic transition peak associated with decomposition was observed at temperatures above 220 °C. The TGA thermogram (Figure 4, bottom) indicates that dehydration starts above 30 °C and the mass loss is completed by 200 °C. The mass loss of 1.92% w/w is well within the expected value for a monohydrate form, i.e., 2.03% w/w. Thus, TGA and DSC data on the obtained crystalline solid venetoclax indicated that this is a hydrated form of venetoclax.

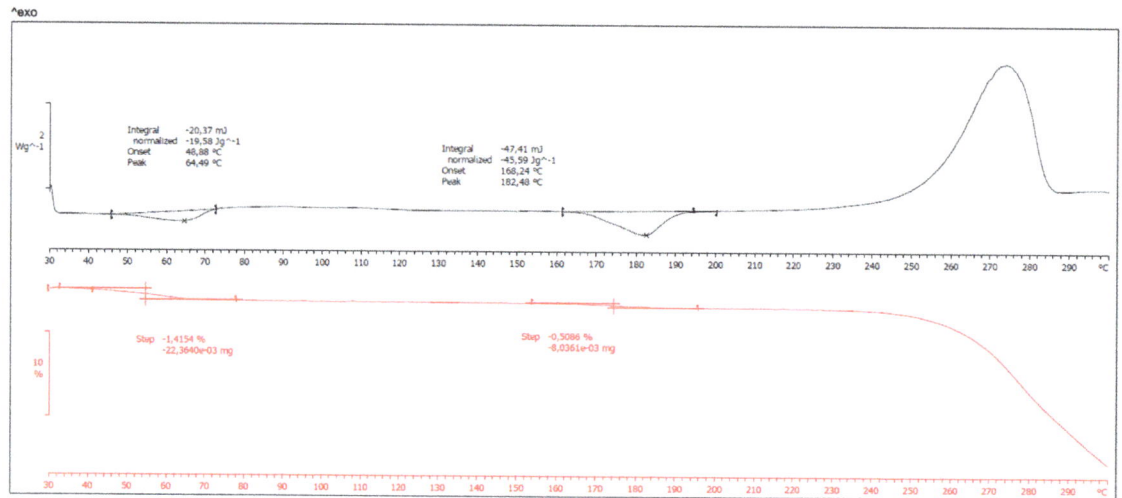

Figure 4. DSC and TGA thermograms of **VEN·H$_2$O**.

3.2.4. Powder X-ray Diffraction Analysis

To investigate whether the analyzed crystal structure is truly representative of the bulk material, the X-ray powder diffraction (*p*-XRD) technique wasperformed at room temperature and compared with the pattern simulated from the crystal structure. As depicted in Figure 5, the experimental *p*-XRD pattern is nearly identical with the corresponding simulated one except for some differences that may be due to the preferential orientation. The studied form has a *p*-XRD comparable to the previously reported monohydrate form in the patent literature [42].

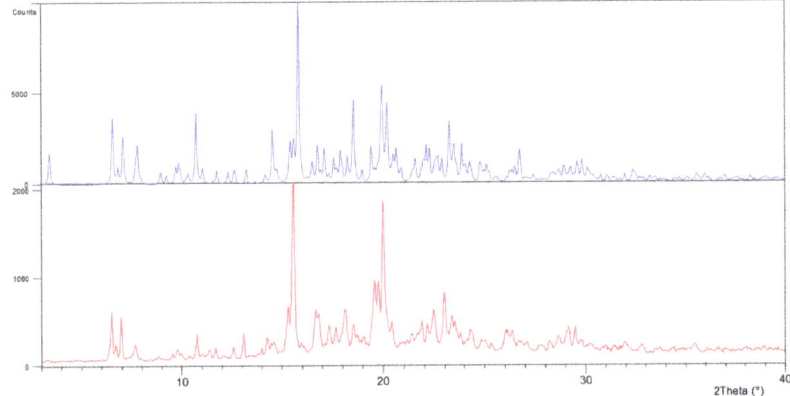

Figure 5. Simulated (blue) and experimental (red) powder X-ray diffraction pattern of **VEN·H$_2$O**.

3.2.5. X-ray Single Crystal Analysis

- Molecular Geometry

Needle-shaped crystals of venetoclax, suitable for single crystal X-ray diffraction, were prepared by crystallization from an ACN-aqueous ammonium bicarbonate buffer system. Thermal analysis and X-ray data indicated that the crystals obtained represented a venetoclax hydrate form [42] that was previously described only in the patent literature and characterized solely with a *p*-XRD analysis. Crystallographic data are listed in Table 1 (see supplementary material for further details). The compound **VEN·H$_2$O** crystalizes in triclinic space group *P*–1 with two crystallographically independent molecules of venetoclax (A and B) and two molecules of interstitial water in the asymmetric unit, with one (O16) being disordered over two positions (Figure 6a). In each molecule (A and B), intramolecular N–H···ONO hydrogen bonding between the amine group (N3, N10) and nitro group, as well as intramolecular N–H···O hydrogen bonding between the amide group (N1, N8) and phenyl oxygen atom (O7, O14), are present and stabilize the molecular structure (Table 2, Figure 6b,c).

Table 2. Hydrogen bonds for **VEN·H$_2$O** [Å and °].

D–H···A	d(D–H)	d(H···A)	d(D···A)	<(DHA)
N1–H1···O7	0.833(17)	1.97(2)	2.602(2)	132(2)
N3–H3···O5	0.848(17)	2.01(2)	2.636(2)	130(2)
N5–H5···N4^i	0.864(17)	2.041(18)	2.891(3)	168(3)
C15–H15···O13^{ii}	1.00	2.55	3.375(3)	139.3
C27–H27A···O4^{iii}	0.99	2.43	3.368(3)	157.1
C29–H29A···O6^{iv}	0.99	2.48	3.456(3)	166.9
C29–H29B···O16B^{ii}	0.99	2.51	3.393(13)	148.8
C31–H31A···O12	0.99	2.50	3.292(3)	136.8
C31–H31A···N9	0.99	2.61	3.310(3)	128.1
C39–H39···O1^{iii}	0.95	2.55	3.244(2)	130.5
C45–H45A···O16B	0.98	2.48	3.429(14)	163.8
N8–H8···O14	0.880(17)	1.90(2)	2.650(3)	141(3)
N10–H10···O12	0.879(18)	2.05(3)	2.665(3)	127(3)
N12–H12A···O11^v	0.870(17)	2.25(2)	3.070(3)	157(3)
C51–H51···O16B	0.95	2.47	3.328(13)	150.3
C61–H61B···O10^{vi}	0.99	2.58	3.330(3)	132.5
C71–H71···O15^{vii}	0.95	2.55	3.483(3)	168.8
O15–H15A···O16A	0.871(10)	2.18(3)	2.890(4)	139(4)
O15–H15A···O16B	0.871(10)	2.03(3)	2.843(14)	156(5)
O15–H15B···O9^{viii}	0.858(3)	2.330(2)	3.170(3)	166.0(2)

Symmetry codes: (i) −*x*, −*y* + 1, −*z*; (ii) *x* − 1, *y*, *z*; (iii) *x* + 1, *y*, *z*; (iv) *x* + 1, *y* − 1, *z*; (v) *x*, *y* + 1, *z*; (vi) −*x*, −*y* + 1, −*z* + 1; (vii) *x* − 1, *y* + 1, *z*; (viii) −*x* + 1, −*y*, −*z* + 1.

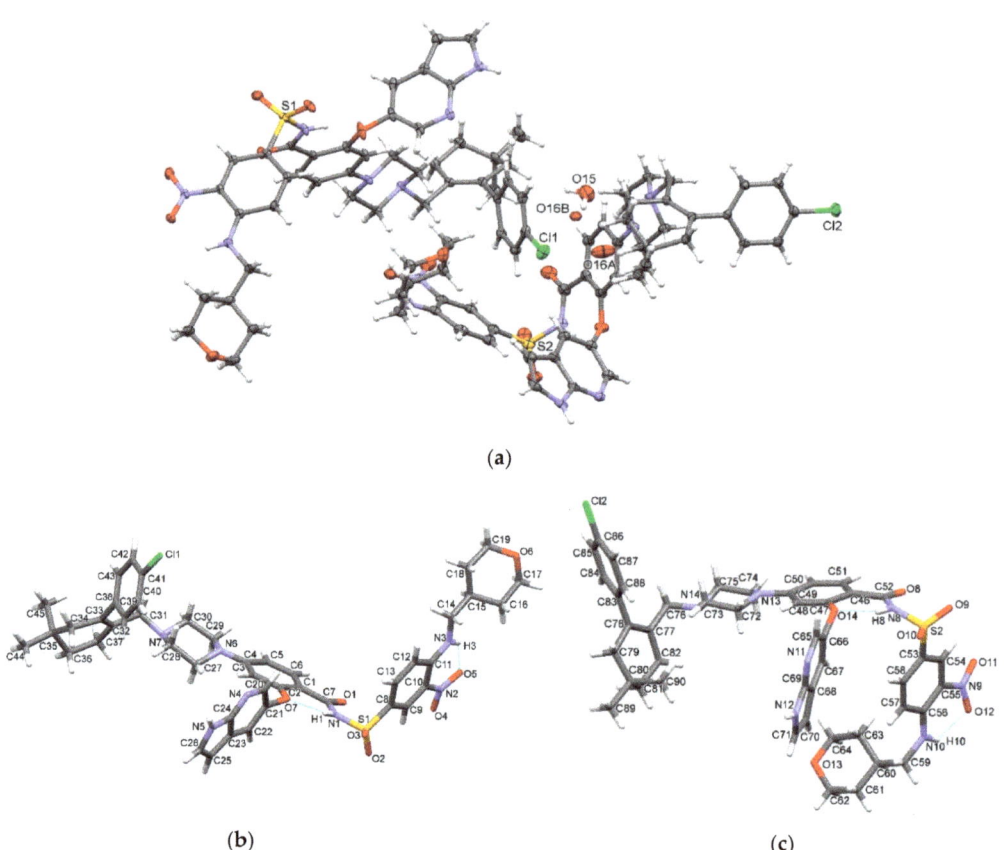

Figure 6. (a) Thermal ellipsoid figure of an asymmetric unit of **VEN·H₂O** drawn at the 30% probability level. Asymmetric unit contains two crystallographically independent molecules of venetoclax and two water molecules (O15, O16 in disorder). (b) Molecule A and (c) molecule B of **VEN·H₂O** with an atom numbering scheme. Intramolecular hydrogen bonds are drawn with dashed blue lines.

The molecular overlay shows that the main difference between molecules A and B is in the orientation of the nitrobenzenesulfonyl moiety with C–S–N–C torsion angle (Φ_1) of 57.09(19)° (molecule A) vs. −57.7(2)° (molecule B) with the additional difference in C–N–C–C torsion angle (Φ_2) of the terminal tetrahydropyranyl substituent of −170.15(18)° (A) vs. 97.6(3)° (B) (Figure 7). Some difference in the inclination of the chlorophenylcyclohexenyl moiety is also evident with the N–C–C–C torsion angle (Φ_3) being 110.2(2)°(A) and 113.7(2)°(B), with the quaternary atom C35 (molecule A) being oriented away from the 1H-pyrrolopyridine moiety, while atom C80 (molecule B) is being oriented toward to this moiety. Furthermore, the difference observed between the two conformations is also due to the inclination of the 1H-pyrrolopyridine-containing substituent in respect of the benzamide scaffold with the C–C–O–C torsion angle (Φ_4) being 18.1(3)° for A and 51.6(3)° for B. In molecule B, the 1H-pyrrolopyridine moiety is thus in close proximity of the nitrobenzenesulfonyl and tetrahydropyranyl rings.

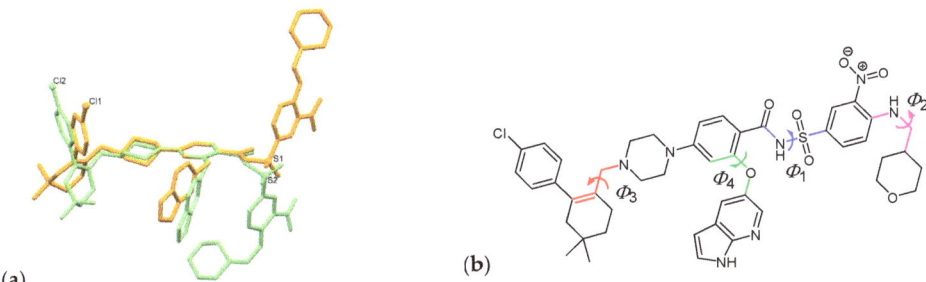

Figure 7. (a) Superposition showing the difference in conformation of venetoclax molecules A (orange) and B (light green). For clarity, hydrogen atoms are omitted, and Cl and S atoms are drawn as small spheres. (b) Selected torsion angles highlighted.

Molecule A forms a hydrogen bonded centrosymmetric dimer via N5–H5···N4^i interactions between adjacent 1H-pyrrolopyridine moieties with the graph-set motif $R_2^2(8)$ [61] (Table 2, Figure 8). Dimers are further connected into a chain along the *a*-axis via C27–H27A···O4^{iii} interactions between the piperazine moiety and nitro group as well as via C39–H39A···O1^{iii} interactions between the chlorophenyl ring and the amide oxygen atom forming a graph-set motif $R_2^2(19)$. This interaction is supported by almost parallel $\pi\cdots\pi$ interactions between each ring of the 1H-pyrrolopyridine moiety and the nitrophenyl ring of the adjacent molecule with a centroid-to-centroid distance of 3.8869(13) and 3.8873(12) Å and ring slippage of 2.037 and 2.016 Å, respectively. Moreover, ONO···π interactions are present between the nitro group and the pyridine ring of the 1H-pyrrolopyridine moiety with an O···π distance of 3.0931(19) Å. The chains are further connected into a layer along the *ab*-plane via C29–H29A···O6^{iv} interactions between the piperazine moiety and the tetrahydropyrane oxygen atom of the adjacent molecule.

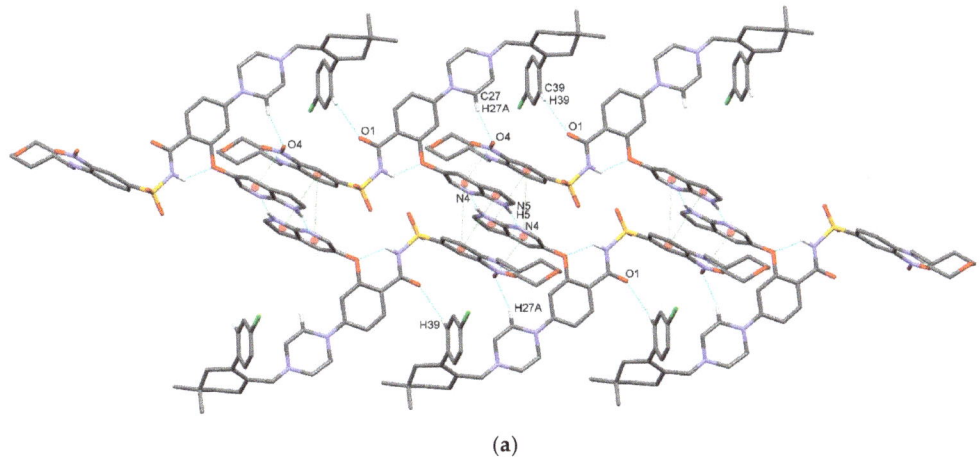

(a)

Figure 8. *Cont.*

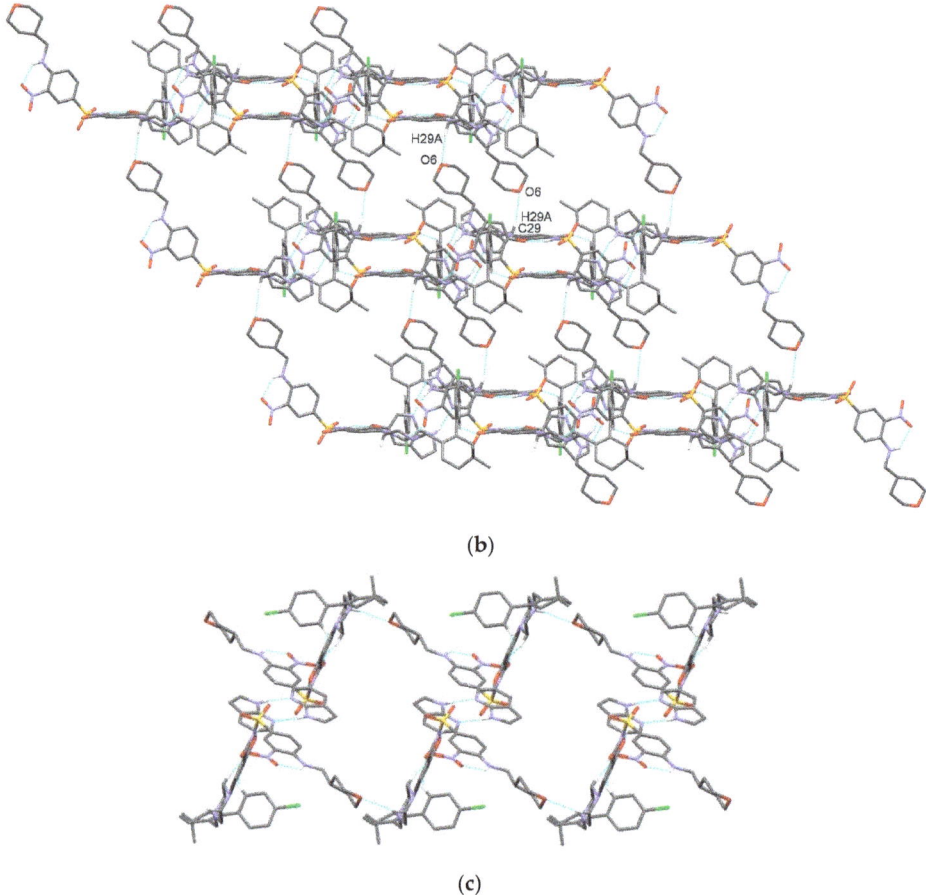

Figure 8. Crystal architecture formed by molecules of A in **VEN·H$_2$O**. (**a**) Hydrogen bonded dimers formed via N5–H5···N4^i interactions connected into a chain along the *a*-axis via C27–H27A···O4^{iii}, π···π, and ONO···π interactions; (**b**) layer formation via C29–H29A···O6^{iv} interactions; and (**c**) view of a layer along the *a*-axis. Hydrogen bonds are drawn by dashed blue lines and π···π and ONO···π interactions by dashed green lines (presented only in (a) for clarity). Hydrogen atoms not involved in the motif shown have been omitted for clarity.

In contrast to molecules of A, where the centrosymmetric hydrogen bonded dimer between the adjacent 1*H*-pyrrolopyridine units is formed, molecules of B form a chain along the *b*-axis through N12–H12···O11^v interactions with the 1*H*-pyrrolopyridine moiety acting as a hydrogen bond donor and the nitro group of the adjacent molecule as a hydrogen bond acceptor (Table 2, Figure 9a). Two such chains are connected into a belt via centrosymmetric C61–H61···O10^{vi} interactions between the tetrahydropyranyl methylene group and the sulfonyl oxygen atom, forming a graph-set motif R$_2^2$(22). The belt structure is supported by π···π interactions between the pyrrole ring of the 1*H*-pyrrolopyridine moiety and the nitrophenyl ring of the adjacent molecule with a centroid-to-centroid distance of 3.860(1) Å and an angle between both rings of 25.4(1)°. The belts are further connected into a layer along the *ab*-plane via C61–H61A···π interactions between the tetrahydropyranyl methylene group and the C46–C51 aromatic system (Figure 9b).

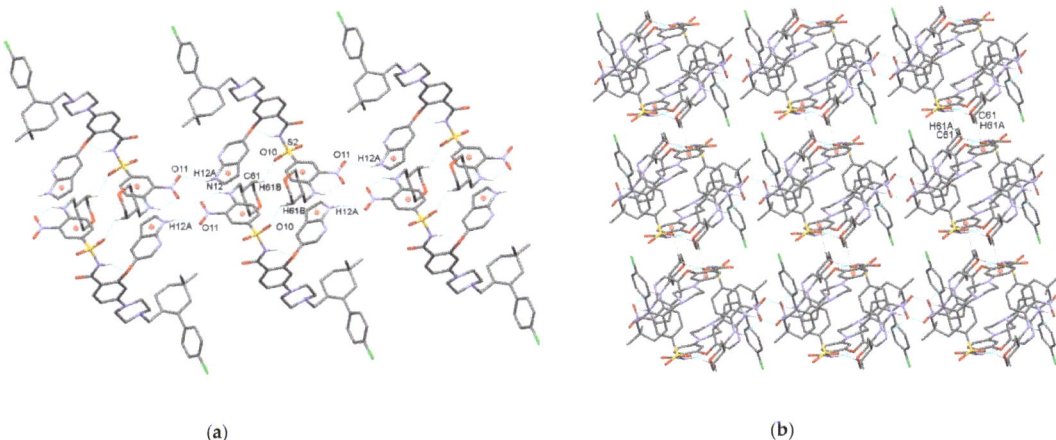

Figure 9. Crystal architecture formed by molecules of B in **VEN·H₂O**. (a) Belt formation along the *b*-axis formed via N12–H12···O11^v, C61–H61B···O10^{vi}, and π···π interactions. (b) Layer formation along the *ab*-plane via C61–H61A···π interactions. Hydrogen bonds are drawn by dashed blue lines and π···π and C–H···π interactions by dashed green lines. Hydrogen atoms not involved in the motif shown have been omitted for clarity.

- Crystal Packing

The supramolecular structure of **VEN·H₂O** is achieved through C–H···O, C–H···π, and C–Cl···π interactions between layers of molecules of A and layers of molecules of B (Table 2, Figure 10). Molecules of A act as hydrogen bond donors and molecules of B as acceptors through C15–H15···O13^{ii} interactions connecting the methine group of a tetrahydropyranyl ring with the oxygen atom of tetrahydropyranyl and through C31–H31A···O12 interactions connecting the methylene unit attached to the piperazine moiety and the nitro group. Furthermore, C37–H37···π interactions connect the methylene unit of the cyclohexenyl ring of molecules of A with the pyrrole ring of molecules of B, while C41–Cl1···π interactions are present between molecules of A and the benzene ring C46–C51 of molecules of B. Furthermore, C87–H87···π interactions connect the chlorobenzene moiety of molecules of B with the benzene ring C1–C6 of molecules of A. Venetoclax crystalizes in a form of monohydrate with two water molecules in the asymmetric unit. These water molecules are also involved in supramolecular aggregation. Water molecule O15 acts as a hydrogen bond donor in the interaction with the disordered water molecule O16 (O15–H15A···O16A, O15–H15A···O16B) and in the interaction with the sulfonyl O9 atom of molecule B as well as a hydrogen bond acceptor in the C71–H71···O15 interaction with the pyrrole ring of molecule B. Hydrogen atoms on the disordered water molecule O16 were not found in the Fourier maps; however, O16B···O9 and O16A···N11 separations of 2.79 and 2.94 Å, respectively, indicate hydrogen bonding interactions with molecules of B. In addition, water molecule O16B is a hydrogen bond acceptor in C29–H29B···O16B, C45–H45A···O16B, and C51–H51···O16B interactions.

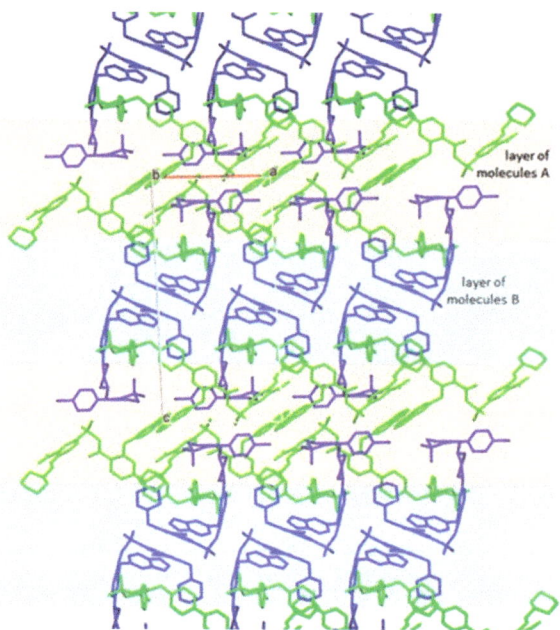

Figure 10. Packing of layers of molecules of A (green) and B (blue).

- Structural comparison between conformations of VEN·H$_2$O and protein:venetoclax complexes

The crystal structure of **VEN·H$_2$O** possesses two crystallographically independent venetoclax molecules with distinctly different conformations. A variety of conformations are possible due to the composition of the molecule containing several rings connected primarily in *para* positions by flexible linkers. Free rotation along the Ar–NH–CH$_2$–R, Ar–CO–NH–SO$_2$–Ar, Ar–O–Ar, and N–CH$_2$–R linkers enables the molecules to adjust to different chemical spaces especially in protein binding sites. We decided to extend our research in order to compare conformations of molecules in **VEN·H$_2$O** with the structures of venetoclax molecules from known crystal structures of protein:venetoclax complexes. **VEN·H$_2$O** was compared with venetoclax molecules in complexes with a BCL-2 antagonist (two crystallographically independent molecules), G101V mutant (two crystallographically independent molecules), G101A mutant, and F104L mutant (two crystallographically independent molecules) [41] since hydrogen bonding and other non-covalent interactions, as well as packing effects, can have a marked influence on the conformation of the venetoclax molecule (Figure 11a). In all the venetoclax structures studied, the intramolecular hydrogen bond N–H···ONO between the amine group (N3, N10 in **VEN·H$_2$O**) and the nitro group is present showing the robustness of this structural motif. On the other hand, the intramolecular hydrogen bond N–H···O between the amide group (N1, N8 in **VEN·H$_2$O**) and the phenyl oxygen atom (O7, O14 in **VEN·H$_2$O**) can be observed only in **VEN·H$_2$O** with a N(H)–C(=O)–C–C(–O) dihedral angle of −5.32 and −7.06° (Figure 11b), respectively, while in all protein:venetoclax complexes, the amide NH group is directed away from the phenyl oxygen atom with dihedral angles in the range 140.7–155.4° in five protein complexes (Figure 11c) and with a dihedral angle of 52.1 and 68.5° in two protein complexes (Figure 11d). The 1*H*-pyrrolopyridine unit in **VEN·H$_2$O** is involved in hydrogen bonding with adjacent molecules, while in all protein:venetoclax structures, it is involved in N–H···O interactions with the carboxylate side arm of the aspartic acid unit of the protein chain. In most protein:venetoclax structures, the carbonyl oxygen atom of the amide unit interacts with the arginine side arm of the adjacent protein and/or water molecule, while sulfonyl oxygen atoms are mostly connected to water molecules and to the glycine NH amide group of the protein chain. Piperazine nitrogen atoms in **VEN·H$_2$O** are not involved in hydrogen bonding; however, in all protein:venetoclax complexes, one nitrogen atom interacts with a water molecule. Since venetoclax molecules in protein complexes are in a markedly different environment with respect to **VEN·H$_2$O**, adopted conformations vary greatly. However, the 1*H*-pyrrolopyridine and nitrobenzene moieties are in close proximity, as is also observed in molecule B of **VEN·H$_2$O**. On the other hand, the chlorobenzene ring in both molecules of **VEN·H$_2$O** is directed in the opposite direction compared to in all of the protein complexes.

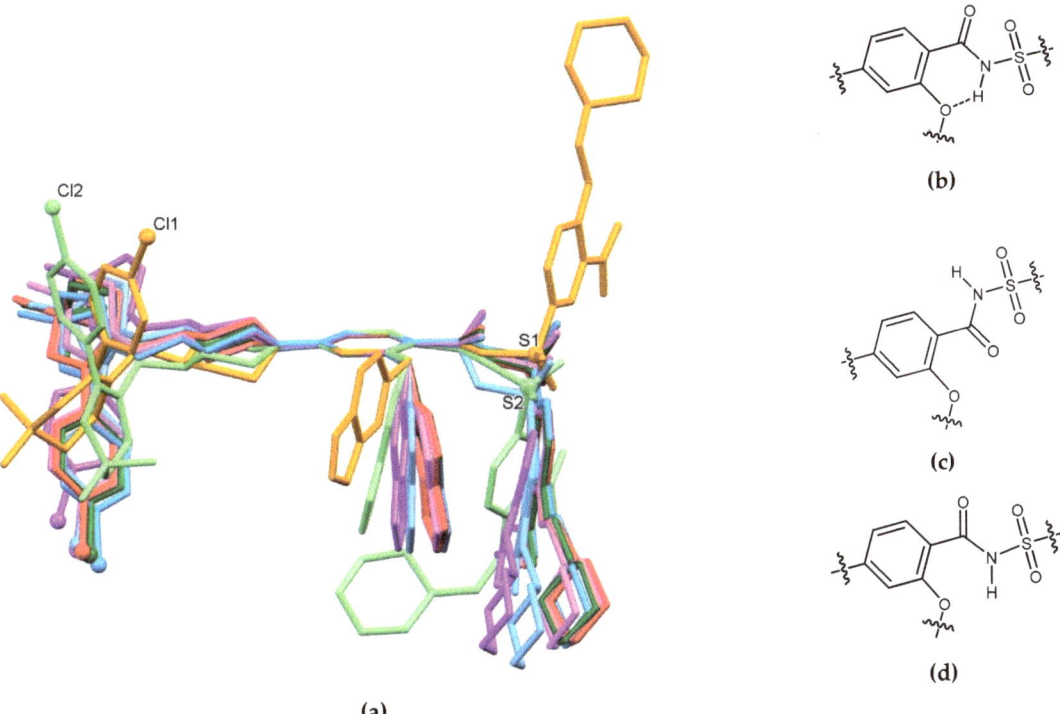

Figure 11. (**a**) Superposition showing the difference in conformation of venetoclax molecules in **VEN·H$_2$O** (A—orange, B—light green) from this work and venetoclax molecules from the BCL-2:venetoclax complex (A—blue, B—light blue), BCL-2 G101V:venetoclax complex (A—red, B—pink), BCL-2 G101A:venetoclax complex (green), and BCL-2 F104L:venetoclax complex (A—magenta, B—light magenta) from Birkinshaw and Czabotar [41]. For clarity, hydrogen atoms are omitted, and Cl and S atoms are drawn as small spheres. Differences in the orientation of the sulfonylamide moiety in (**b**) **VEN·H$_2$O** versus (**c**) most of the protein:venetoclax complexes and (**d**) molecules of B in BCL-2 and in BCL-2 G101A.

4. Conclusions

In this report, we present the first crystal structure of venetoclax, a B-cell lymphoma-2 selective inhibitor used for the treatment of chronic lymphocytic leukemia, small lymphocytic lymphoma, and acute myeloid leukemia. The X-ray single crystal structural analysis revealed the formation of venetoclax hydrate (**VEN·H$_2$O**) crystalizing in triclinic space group *P*–1 with two crystallographically independent molecules of venetoclax (A and B) and two molecules of interstitial water in the asymmetric unit. Two intramolecular N–H···O hydrogen bonds are present in both molecules, and a molecular overlay shows differences in their molecular conformations. Differences are also shown in respect to venetoclax molecules from known crystal structures of protein:venetoclax complexes with BCL-2 antagonist and BCL-2 mutants. In **VEN·H$_2$O**, molecules of A form hydrogen bonded layers via a series of N–H···N, C–H···O, ONO···π, and π···π interactions, as well as molecules of B via N–H···N, C–H···O, C–H···π, and π···π interactions. The supramolecular structure of **VEN·H$_2$O** is achieved through various C–H···O, C–H···π, and C–Cl···π interactions between layers of molecules of A and layers of molecules of B as well as through the O–H···O and C–H···O interactions involving the hydrate molecules. The obtained crystals were additionally characterized with spectroscopic techniques, such as IR and Raman, as well as with thermal analysis.

Supplementary Materials: CCDC 2063224 contains the supplementary crystallographic data for this paper. These data can be obtained free of charge via www.ccdc.cam.ac.uk/data_request/cif or by emailing data_request@ccdc.cam.ac.uk or by contacting The Cambridge Crystallography Data Centre, 12 Union Road, Cambridge CB2 1EZ, UK; fax: +44 1223 336033.

Author Contributions: Conceptualization, Z.Č.; methodology, N.Ž., Z.Č., and F.P.; validation, Z.Č. and F.P.; formal analysis, F.P. and Z.Č.; investigation, N.Ž., Z.Č., and F.P.; resources, Z.Č.; data curation, Z.Č. and F.P.; writing—original draft preparation, Z.Č. and F.P.; writing—review and editing, N.Ž., Z.Č., and F.P.; visualization, Z.Č. and F.P.; supervision, Z.Č.; project administration, Z.Č.; funding acquisition, Z.Č. All authors have read and agreed to the published version of the manuscript.

Funding: This research was funded by Lek Pharmaceuticals d.d. The APC was funded by Lek Pharmaceuticals d.d.

Data Availability Statement: All the data supporting the findings of this study are available within the article and supplementary materials.

Acknowledgments: Authors gratefully acknowledge D. Lipovec for technical assistance in crystallization experiments; H. Cimerman for the acquisition of IR and Raman spectra as well as for the DCS and TGA measurements; and the EN-FIST Centre of Excellence, Ljubljana, Slovenia, for using the SuperNova diffractometer.

Conflicts of Interest: The authors declare no conflict of interest. The funders had no role in the design of the study; in the collection, analyses, or interpretation of data; in the writing of the manuscript, or in the decision to publish the results.

References

1. Lutz, R.J. Role of the BH3 (Bcl-2 homology 3) domain in the regulation of apoptosis and Bcl-2-related proteins. *Biochem. Soc. Trans.* **2000**, *28*, 51–56. [CrossRef] [PubMed]
2. Petch, A.; Al-Rubeai, M. The Bcl-2 family. In *Cell Engineering: Apoptosis*; Al-Rubeai, M., Fussenegger, M., Eds.; Springer Netherlands: Dordrecht, The Netherlands, 2004; Volume 4, pp. 25–47. ISBN 978-1-4020-2217-3. [CrossRef]
3. Ku, B.; Liang, C.; Jung, J.U.; Oh, B.H. Evidence that inhibition of BAX activation by BCL-2 involves its tight and preferential interaction with the BH3 domain of BAX. *Cell Res.* **2011**, *21*, 627–641. [CrossRef] [PubMed]
4. García-Sáez, A. The secrets of the Bcl-2 family. *Cell Death Differ.* **2012**, *19*, 1733–1740. [CrossRef] [PubMed]
5. Lopez, J.; Tait, S. Mitochondrial apoptosis: Killing cancer using the enemy within. *Br. J. Cancer* **2015**, *112*, 957–962. [CrossRef]
6. Delbridge, A.R.D.; Strasser, A. The BCL-2 protein family, BH3-mimetics and cancer therapy. *Cell Death Differ.* **2015**, *22*, 1071–1080. [CrossRef]
7. Dai, H.; Meng, X.W.; Kaufmann, S.H. Mitochondrial apoptosis and BH3 mimetics. *F1000Research* **2016**, *5*, 2804. [CrossRef] [PubMed]
8. Mandal, T.; Shin, S.; Aluvila, S.; Chen, H.C.; Grieve, C.; Choe, J.Y.; Cheng, E.H.; Hustedt, E.J.; Oh, K.J. Assembly of Bak homodimers into higher order homooligomers in the mitochondrial apoptotic pore. *Sci. Rep.* **2016**, *6*, 30763. [CrossRef]
9. Delbridge, A.R.D.; Grabow, S.; Strasser, A.; Vaux, D.L. Thirty years of BCL-2: Translating cell death discoveries into novel cancer therapies. *Nat. Rev. Cancer* **2016**, *16*, 99–109. [CrossRef]
10. Adams, J.M.; Cory, S. The BCL-2 arbiters of apoptosis and their growing role as cancer targets. *Cell Death Differ.* **2018**, *25*, 27–36. [CrossRef]
11. Kalkavan, H.; Green, D.R. MOMP, cell suicide as a BCL-2 family business. *Cell Death Differ.* **2018**, *25*, 46–55. [CrossRef]
12. Montero, J.; Letai, A. Why do BCL-2 inhibitors work and where should we use them in the clinic? *Cell Death Differ.* **2018**, *25*, 56–64. [CrossRef] [PubMed]

13. Kale, J.; Osterlund, E.J.; Andrews, D.W. BCL-2 family proteins: Changing partners in the dance towards death. *Cell Death Differ.* **2018**, *25*, 65–80. [CrossRef] [PubMed]
14. Campbell, K.J.; Tait, S.W.G. Targeting BCL-2 regulated apoptosis in cancer. *Open Biol.* **2018**, *8*, 180002. [CrossRef] [PubMed]
15. Ngoi, N.Y.L.; Choong, C.; Lee, J.; Bellot, G.; Wong, A.L.; Goh, B.C.; Pervaiz, S. Targeting mitochondrial apoptosis to overcome treatment resistance in cancer. *Cancers* **2020**, *12*, 574. [CrossRef] [PubMed]
16. Explore BCL-2. Available online: https://www.genentechoncology.com/pathways/cancer-tumor-targets/bcl-2.html (accessed on 1 January 2021).
17. Srivastava, R.K.; Sasaki, C.Y.; Hardwick, J.M.; Longo, D.L. Bcl-2–mediated drug resistance: Inhibition of apoptosis by blocking nuclear factor of activated T lymphocytes (Nfat)-induced FAS ligand transcription. *J. Exp. Med.* **1999**, *190*, 253–266. [CrossRef]
18. Reed, J.C. BCL-2: Prevention of apoptosis as a mechanism of drug resistance. *Oncol. Clin. N. Am.* **1995**, *9*, 451–473. [CrossRef]
19. Reed, J.C.; Miyashita, T.; Takayama, S.; Wang, H.-G.; Sato, T.; Krajewski, S.; Aimé-Sempé, C.; Bodrug, S.; Kitada, S.; Hanada, M. BCL-2 family proteins: Regulators of cell death involved in the pathogenesis of cancer and resistance to therapy. *J. Cell. Biochem.* **1996**, *60*, 23–32. [CrossRef]
20. Flemming, A. Reversing resistance. *Nat. Rev. Drug. Discov.* **2008**, *7*, 119. [CrossRef]
21. D'Aguanno, S.; Del Bufalo, D. Inhibition of anti-apoptotic Bcl-2 proteins in preclinical and clinical studies: Current overview in cancer. *Cells* **2020**, *9*, 1287. [CrossRef]
22. Lin, V.S.; Xu, Z.-F.; Huang, D.C.S.; Thijssen, R. BH3 mimetics for the treatment of B-cell malignancies—Insights and lessons from the clinic. *Cancers* **2020**, *12*, 3353. [CrossRef]
23. Liu, Q.; Wang, H.-G. Anti-cancer drug discovery and development. *Commun. Integr. Biol.* **2012**, *5*, 557–565. [CrossRef] [PubMed]
24. Mullard, A. Pioneering apoptosis-targeted cancer drug poised for FDA approval. *Nat. Rev. Drug Discov.* **2016**, *15*, 147–149. [CrossRef] [PubMed]
25. Adams, C.M.; Clark-Garvey, S.; Porcu, P.; Eischen, C.M. Targeting the Bcl-2 family in B cell lymphoma. *Front. Oncol.* **2019**, *8*, 636. [CrossRef] [PubMed]
26. Sillar, J.R.; Enjeti, A.K. Targeting apoptotic pathways in acute myeloid leukaemia. *Cancers* **2019**, *11*, 1660. [CrossRef]
27. Carneiro, B.A.; El-Deiry, W.S. Targeting apoptosis in cancer therapy. *Nat. Rev. Clin. Oncol.* **2020**, *17*, 395–417. [CrossRef]
28. Souers, A.J.; Leverson, J.D.; Boghaert, E.R.; Ackler, S.L.; Catron, N.D.; Chen, J.; Dayton, B.D.; Ding, H.; Enschede, S.H.; Fairbrother, W.J.; et al. ABT-199, a potent and selective BCL-2 inhibitor, achieves antitumor activity while sparing platelets. *Nat. Med.* **2013**, *19*, 202–208. [CrossRef]
29. Deeks, E.D. Venetoclax: First global approval. *Drugs* **2016**, *76*, 979–987. [CrossRef]
30. King, A.C.; Peterson, T.J.; Horvat, T.Z.; Rodriguez, M.; Tang, L.A. Venetoclax: A first-in-class oral BCL-2 Inhibitor for the management of lymphoid malignancies. *Ann. Pharmacother.* **2017**, *51*, 410–416. [CrossRef]
31. Žigart, N.; Časar, Z. A literature review of the patent publications on venetoclax—A selective Bcl-2 inhibitor: Discovering the therapeutic potential of a novel chemotherapeutic agent. *Expert Opin. Ther. Pat.* **2019**, *29*, 487–496. [CrossRef]
32. Korycka-Wolowiec, A.; Wolowiec, D.; Kubiak-Mlonka, A.; Robak, T. Venetoclax in the treatment of chronic lymphocytic leukemia. *Expert Opin. Drug Metab. Toxicol.* **2019**, *15*, 353–366. [CrossRef]
33. Blair, H.A. Venetoclax: A review in previously untreated chronic lymphocytic leukaemia. *Drugs* **2020**, *80*, 1973–1980. [CrossRef] [PubMed]
34. Guerra, V.A.; DiNardo, C.; Konopleva, M. Venetoclax-based therapies for acute myeloid leukemia. *Best Pract. Res. Clin. Haematol.* **2019**, *32*, 145–153. [CrossRef]
35. DiNardo, C.D.; Jonas, B.A.; Pullarkat, V.; Thirman, M.J.; Garcia, J.S.; Wei, A.H.; Konopleva, M.; Döhner, H.; Letai, A.; Fenaux, P.; et al. Azacitidine and venetoclax in previously untreated acute myeloid leukemia. *N. Engl. J. Med.* **2020**, *383*, 617–629. [CrossRef]
36. Venclexta FDA Approval History. Available online: https://www.drugs.com/history/venclexta.html (accessed on 7 February 2021).
37. FDA Grants Regular Approval to Venetoclax in Combination for Untreated Acute Myeloid Leukemia. Available online: https://www.fda.gov/drugs/drug-approvals-and-databases/fda-grants-regular-approval-venetoclax-combination-untreated-acute-myeloid-leukemia (accessed on 7 February 2021).
38. FDA Approves Venetoclax for CLL or SLL, with or Without 17 p Deletion, After One Prior Therapy. Available online: https://www.fda.gov/drugs/resources-information-approved-drugs/fda-approves-venetoclax-cll-or-sll-or-without-17-p-deletion-after-one-prior-therapy (accessed on 7 February 2021).
39. FDA Approves New Drug for Chronic Lymphocytic Leukemia in Patients with a Specific Chromosomal Abnormality. Available online: https://www.fda.gov/news-events/press-announcements/fda-approves-new-drug-chronic-lymphocytic-leukemia-patients-specific-chromosomal-abnormality (accessed on 7 February 2021).
40. Clinical Trials Using Venetoclax. Available online: https://www.cancer.gov/about-cancer/treatment/clinical-trials/intervention/Venetoclax (accessed on 7 February 2021).
41. Birkinshaw, R.W.; Gong, J.N.; Luo, C.S.; Lio, D.; White, C.A.; Anderson, M.A.; Blombery, P.; Lessene, G.; Majewski, I.J.; Thijssen, R.; et al. Structures of BCL-2 in complex with venetoclax reveal the molecular basis of resistance mutations. *Nat. Commun.* **2019**, *10*, 2385. [CrossRef]
42. Catron, N.D.; Chen, S.; Gong, Y.; Zhang, G.G. Salts and Crystalline Forms of an Apoptosis-Inducing Agent. International Patent Application WO12071336 A1, 31 May 2012.

43. Potarine Juhasz, Z.; Struba, S.; Nemethne Racz, C.; Toth, Z.G.; Szilagyi, A.; Kerti-Ferenczi, R.; Molnar, S.J.; Pasztor Debreczeni, N.; Hajko, J. Solid State Forms of Venetoclax and Processes for Preparation of Venetoclax. International Patent Application WO17156398 A1, 14 September 2017.
44. Vadali, L.R.; Gottumukkala, N.; Sangvikar, Y.; Jayachandra, S.B.; Jaldu, R. Polymorphic Forms of Venetoclax. WO19135253 A1, 11 July 2019.
45. Datta, S.; Grant, D.J.W. Crystal Structures of Drugs: Advances in Determination, Prediction and Engineering. *Nat. Rev. Drug Discov.* **2004**, *3*, 42–57. [CrossRef] [PubMed]
46. Rychkov, D.A.; Arkhipov, S.G.; Boldyreva, E.V. Simple and efficient modifications of well known techniques for reliable growth of high-quality crystals of small bioorganic molecules. *J. Appl. Cryst.* **2014**, *47*, 1435–1442. [CrossRef]
47. Growing Crystals for X-ray Diffraction Analysis. Available online: https://www.jove.com/v/10216/growing-crystals-for-x-ray-diffraction-analysis (accessed on 14 February 2021).
48. Brameld, K.A.; Kuhn, B.; Reuter, D.C.; Stahl, M. Small molecule conformational preferences derived from crystal structure data. A medicinal chemistry focused analysis. *J. Chem. Inf. Model.* **2008**, *48*, 1–24. [CrossRef]
49. Groom, C. Small Molecule Crystal Structures in Drug Discovery. In *Multifaceted Roles of Crystallography in Modern Drug Discovery. NATO Science for Peace and Security Series A: Chemistry and Biology*; Scapin, G., Patel, D., Arnold, E., Eds.; Springer: Dordrecht, The Netherlands, 2015; pp. 107–114. [CrossRef]
50. Liebeschuetz, J.; Hennemann, J.; Olsson, T.; Groom, C.R. The good, the bad and the twisted: A survey of ligand geometry in protein crystal structures. *J. Comput. Aided. Mol. Des.* **2012**, *26*, 169–183. [CrossRef]
51. Zheng, Y.; Tice, C.M.; Singh, S.B. Conformational control in structure-based drug design. *Bioorg. Med. Chem. Lett.* **2017**, *27*, 2825–2837. [CrossRef]
52. Friedrich, N.-O.; Simsir, M.; Kirchmair, J. How diverse are the protein-bound conformations of small-molecule drugs and cofactors? *Front. Chem.* **2018**, *6*, 68. [CrossRef] [PubMed]
53. Jarvis, A.; Ouvry, G. Essential ingredients for rational drug design. *Bioorg. Med. Chem. Lett.* **2019**, *29*, 126674. [CrossRef] [PubMed]
54. Taylor, R.; Wood, P.A. A million crystal structures: The whole is greater than the sum of its parts. *Chem. Rev.* **2019**, *119*, 9427–9477. [CrossRef] [PubMed]
55. Agilent Technologies Ltd. *CrysAlisPro, Version 1.171.36.28*; Agilent Technologies: Yarnton, UK, 2013; Available online: https://www.agilent.com/cs/library/usermanuals/Public/CrysAlis_Pro_User_Manual.pdf (accessed on 7 February 2021).
56. Sheldrick, G.M. SHELXT—Integrated space-group and crystal-structure determination. *Acta Crystallogr.* **2015**, *A71*, 3–8. [CrossRef] [PubMed]
57. Sheldrick, G.M. Crystal structure refinement with SHELXL. *Acta Crystallogr.* **2015**, *C71*, 3–8. [CrossRef]
58. Dolomanov, O.V.; Bourhis, L.J.; Gildea, R.J.; Howard, J.A.K.; Puschmann, H. OLEX2: A complete structure solution, refinement and analysis program. *J. Appl. Crystallogr.* **2009**, *42*, 339–341. [CrossRef]
59. Žigart, N.; Črnugelj, M.; Ilaš, J.; Časar, Z. On the stability and degradation pathways of venetoclax under stress conditions. *Pharmaceutics* **2020**, *12*, 639. [CrossRef]
60. Žigart, N.; Časar, Z. Development of a stability-indicating analytical method for determination of venetoclax using AQbD principles. *ACS Omega* **2020**, *5*, 17726–17742. [CrossRef] [PubMed]
61. Bernstein, J.; Davis, R.E.; Shimoni, L.; Chang, N.L. Patterns in hydrogen bonding: Functionality and graph set analysis in crystals. *Angew. Chem. Int. Ed.* **1995**, *34*, 1555–1573. [CrossRef]

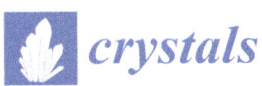

Article

Synthesis, Crystal Structure and Solid State Transformation of 1,2-Bis[(1-methyl-1*H*-imidazole-2-yl)thio]ethane

Leo Štefan [1],*, Dubravka Matković-Čalogović [2], Darko Filić [3] and Miljenko Dumić [4]

1. JGL d.d., Jadran Galenski Laboratorij, 51000 Rijeka, Croatia
2. Department of Chemistry, Faculty of Science, University of Zagreb, 10000 Zagreb, Croatia; dubravka@chem.pmf.hr
3. Fidelta d.o.o., 10000 Zagreb, Croatia; darko.filic@fidelta.eu
4. Department of Biotechnology, University of Rijeka, 51000 Rijeka, Croatia; mdumic@biotech.uniri.hr
* Correspondence: leo.stefan@jgl.hr; Tel.: +385-98-214-996

Received: 13 July 2020; Accepted: 28 July 2020; Published: 3 August 2020

Abstract: The spontaneous *S*-alkylation of the thyreostatic drug methimazole (1-methyl-1,3-dihydro-1*H*-imidazole-2-thione, **1**) with 1,2-dichloroethane at room temperature, in dark or light conditions, led to the formation of its related substance 1,2-bis[(1-methyl-1*H*-imidazole-2-yl)thio]ethane, $C_{10}H_{14}N_4S_2$ (**2a**), primarily isolated in the form of dihydrochloride tetrahydrate $[C_{10}H_{16}N_4S_2]Cl_2·4(H_2O)$ (**2b**), which crystallized in the monoclinic $P2_1/c$ space group. Neutralization of **2b**, followed by crystallization from the acetone/water mixture, produced dihydrate $C_{10}H_{14}N_4S_2·2(H_2O)$ (**2c**), which crystallized in the trigonal R-3 space group. Six water molecules in **2c** are H-bonded mutually and to the nitrogen atoms of six molecules of **2a**. DSC and TGA showed that **2c** melts at 65 °C and loses water up to 120 °C. By cooling to room temperature, anhydrous **2a** was obtained. Single crystals of **2a** that are suitable for X-ray structure analysis were obtained by neutralization of **2b**, followed by crystallization from dry dichloromethane. Anhydrous **2a** crystallizes in the monoclinic $P2_1/c$ space group. The dehydration of **2c** led to the formation of the anhydrous product **2a**, which is identical to the one obtained by crystallization, as was found by complementary solid-state techniques. No intermediate monohydrate or hemihydrate phases were detected. Powder diffraction showed the same pattern of **2c** via both preparation procedures. The structures of all the forms were elucidated by spectroscopy, microscopy and thermal methods and confirmed by single crystal X-ray analysis.

Keywords: methimazole; 1,2-bis[(1-methyl-1*H*-imidazole-2-yl)thio]ethane; solid-state forms; hydrates; dehydration

---

1. Introduction

Methimazole (1-methyl-1,3-dihydro-1*H*-imidazole-2-thione, **1**), a well-known commercially available thyreostatic drug [1], has an ambidentate heterocyclic anion of the type [N-C-S] and was used as the terminal group in the synthesis of noncyclic crown ethers as scorpionate ligands in diverse aspects of the coordination chemistry [2,3].

Among the bridged bis(methimazole) compounds, 1,2-bis[(1-methyl-1*H*-imidazole-2-yl)thio]methane (**A**) and an analogous ethane derivative 1,2-bis[(1-methyl-1*H*-imidazole-2-yl)thio]ethane (**2a**) were synthesized from **1** and dichloromethane or 1,2-dibromoethane. Synthesis was performed in the presence of a strong base, without or under phase-transfer conditions at an elevated temperature [4,5]. In the context of the pharmaceutical purity profile, these compounds are considered as potential methimazole related substances [6], especially if common solvents, e.g., dichloromethane (DCM) and 1,2-dichloroethane (DCE), are used in the synthetic transformations, isolation, purification and methimazole analytics.

Therefore, it was important to understand their behaviour from a chemical, structural and solid-state point of view. To evaluate these factors, we carried out a preliminary stability study of **1** in DCM and DCE in daylight or dark, at ambient humidity and room temperature.

2. Results and Discussion

2.1. Synthesis of Bis Derivative 2

Solutions of **1** in DCM or DCE were left without stirring in daylight or dark, at ambient humidity and at room temperature for 15 days. According to the TLC analysis, no changes of **1** were observed in DCM solutions. However, in both DCE solutions (i.e., in light and dark) spontaneous S-bis alkylation of **1** by 1,2-dichloroethane led to the formation of colourless plate shaped crystals of 1,2-bis[(1-methyl-1*H*-imidazole-2-yl)thio]ethane in the form of dihydrochloride tetrahydrate (**2b**) with a 30% yield; mp. (DSC, onset): 208 °C. Purity by HPLC: 98%. Upon its neutralization, extraction, evaporation of the solvent and crystallization of the crude residue from the dry dichloromethane under low humidity conditions of the anhydrous 1,2-bis[(1-methyl-1*H*-imidazole-2-yl)thio]ethane **2a** was obtained with an 84% yield, mp. (DSC, onset): 89 °C (lit: 88–90 °C, [5]).

However, if crystallization of the crude residue is attempted from the acetone/water (1/1) mixture, 1,2-bis[(1-methyl-1*H*-imidazole-2-yl)thio]ethane dihydrate (**2c**) is obtained with a 78% yield; mp. (DSC, onset): 65 °C. The same product was obtained by the crystallization of pure **2a** from the acetone/water (1/1) mixture. Anhydrous from **2a** was also prepared by drying the dihydrate **2c** (Scheme 1).

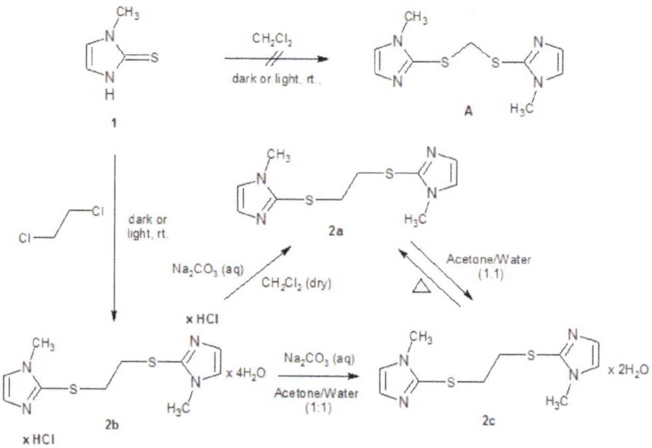

Scheme 1. Synthesis of 1,2-bis[(1-methyl-1*H*-imidazole-2-yl)thio]—derivatives **A** and **2** (**2a–2c**).

2.2. Characterization of 1,2-Bis[(1-methyl-1H-imidazole-2-yl)thio]ethane Forms 2a–2c

All the studied forms, **2a–2c**, were elucidated using spectroscopy, microscopy, thermal and complementary analytical methods. Their structures were confirmed by the single crystal X-ray diffraction analysis.

Proton chemical shifts of dihydrochloride tetrahydrate **2b**, recorded in D_2O, were different in comparison to the previously reported data for **2a** in $CHCl_3$-C_6H_6 [5], while relative integrations indicated protonation of the imidazole ring and confirmed the proposed structure (Figure 1). Mass spectra recorded in the positive mode indicated the most abundant ion at 255.0743 m/z, which was attributed to the base peak of **2a**, corresponding to $[M+H-2HCl]^+$. Additionally, two formed fragments at 141.0486 m/z and 114.0249 m/z indicated cleavage of the thioethyl group. However, DSC showed an endothermic loss of volatile solvents between 35 and 70 °C. In addition, mass loss by TGA of 3.8% and chloride content of 18%, determined by ionic chromatography, indicated that the product crystallized as a dihydrochloride tetrahydrate. The hypothesis was confirmed by single crystal X-ray diffraction analysis.

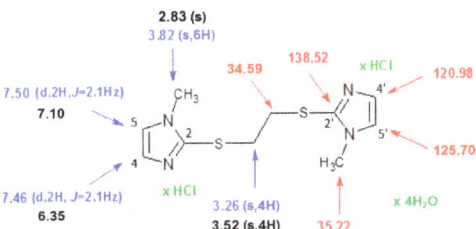

Figure 1. ^{1}H (600 MHz) (blue), ^{13}C (151 MHz) (red) NMR in D$_2$O of **2b** and ^{1}H (black) NMR in CDCl$_3$-C$_6$D$_6$ of **2a** [5].

The molecular structure of **2b** consisted of two cationic imidazolyl groups bounded to the S-atoms of the dithioethyl group (Figure 2a). Each chloride anion was a hydrogen bond acceptor from the protonated imidazole nitrogen atom N2 and two water molecules (Figure 2b, Table 1). The two water molecules were also connected by hydrogen bonds. Through these hydrogen bonds, the cations, chloride anions and water molecules were interconnected into a 3D network.

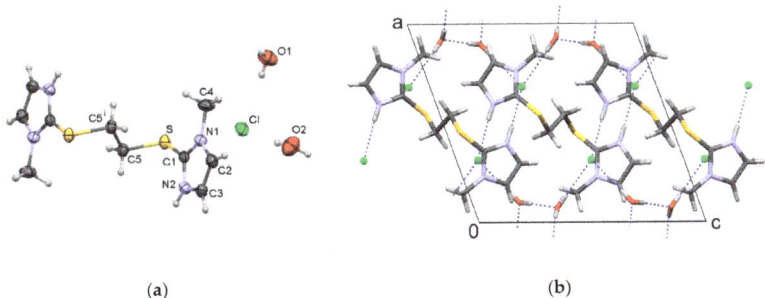

Figure 2. (**a**) Molecular structure of **2b** with the atomic numbering scheme; symmetry code (i) 1 − x, −y, −z, and (**b**) packing diagram of **2b** viewed along the *b*-axis. Hydrogen bounds are marked by dashed blue lines.

Table 1. Distances and angles of the hydrogen bonds in **2b** and **2c**.

Form	Donor-H···Acceptor	d(D-H)/Å	d(H-A)/Å	d(D···A)/Å	<d(D-H···A)/°
2b	N2-H2···Cl [a]	0.86	2.26	3.112 (2)	172
	O1-H11···O2 [b]	0.78 (4)	1.98 (4)	2.749 (5)	169 (5)
	O1-H12···Cl [c]	0.75 (5)	2.44 (5)	3.190 (4)	178 (6)
	O2-H21···Cl	0.78 (6)	2.42 (6)	3.198 (4)	174 (5)
	O2-H22···O1	0.83 (3)	1.93 (3)	2.756 (5)	172 (3)
2c	O1-H1···N2 [d]	0.81 (3)	2.03 (3)	2.827 (3)	167 (4)
	O1-H12···O1 [e]	0.87 (4)	1.92 (4)	2.787 (4)	176 (4)
	C4-4B···O1 [f]	0.96	2.58	3.489 (4)	157

Transformation of the asymmetric unit: (**a**) 1 − x, −1/2 + y, 1/2 − z; (**b**) −x, 1/2 + y, 1/2 −z; (**c**) x, 3/2 − y, 1/2 + z; (**d**) −x + y, −x, z; (**e**) y, −x + y, −z; (**f**) 1/3 − x + y, 2/3 −x, −1/3 + z.

Proton and carbon chemical shifts in the NMR spectra of **2a** in DMSO-d6 exhibited similar values to those in **2b**, and experimental MS data matched the theoretical data. After several attempts, we obtained good quality, single crystals by crystallisation from dry dichloromethane at dry conditions (see experimental section) that allowed us to confirm the anhydrous structure of **2a**, which crystallized in the monoclinic P2$_1$/c space group.

There are no hydrogen bounds in the structure of **2a**, only van der Waals forces connect the molecules (Figure 3).

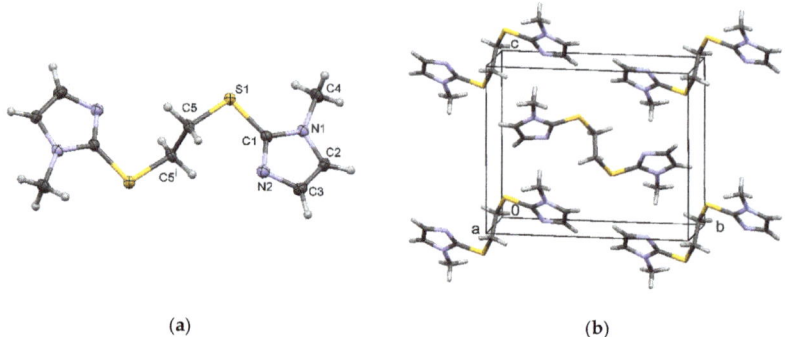

(a) (b)

Figure 3. (a) Molecular structure of **2a** with the atomic numbering scheme; symmetry code (i) 1 − x, −y, −z, and (b) packing diagram of **2a**.

Crystals of **2c** showed the TLC Rf value of 0.59, which was the same as **2a** and **2b**, and a TGA volatile content of 11.31%, indicating the solvated form of the same substance. The structure was solved by the single crystal X-ray diffraction analysis, showing that the dihydrate **2c** crystallizes in the trigonal R -3 space group. Six water molecules were mutually interconnected by hydrogen bonds, forming a hexagon in the chair conformation, which is the most common conformation for a cluster of six water molecules. The R6 motif is usually formed by water molecules related by a centre of symmetry [7]. In **2c**, one water molecule formed the R6 pattern by the -3 symmetry element ($R_6^6(12)$ by the graph-set notation). The water molecule was an acceptor of a hydrogen bond from N2 and a weak one from C4, thus forming a 3D network (Figure 4, Table 1).

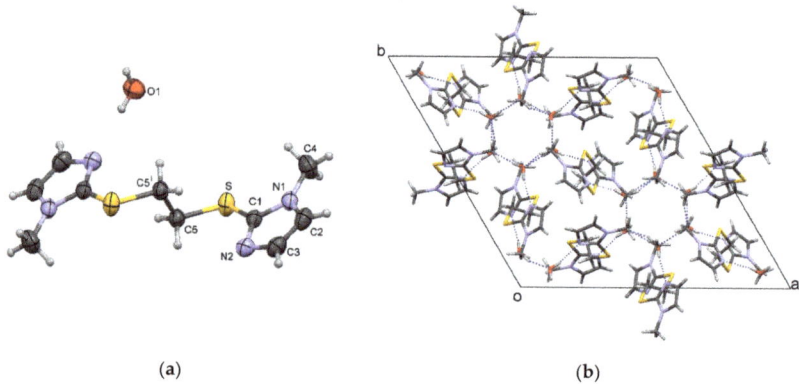

(a) (b)

Figure 4. (a) Molecular structure with the atomic numbering scheme; symmetry code (i) 2/3 − x, 1/3 − y, 4/3 − z, and (b) packing diagram of **2c** viewed along the *c*-axis. Hydrogen bonds are marked with blue dashed lines.

The molecular structure of 1,2-bis[(1-methyl-1*H*-imidazole-2-yl)thio]ethane consisted of two imidazole groups bounded to the S-atoms of the dithioethyl group (**2a, 2c**). The imidazole groups were protonated in **2b**. In all three structures, the ethane moiety lied at the centre of symmetry, and thus only half of the molecule was in the asymmetric unit. Therefore, the imidazole groups were parallel. The difference in the three structures was found in the orientation of the imidazole group, i.e., rotation about the S-C1 bond resulting in different C5-S-C1-N1 torsion angles (−173.8(2)°, −113.4(2)° and 151.8(2)°, in **2a**, **2b** and **2c**, respectively (Figure 5).

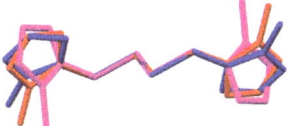

Figure 5. Molecule overlay of **2a** (blue), **2b** (magenta) and **2c** (red). Atoms C5 and S and their pairs related by the inversion centre were used for the overlay. Hydrogen atoms are omitted for clarity.

2.3. Dehydration Behaviour of Dihydrate 2c and Its Transformation to the Anhydrous Form 2a

Hydrates are the most common type of solvated organic compounds [8], and understanding their dehydration pathways, as a widespread but not properly understood phenomenon, is critical for designing optimal properties for materials, particularly in the case of pharmaceutical solids [9]. Several schemes for the classification of hydrates have been proposed [10–13], but in general, dehydration results in three types of crystallographic behaviour: a) material where the crystal structure changes (different powder pattern) after dehydration, i.e., as in the present study, contrary to b) material that undergoes only a slight change in crystal structure (related XRPD pattern) after dehydration, like some azithromycin solvates [14], or c) material that becomes amorphous after dehydration, like some other azithromycin solvates [15].

The dehydration process of **2c** had a markedly different crystal structure of the anhydrous form **2a** and has been studied using different experimental techniques. The dihydrate **2c** was heated below the melting point, at around 55 °C and at reduced pressure of 200 mbar to a constant mass. A significant rate of the dehydration process was detected after 30 min by the formation of opaque crystals. The process was completed after 60 min.

DSC measurement of the selected samples showed, after 30 min, endothermic events belonging to the melting of **2c** and **2a**, indicating the coexistence of both forms in the sample (Figure 6, iii), and finally, after 60 min, only a single endothermic event at 90 °C, belonging to the melting of the anhydrous form **2a** (Figure 6, iv). Unfortunately, no sign of recrystallization was detected.

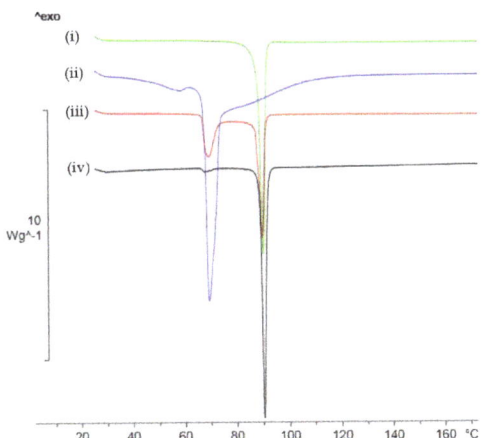

Figure 6. Selected DSC thermograms showing solid state transformation of the dihydrate **2c** to the anhydrous form **2a** recorded under a heating rate of 10 °C/min and N_2 purge in a pierced lid crucible; (i) anhydrous form **2a**; (ii) dihydrate **2c**; (iii) product after heating **2c** at 55 °C/200 mbar for 30 min, and (iv) product after heating **2c** at 55 °C/200 mbar for 60 min.

Finally, the XRPD powder pattern of the dried sample was different from the powder pattern of dihydrate **2c** and identical to the calculated powder pattern of anhydrous **2a** prepared by crystallization (Figure 7), confirming that **2a** is also the final product of dihydrate **2c** dehydration.

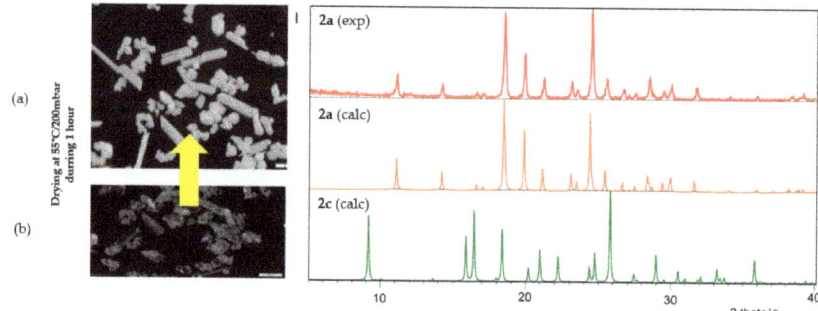

Figure 7. Photomicrographs of: (**a**) anhydrous **2a** after drying of **2c** during 60 min at 55 °C /200mbar; (**b**) starting dihydrate **2c** and the related PXRD patterns.

Additional studies were performed under atmospheric pressure to determine whether dehydration of **2c** to **2a** proceeds via a metastable monohydrate intermediate, as in lisinopril dihydrate [16], or as a hemihydrate, such as ondansetron hydrochloride dihydrate [17].

The TGA thermogram of **2c** showed a single thermal event in the range 40–110 °C with a mass loss of 11.31%, corresponding to the loss of two water molecules. This was in agreement with the DSC thermogram showing only a sharp endothermic event with an onset at 65 °C, corresponding to the melting of **2c**. Additional exothermic processes of recrystallization and endothermic of melting were not detected (Figure 8).

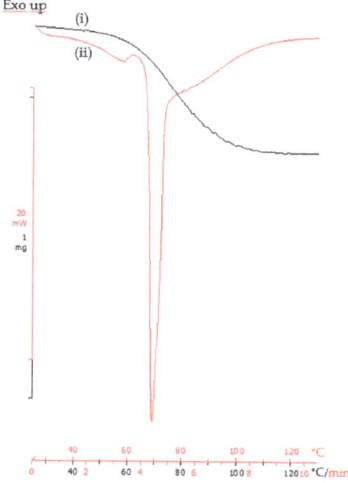

Figure 8. TGA (i) and DSC (ii) analysis of dihydrate **2c** in perforated crucibles under a heating rate of 10 °C/min and N_2 purge.

The changes upon dehydration of **2c** were monitored by the combination of hot stage microscopy (HSM) with DSC at a heating/cooling rate of 10 °C/min (Figure 9). Melting started at 40 °C until completed at around 65 °C (step i). Immediately after the melting point, the melt of **2c** was cooled to room temperature, resulting in a glassy product, and no further crystallisation was observed after prolonged standing. However, if **2c** was heated to 80 °C and immersed in oil during the HSM experiment, followed by cooling, recrystallization of the dihydrate **2c** was observed due to the conditions that inhibited efficient water removal. However, if the sample was heated over melting, up to 95 °C, in an open pan followed by cooling to room temperature, spontaneous crystallisation occurred, and according to XRPD, the obtained product was a mixture of the dihydrate **2c** and the anhydrous form **2a**.

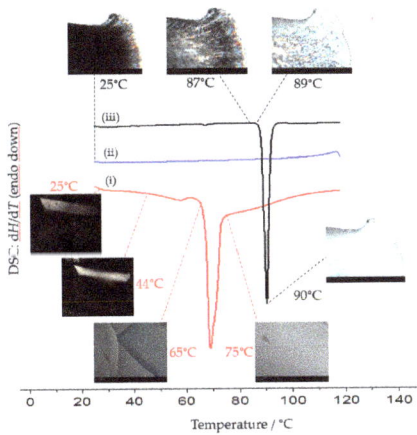

Figure 9. Selected DSC thermograms and HSM micrographs of dihydrate **2c**, recorded using a heating/cooling rate of 10 °C/min with perforated DSC crucibles: (i) dihydrate **2c** heating step up to 120 °C; (ii) cooling step to room temperature, and (iii) heating step of the recrystallized anhydrous form **2a**, i.e., re-run (re-heating) of the sample in the bottom thermogram.

In contrast, when the melt of **2c** was heated to 120 °C and cooled to room temperature, according to the XRPD slow nucleation and growth process of the anhydrous form **2a** occurred after prolonged standing indicating complete dehydration (step ii). In the re-run the sample melting started at 89 °C until completed at around 90 °C (step iii), i.e., at the melting point of the anhydrous form **2a**. However, no additional exothermic and endothermic events or changes in XRPD, which could indicate the formation of potential intermediary monohydrate or hemihydrate phases, were observed.

Dehydration of **2c** in vacuo favours rapid water removal below the melting point, without the appearance of a liquid or melt phase. Removal of water molecules from **2c** under these conditions resulted in the solid-solid rearrangement of the molecules in the crystal lattice, leading to anhydrous **2a**. On the contrary, crystallization of **2a** from the melt of dihydrate **2c** under atmospheric pressure only occurred when all the residual water was removed from the sample (at 120 °C). When a sample of melted **2c** was only heated to 95 °C, concomitant crystallization of **2a** and **2c** was observed, and this was identical to the partial dehydration of **2c** after 30 min under reduced pressure.

Finally, we can conclude that the dehydration at both conditions, i.e., under reduced and atmospheric pressure, proceeds to the anhydrous form **2a** and it is in accordance with the well-known fact that dehydration processes are greatly dependent on the atmospheric environment [11,18].

3. Materials and Methods

3.1. General

Methimazole **1** 99%, Ph Eur quality, was purchased from CU Chemie Ueticon, Lahr, Germany (water content 0.4%), 1,2-dichloroethane (Fisher, Hampton, NH, USA) (water content, 0.02%), dichloromethane (Merck KGaA, Darmstadt, Germany) acetone (Sigma, St. Louis, MO, USA) (water content, 0.2%), methanol dried (Merck KGaA, Darmstadt, Germany), water was purified in a house system (Thornton

2000CRS, Mettler Toledo, Colombus, OH, USA) and was of HPLC grade. Dichloromethane was dried under anhydrous sodium sulphate and distilled prior to use. All other used chemicals were of analytical grade. pH measurements were performed using Mettler Toledo (Columbus, OH, USA) Seven Multi pH meter, and prior to measurement, it was calibrated in six points. Ionic chromatography measurements were performed on Thermo (Waltham, MA, USA) ionic chromatography using LC chlorine standard. HPLC analysis was performed on an Agilent Technologies (Santa Clara, CA, USA) HPLC instrument under gradient elution at a flow rate of 0.6 mL/min using mobile phase A (ammonium acetate, Merck KGaA, Darmstadt, Germany buffer) and mobile phase B (acetonitrile, Merck KGaA, Darmstadt, Germany) at the Zorbax C18 column. The effluent was monitored using the Agilent DAD/UV detector. ^{1}H NMR and ^{13}C NMR spectra were recorded on a Bruker (Billerica, MA, USA) Advance 600 and 150, respectively, with DMSO-d_6 or D_2O as a solvent. Mass spectra were recorded on an Agilent 6550 iFunnel quadrupole time-of-flight mass spectrometer equipped with dual AJS ESI source (Agilent Technologies Santa Clara, CA, USA). Hot stage microscopy was carried out using an Olympus (Shinjuku City, Tokyo, Japan) BX51 microscope combined with a Linkam THMS 600 hot stage (Linkam Scientific Instruments, Waterfield, UK) and a digital camera (QImaging, Surrey, Canada) for image capture. A small amount of the sample was placed onto a glass slide and viewed with 100x magnification and partially polarised light. It was simultaneously being heated from ambient temperature at a rate of 10 °C/min. Thermal analysis was performed using a Mettler DSC 1 instrument (Mettler Toledo, Greifensee, Swizerland) in aluminium pans with a pierced lid at a heating rate of 10 °C/min under the inert nitrogen atmosphere with a flow rate of 55 mL/min. Temperature calibration was performed using the indium metal standard. TGA data were collected on a Mettler Toledo (Greifensee, Switzerland)) TGA/SDTA 851e system. The sample was loaded onto a pre-tared alumina crucible and was heated at a heating rate 10 °C/min over the temperature range 25–300 °C. A nitrogen purge at 50 mL/min was maintained over the sample. The instrument was temperature calibrated using certified $NiMn_3Al$ and nickel. All weighing operations were carried using Mettler Toledo (Greifensee, Switzerland)) balance, daily calibrated according to the internal program.

3.2. Synthesis of 1,2-Bis[(1-methyl-1H-imidazole-2-yl)thio]ethane Dihydrochloride Tetrahydrate (2b)

Method (A) Methimazole (100 mg, 0.87 mmol) was dissolved in 10 mL of 1,2-dichloroethane. The solution was left without stirring for 15 days in the dark at room temperature in a humidity non-controlled environment. The precipitated product was collected using vacuum suction and rinsed few times with cold 1,2-dichloroethane, yielding 1,2-bis[(1-methyl-1*H*-imidazole-2-yl)thio]ethane dihydrochloride tetrahydrate (**2b**, 53 mg, 31%) in the form of colourless plate shape crystals. Melting point (DSC, onset): 208 °C, MS-QTOF: [M+H-2HCl]$^+$ 255.0743, [M-2HCl] 254.066, $C_{10}H_{14}N_4S_2$. ^{1}H NMR (D_2O, 600 MHz/ppm): N-CH$_3$ (s, 6H), 3.82, H-C4 (d, 2H) 7.46, J = 2.1 Hz, H-C5 (d, 2H) 7.50, J = 2.1 Hz, S-CH$_2$ (s, 4H) 3.26. ^{13}C NMR (D_2O, 151 MHz/ppm): N-CH$_3$ 35.22, C4 120.98, C5 125.70, C2 138.52, S-CH$_2$ 34.59, Purity (HPLC): 98%, RRT: 20.518. Ionic chromatography: experimentally determined percentage of Cl ions (19%) corresponded to the theoretical value (18%) within the experimental error. The structure of **2b** was confirmed by single crystal X-ray diffraction analysis.

Method (B) Methimazole (100 mg, 0.87 mmol) was dissolved in 10 mL of 1,2-dichloroethane. The solution was left without stirring for 15 days in daylight and room temperature in a humidity non-controlled environment. The precipitated product was collected using vacuum suction and rinsed a few times with cold 1,2-dichloroethane, yielding dihydrochloride tetrahydrate **2b** (52 mg, 30%) in the form of colourless plate shaped crystals. Melting point (DSC, onset): 208 °C. The NMR spectra and XRPD diffractogram of the prepared sample were identical to the spectra and diffractogram of the **2b** sample obtained by Method A.

3.3. Synthesis of Anhydrous 1,2-Bis[(1-methyl-1H-imidazole-2-yl)thio]ethane (2a)

Method (A) Dihydrochloride tetrahydrate **2b** (300 mg) was dissolved in 30 mL of water and neutralized with 1M Na_2CO_3 to pH 7.0, followed by extraction with dichloromethane (3 × 10 mL), washed with brine and dried with anhydrous Na$_2$SO$_4$. Evaporation of the solvent in vacuo to dryness yielded crude 1,2-bis[(1-methyl-1H-imidazole-2-yl)thio]ethane (**2a**, 160 mg, 84%) in a form of white powder. Recrystallization of dry crude **2a** from dry dichloromethane under low humidity conditions gave pure anhydrous **2a**. Melting point (DSC, onset): 89 °C (lit: 88–90 °C) [5], ^{1}H NMR (DMSO-d_6, 600 MHz/ppm): N-CH$_3$ (s, 6H) 3.57, H-C4 (d, 2H) 7.24 J = 1.2 Hz, H-C5 (d, 2H) 6.94 J = 1.2 Hz, S-CH$_2$ (s, 4H) 3.21; ^{13}C NMR (DMSO-d_6, 151 MHz/ppm): N-CH$_3$ 32.79, C4 123.29, C5 128.53, C2 139.23, S-CH$_2$ 33.30. The structure of **2a** was confirmed by single crystal X-ray diffraction analysis.

Method (B) Dihydrate **2c** (100 mg) was dried under reduced pressure of 200 mbar at 55 °C for 60 min and anhydrous form **2a** (71 mg, 81%) was obtained. DSC thermogram and XRPD diffractogram of the obtained sample were identical to the thermogram and diffractogram of the **2a** sample obtained by Method A.

3.4. Synthesis of 1,2-Bis[(1-methyl-1H-imidazole-2-yl)thio]ethane Dihydrate (2c)

Method (A) Crude **2a** obtained by neutralization of dihydrochloride tetrahydrate **2b** (160 mg) was dissolved in an acetone/water mixture (1:1). After prolonged standing of the solution without stirring at room temperature, crystals of the pure dihydrate form **2c** (133 mg, 73%) were obtained. Melting point (DSC, onset, 65 °C). Structure of **2c** was confirmed by the single crystal X-ray diffraction analysis.

Method (B) Pure anhydrous form **2a** (300 mg) was dissolved in an acetone/water mixture (1:1). After prolonged standing of the solution without stirring at room temperature, pure crystals of the dihydrate form **2c** (238 mg, 70%) were obtained. DSC thermogram and XRPD diffractogram of the so obtained sample were identical to the thermogram and diffractogram of the **2c** sample obtained by Method A.

3.5. Powder X-ray Diffraction

X-ray powder diffraction (XRPD) data were collected at room temperature using copper Kα radiation on a PANalytical X'Pert Pro powder diffractometer model PW3050/60 (PANalytical, Almelo, The Netherland) in Bragg-Brentano geometry equipped with a X'celerator detector. The sample was prepared by mounting a sample on a wafer (zero background) plate and scanned from 3 to 40° 2θ using the following acquisition parameters: generator tension 45 kV, generator current 40 mA, step size 0.0167°, scan speed 0.011°/second, number of steps 2214 and total collection time 60 min, scan speed 0.05°/second, number of steps 2214 and total collection time 13 min.

3.6. Single Crystal X-ray Diffraction Analysis and Structure Determination

Suitable single crystals were selected and mounted in air onto thin glass fibres. Diffraction data of **2b** and **2c** were collected at room temperature, while data from the anhydrous form **2a** were collected at 150 K on an Oxford Diffraction Xcalibur four-circle kappa geometry diffractometer with Xcalibur Sapphire 3 CCD detector, using graphite monochromated MoKα (λ = 0.71073 Å) radiation.

The essential crystallographic data from the solid forms **2a**, **2b** and **2c** are presented in Table 2.

Data reduction, correction for the Lorentz-polarization factor, scaling and multi-scan absorption correction was performed using the CrysAlisPro software package [19]. Solution, refinement and analysis of the structures were done using the programs integrated in the WinGX system [20]. The structures were solved by direct methods implemented in SHELXS [21,22]. Refinement by the full-matrix least-squares methods, based on F^2 against all reflections, was performed by SHELXL [21,22], including anisotropic displacement parameters for all non-H atoms. Hydrogen atoms bound to C and N (in **2b**) atoms were modelled by the riding model using the AFIX routine, while those bound to water oxygen atoms were located in the difference Fourier maps and refined isotropically. Analysis of the molecular geometry and hydrogen bonds was performed by PLATON [23]. The molecular graphics were done with MERCURY (Version 4.1.0) [24]. The crystal parameters, data collection and refinement results are summarized in Table 2. CCDC deposition numbers 2013658 (**2a**), 2013659 (**2b**) and 2013660 (**2c**) contain the supplementary crystallographic data for this paper. These data can be obtained free of charge via http://www.ccdc.cam.ac.uk/conts/retrieving.html (or from the CCDC, 12 Union Road, Cambridge CB2 1EZ, UK; Fax: +44 1223 336033; E-mail: deposit@ccdc.cam.ac.uk)

Table 2. Essential crystallographic data for **2a**, **2b** and **2c**.

Compound	2a	2b	2c
Chemical formula	$C_{10}H_{14}N_4S_2$	$[C_{10}H_{16}N_4S_2]Cl_2 \cdot 4(H_2O)$	$C_{10}H_{14}N_4S_2 \cdot 2(H_2O)$
Formula weight	254.37	399.35	290.40
Crystal system	Monoclinic	Monoclinic	Trigonal
Space group	$P\,2_1/c$	$P\,2_1/c$	$R\text{-}3$
$a/Å$	4.7035 (7)	11.1667 (10)	19.3142 (13)
$b/Å$	12.3772 (14)	7.7629 (7)	19.3142 (13)
$c/Å$	10.3316 (11)	11.8970 (13)	10.3283 (5)
$\alpha/°$	90	90	90
$\beta/°$	92.772 (14)	109.637 (11)	90
$\gamma/°$	90	90	180
Z	2	2	9
$F\,(000)$	268	420	1386
T/K	150	292	292
$V/Å^3$	600.76 (13)	971.32 (18)	3336.75 (5)
$D_x/\text{g.cm}^3$	1.406	1.365	1.301
S	0.933	0.900	1.047
R	0.0493	0.049	0.0398
$wR\,(F^2)$	0.1063	0.1272	0.0994
No. of reflections	972	2329	1448
CCDC	2013658	2013659	2013660

4. Conclusions

The presented research confirmed the great reactivity of methimazole in the 1,2-dichloroethane solution under mild conditions, leading to its spontaneous *S*-bis alkylation to 1,2-bis[(1-methyl-1*H*-imidazole-2-yl)thio]ethane in the form of dihydrochloride tetrahydrate (**2b**). Therefore, the use of 1,2-dichloroetane should be avoided when working with methimazole. Dihydrochloride tetrahydrate 2b, anhydrous **2a**, and dihydrate **2c** crystal forms were prepared and their structures were confirmed by the single crystal X-ray diffraction analysis. Dehydration process of the dihydrate **2c**, studied using complementary solid-state techniques, led to the formation of the anhydrous product **2a**, which was identical to the one obtained by crystallization. No intermediate monohydrate or hemihydrate phases were detected.

Author Contributions: Conceptualization, L.Š. and M.D.; investigation, L.Š., D.M.-Č., D.F.; data curation, L.Š., D.M.-Č., and M.D.; writing—original draft preparation L.Š. and M.D.; writing-review and editing L.Š., D.M.-Č., D.F. and M.D.; supervision M.D. All authors have read and agreed to the published version of the manuscript.

Funding: This research received no external funding.

Acknowledgments: The authors appreciate Lara Saftić Martinović (U. of Rijeka, Department for Biotechnology) for recording HR-MS spectra and deep discussion, Ivica Đilović (U. of Zagreb, Faculty of Science, Department of Chemistry) for single crystal data collection of 2a and Ana Čikoš (Institute Ruđer Bošković, Center for NMR, Zagreb) for recording NMR spectra and deep discussion.

Conflicts of Interest: The authors declare no conflict of interest.

References

1. Aboul-Enein, H.Y.; Al-Badr, A.A. Analytical Profile of Methimazole. In *Analytical Profiles of Drug Substances*; Florey, K., Ed.; Academic Press: New York, NY, USA, 1979; Volume 8, pp. 351–370.
2. Qingjian, L.; Mingli, S. Synthesis of noncyclic crown ethers with methimazole heterocycle as a terminal group. *Youji Huaxue* **1992**, *12*, 509–513.

3. Qingjian, L.; Mingli, S.; Chongqiu, J.; Fengling, L. Syntheses and coordination properties of bridged bis(methimazole) compounds. *Gaodeng Xuexiao Huaxue Xuebao* **1992**, *13*, 328–331.
4. Silva, R.M.; Smith, M.D.; Gardinier, J.R. Unexpected New Chemistry of the Bis(thioimidazolyl)methanes. *J. Org. Chem.* **2005**, *70*, 8755–8763. [CrossRef] [PubMed]
5. Hassanaly, P.; Dou, H.J.M.; Metzger, J.; Assef, G.; Kister, J.S. Alkylation of 2-Thioxo-2,3-dihydroimidazole and its 1-Methyl Derivative under Phase-Transfer Conditions. *Synthesis* **1997**, *4*, 253–254.
6. Pilaniya, K.; Chandrawanshi, H.K.; Pilaniya, U.; Manchandani, P.; Jain, P.; Singh, N. Recent trends in the impurity profile of pharmaceuticals. *J. Adv. Pharm. Technol. Res.* **2010**, *1*, 302–310.
7. Infantes, L.; Motherwell, S. Water clusters in organic molecular crystals. *Cryst. Eng. Comm.* **2002**, *4*, 454–461. [CrossRef]
8. Aaltonen, J.; Allesø, M.; Mirza, S.; Koradia, V.; Gordon, K.C.; Rantanen, J. Solid form screening—A review. *Eur. J. Pharm. Biopharm.* **2009**, *71*, 23–37. [CrossRef]
9. Larsen, A.S.; Ruggiero, M.T.; Johansson, K.E.; Zeitler, J.A.; Rantanen, J. Tracking Dehydration Mechanisms in Crystalline Hydrates with Molecular Dynamics Simulations. *Cryst. Growth Des.* **2017**, *17*, 5017–5022. [CrossRef]
10. Galwey, A.K. Structure and order in thermal dehydration of crystalline solids. *Thermochim. Acta* **2000**, *355*, 181–238. [CrossRef]
11. Petit, S.; Coquerel, G. Mechanism of Several Solid–Solid Transformations between Dihydrated and Anhydrous Copper (II) 8-Hydroxyquinolinates. Proposition for a Unified Model for the Dehydration of Molecular Crystals. *Chem. Mater.* **1996**, 2247–2258. [CrossRef]
12. Morris, K.R. Structural Aspects of Hydrates and Solvates. In *Polymorphism in Pharmaceutical Solids*; Brittain, H.G., Ed.; Marcel Dekker Inc.: New York, NY, USA, 1999; pp. 125–182.
13. Mimura, H.; Kitamura, S.; Kitagawa, T.; Kohda, S. Characterization of the non-stoichiometric and isomorphic hydration and solvation in FK041 clathrate. *Colloids Surf. B: Biointerfaces* **2002**, *26*, 397–406. [CrossRef]
14. Dumić, M.; Vinković, M.; Orešić, M.; Meštrović, E.; Danilovski, A.; Dumbović, A.; Knežević, Z.; Lazarevski, G.; Filić, D.; Činčić, D.; et al. Isostructural Pseudopolymorphs of 9-Deoxo-9a-aza-9a-methyl-9a-homoerithromycin A. U.S. 7,569,549 B2, 4 August 2009.
15. Dumić, M.; Vinković, M.; Orešić, M.; Meštrović, E.; Danilovski, A.; Dumbović, A.; Knežević, Z.; Lazarevski, G.; Filić, D.; Činčić, D.; et al. Novel Amorphous 9-Deoxo-9a-aza-9a-methyl-9a-homoerithromycin A, Process for Preparing the Same, and Uses Thereof. U.S. 6,936,591 B2, 30 August 2005.
16. Fujii, K.; Uekusa, H.; Itoda, N.; Yonemochi, E.; Terada, K. Mechanism of Dehydration–Hydration Processes of Lisinopril Dihydrate Investigated by ab Initio Powder X-ray Diffraction Analysis. *Cryst. Growth Des.* **2012**, *12*, 6165–6172. [CrossRef]
17. Mizoguchi, R.; Uekusa, H. Elucidating the Dehydration Mechanism of Ondansetron Hydrochloride Dihydrate with a Crystal Structure. *Cryst. Growth Des.* **2018**, *18*, 6142–6149. [CrossRef]
18. Byrn, S.R.; Pfeiffer, R.R.; Stowell, J.G. *Solid-State Chemistry of Drugs*, 2nd ed.; SSCI Inc.: West Lafayette, IN, USA, 1999; p. 292.
19. *CrysAlisPro Software System*, version 1.171.39.46; Rigaku Oxford Diffraction: Oxford, UK, 2018.
20. Farrugia, L.J. WinGX and ORTEP for Windows: An update. *J. Appl. Cryst.* **2012**, *45*, 849–854. [CrossRef]
21. Sheldrick, G.M. A short history of SHELX. *Acta Cryst.* **2008**, *64*, 112–122. [CrossRef] [PubMed]
22. Sheldrick, G.M. Crystal structure refinement with SHELXL. *Acta Cryst.* **2015**, *71*, 3–8.
23. Spek, A.L. Structure validation in chemical crystallography. *Acta Cryst.* **2009**, *65*, 148–155. [CrossRef] [PubMed]
24. Macrae, C.F.; Bruno, I.J.; Chisholm, J.A.; Edgington, P.R.; McCabe, P.; Pidcock, E.; Rodriguez-Monge, L.; Taylor, R.; Van De Streek, J.; Wood, P.A. *Mercury CSD 2.0*—New features for the visualization and investigation of crystal structures. *J. Appl. Cryst.* **2008**, *41*, 466–470. [CrossRef]

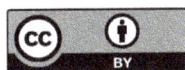

© 2020 by the authors. Licensee MDPI, Basel, Switzerland. This article is an open access article distributed under the terms and conditions of the Creative Commons Attribution (CC BY) license (http://creativecommons.org/licenses/by/4.0/).

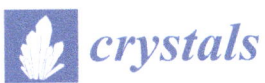

Article

Design, Synthesis, Crystal Structure, and Fungicidal Activity of Two Fenclorim Derivatives

Ke-Jie Xiong and Feng-Pei Du *

Department of Applied Chemistry, College of Science, China Agricultural University, Beijing 100193, China; kejieailan@163.com
* Correspondence: dufp@cau.edu.cn; Tel.: +86-10-62732507

Received: 21 June 2020; Accepted: 4 July 2020; Published: 7 July 2020

Abstract: Two fenclorim derivatives (compounds **6** and **7**) were synthesized by linking active sub-structures using fenclorim as the lead compound. The chemical structures of the two compounds were confirmed by NMR spectroscopy, high resolution mass spectrometry, and X-ray diffraction analysis. Their fungicidal activity against six plant fungal strains was tested. Compounds **6** and **7** both crystallized in the monoclinic system, with a $P2_1/c$ space group (a = 8.4842(6) Å, b = 24.457(2) Å, c = 8.9940(6) Å, V = 1855.0(2) Å^3, Z = 4) and Cc space group (a = 10.2347(7) Å, b = 18.3224(10) Å, c = 7.2447(4) Å, V = 1357.50(14) Å^3, Z = 4), respectively. The crystal structure of compound **6** was stabilized by C–H···N and C–H···O hydrogen bonding interactions and N–H···N hydrogen bonds linked the neighboring molecules of compound **7** to form a three-dimensional framework. Compound **6** displayed the most excellent activity, which is much better than that of pyrimethanil against *Botrytis cinerea* in vivo. Additionally, compound **6** exhibited greater in vitro activity against *Pseudoperonospora cubensis* compared to that of pyrimethanil. Moreover, compound **7** exhibited strong fungicidal activity against *Erysiphe cichoracearum* at 50 mg/L in vitro, while pyrimethanil did not. Compounds **6** and **7** could be used as new pyrimidine fungicides in the future.

Keywords: synthesis; crystal structure; fenclorim; antifungal activity; pyrimidine

1. Introduction

Plant diseases caused by fungi can significantly affect the growth and development of crops such as potato, soybean, and rice, and reduce the yield (20% perennial yield losses and 10% postharvest losses) of crop plants globally [1–4]. Meanwhile, fungal plant diseases also cause fresh fruit yield loss due to the shortening of storage times and secretion of fungal toxins that can damage human health [5,6]. Chemically synthesized fungicides are a major tool that producers use to protect against plant diseases. However, long-term and unreasonable application of fungicides has led to the emergence of resistance [7–11]. Hence, novel and efficient fungicides are necessary to solve problems arising from current fungicide resistance.

Fenclorim (4,6-dichloro-2-phenyl-pyrimidine, Figure 1a) is a commercial herbicide safener, which could alleviate the injury caused by chloroacetanilide herbicides, especially pretilachlor, without affecting their herbicide activity [12,13]. Zheng et al. [12] showed that fenclorim exhibited excellent in vivo fungicidal activity against *Sclerotinia sclerotiorum*, *Fusarium oxysporum*, *Fusarium graminearum*, and *Thanatephorus cucumeris*, and could be used as a lead compound to design novel pyrimidine-type fungicides. A fenclorim derivative, named *N*-(4,6-dichloropyrimidine-2-yl) benzamide, was synthesized by inserting an amide group between the phenyl ring and the pyrimidine ring in fenclorim to study the activity relationship (SAR) against fenclorim. This derivative displayed greater fungicidal activity than that of lead fenclorim and the positive control of pyrimethanil against *Sclerotinia sclerotiorum* and *Fusarium oxysporum*, with in vivo IC$_{50}$ values of 1.23 and 9.97 mg/L, respectively. These results indicate that the modification of fenclorim can produce highly active fungicidal compounds and that fenclorim provides broad potential as a lead compound for screening fungicides.

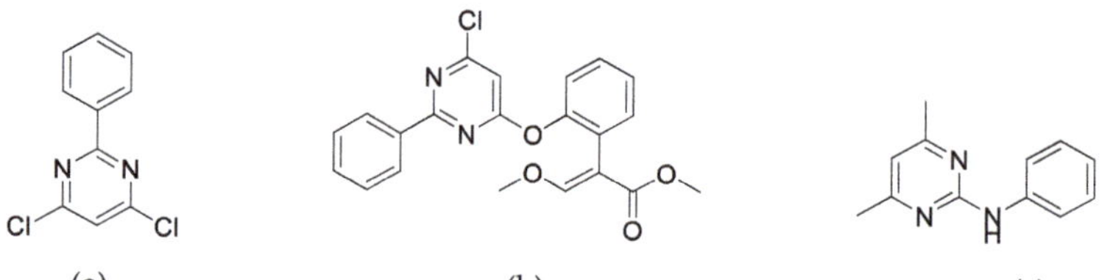

Figure 1. Chemical structure of fenclorim (**a**), azoxystrobin (**b**), and pyrimethanil (**c**).

Azoxystrobin (Figure 1b) and pyrimethanil (Figure 1c) are commercial pyrimidine fungicides. Azoxystrobin, named methyl (*E*)-2-{[6-(2-cyanophenoxy)-4-pyrimidinyl]oxy}-alpha-(methoxy methylene)benzeneacetate, belongs to the strobilurin fungicides, and was commercialized in 1996. Azoxystrobin stably held 23–25% of the fungicide market share until 2016. Azoxystrobin is a broad-spectrum fungicide and that displays strong activity against plant fungi such as ascomycetes, deuteromycetes, and oomycetes in crop plants, vegetables, and fruits [14]. Azoxystrobin causes the mitochondrial respiration of pathogenic fungi to be hindered, by binding to the Q_0 site of cytochrome bc1 enzyme complex to block electron transfer and freeze adenosine triphosphate (ATP) production [15]. Pyrimethanil, named 4,6-dimethyl-*N*-phenylpyrimidin-2-amine, was commercialized in 1991 and controlled plant fungi such as pear scab (*Venturia pirina*) and gray mold (*Botrytis cinerea*) in agricultural product [16]. It acts as an athogenesis inhibitor to inhibit the secretion of cell wall degrading enzymes in plant fungi [17].

The linking of active sub-structures to compounds is a common method for identifying novel pesticides [18–20]. Here, in order to find new fungicide candidates with high efficiency, two fenclorim derivatives (compound 6 and 7) were synthesized via the linking of active sub-structures. This was achieved by combining the (*Z*)-methyl 2-iodo-3-methoxyacrylate group substituted phenoxy group (red) in azoxystrobin and the aminophenyl group (pink) in pyrimethanil (Scheme 1). The chemical structures of compounds **6** and **7** were confirmed by NMR spectroscopy, high-resolution mass spectrometry (HRMS) and X-ray diffraction analysis. Their fungicidal activity against *Botrytis cinerea* (*B. cinerea*), *Pseudoperonospora cubensis* (*P. cubensis*), *Erysiphe cichoracearum* (*E. cichoracearum*), *Blumeria graminis* (*B. graminis*), *Rhizoctonia solani* (*R. solani*), and *Puccinia polysora* (*P. polysora*) were evaluated. These results provide useful guidance for designing novel fungicides using fenclorim as a lead compound.

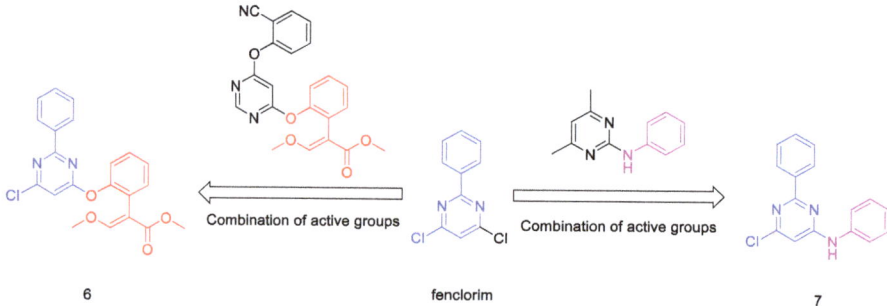

Scheme 1. Design strategies for compounds **6** and **7**.

2. Materials and Methods

2.1. Chemicals

All chemicals used in this research, including reagents and starting materials, were obtained from the Jilin Chinese Academy of Sciences, Yanshen Technology Co., Ltd., Jilin, China. ^{1}H and ^{13}C NMR spectra were recorded using a Bruker Avance-300 spectrometer (Bruker AXS, Karlsruhe, BW, Germany) operating at 300 MHz (^{1}H) and 75 MHz (^{13}C), respectively, with chemical shifts reported in ppm (δ). Deuterated chloroform (CDCl$_3$) was used as the solvent and tetramethylsilane (TMS) was used as the internal standard. HRMS analysis data was obtained on an FTICR-MS Varian 7.0 T FTICR-MS instrument (Varian IonSpec, Lake Forest, CA, USA). Melting points were measured using a Hanon MP100 automatic melting point instrument (Jinan Hanon Instruments Co., Ltd., Jinan, Shandong, China) using an open capillary tube. X-ray crystal structures of compounds **6** and **7** were measured using a Bruker SMART APEX II X-ray single-crystal diffractometer (Bruker AXS, Karlsruhe, BW, Germany). Reagents obtained from commercial sources were used without further purification.

2.2. Synthetic Procedure

Target compounds 6 and 7 were synthesized based on methods reported in the literature [21–23]. The synthetic routes of target compounds **6** and **7** are described in Scheme 2; Scheme 3.

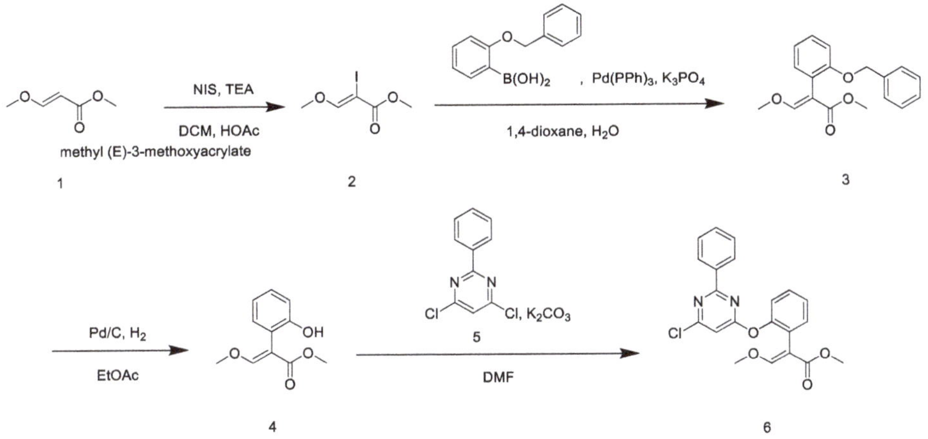

Scheme 2. The synthetic route of target compound **6**.

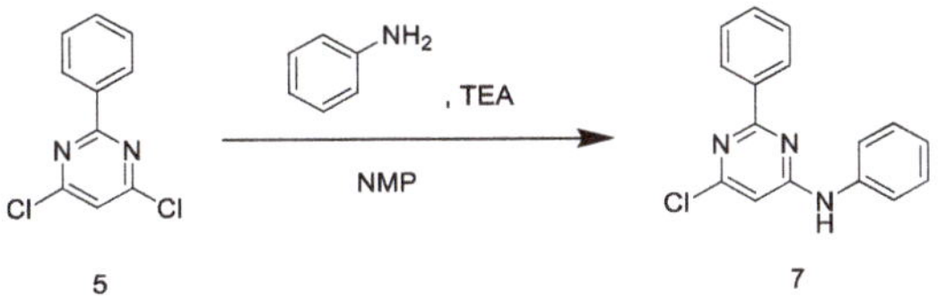

Scheme 3. The synthetic route of target compound **7**.

2.2.1. Synthesis of (Z)-methyl 2-iodo-3-methoxyacrylate (2)

A mixture of **1** (1.00 g, 8.61 mmol), N-iodosuccinimide (NIS, 2.32 g, 10.33 mmol), glacial acetic acid (0.98 mL, 17.22 mmol), and dichloromethane (15 mL) was stirred at 20 °C for 24 h. Afterwards, triethylamine (TEA, 4.2 mL, 30 mmol) was added dropwise. The reaction mixture was then stirred at

20 °C for another 12 h and water (30 mL) was added to quench the reaction. The mixture was extracted with dichloromethane (20 mL) twice. The organic extract was washed with saturated aqueous sodium thiosulfate (30 mL) twice, saturated aqueous sodium bicarbonate (30 mL) twice, and water (30 mL) twice. The mixtures were dried using anhydrous sodium sulfate and concentrated under vacuum. The residue was further purified by silica gel column chromatography (1:6 ethyl EtOAc /hexane) to obtain 3 (white solid, 1.56 g, 75.1%).

2.2.2. (E)-Methyl-3-methoxy-2-(2-phenoxyphenyl)acrylate (3)

A mixture of intermediate 2 (1.00 g, 4.13 mmol), arylboronic acid (1.23 g, 5.37 mmol), Pd(PPh$_3$)$_4$ (0.24 g, 0.21 mmol) and K$_3$PO$_4$ (2.63 g, 12.40 mmol) was dissolved into a mixture of 6 mL dioxane and 2 mL water, and this mixture was stirred under nitrogen atmosphere at 90 °C for 10 h. Then, the reaction mixture was cooled down, poured into ice water (100 mL) and extracted with EtOAc (30 mL) twice. The mixture was dried using anhydrous sodium sulfate and the solvent was evaporated under vacuum. Next, the residue was purified by silica gel column chromatography (1:8 EtOAc /hexane) to obtain 4 (white solid, 1.56 g, 90.3%).

2.2.3. (E)-Methyl-3-methoxy-2-(2-hydroxyphenyl)acrylate (4)

A mixture of 10 wt. % Pd/C (0.18 g, 0.085 mmol) was added into a solution of compound 4 (1.00 g, 3.36 mmol) in 30 mL EtOAc. The mixed solution was then stirred under a H$_2$ atmosphere (1 atm) at 35 °C for 12 h. Then, the reaction mixture was filtered and the filtrate was concentrated under vacuum. The residue was further purified by silica gel column chromatography (1:3 EtOAc /hexane) to afford 4 (1.34 g, 95.4%).

2.2.4. Methyl (E)-2-{2-[(6-chloro-2-phenylpyrimidin-4-yl)oxy]phenyl}-3-methoxyacrylate (6)

A mixture of intermediate 4 (1.00 g, 4.80 mmol), fenclorim 5 (2.16 g, 9.60 mmol), and K$_2$CO$_3$ (1.33 g, 9.60 mmol) was dissolved in dry dimethylformamid (DMF, 50 mL) at 0 °C under nitrogen atmosphere. The mixture was then stirred at this temperature for a further 12 h. The mixture was then poured into ice water (100 mL) and extracted with EtOAc (20 mL) twice. The organic extract was evaporated under vacuum and the residue was purified by silica gel column chromatography (1:7 EtOAc /hexane) to afford compound 6 (2.99 g, 79%). Compound 6 was a white solid with the following characteristics: m.p. 121–122 °C; ^{1}H NMR (300 MHz, CDCl$_3$) δ [ppm]: 3.54 (s, 3H, OCH$_3$), 3.67 (s, 3H, OCH$_3$), 6.63 (s, 1H, PyH), 7.24–7.26 (m, 2H, ArH), 7.32–7.35 (m, 2H, ArH), 7.39–7.44 (m, 4H, ArH+CH), 8.28–8.32 (m, 2H, ArH); ^{13}C NMR (75 MHz, CDCl$_3$) δ [ppm]:170.5, 167.4, 165.0, 162.0, 161.0, 150.3, 135.7, 132.7, 131.6, 129.1, 128.7, 128.5, 126.1, 125.9, 122.0, 107.2, 104.5, 61.8, 50.8 HRMS (ESI+) m/z: 397.0950 ([M+H]$^+$); found: 397.0946.

2.2.5. 6-chloro-N-2-diphenylpyrimidin-4-amine (7)

A mixture of fenclorim 5 (1.00 g, 4.44 mmol), phenylamine (0.34 g, 3.70 mmol) and TEA (0.50 g, 4.44 mmol), was dissolved in dry N-methylpyrrolidin-2-one (NMP, 20 mL) at 120 °C under nitrogen atmosphere for 24 h. The mixture was then cooled to room temperature, and a mixture of EtOAc (20 mL) and saturated sodium chloride solution (20 mL) was added. Then, this mixture was stirred for 30 min. The organic layer was separated, dried using anhydrous sodium sulfate, filtered, and concentrated under a vacuum. Next, the residue was purified using silica gel column chromatography (1:6 EtOAc/hexane) to obtain compound 7 (0.90 g, 72%). Compound 7 was a white solid with the following characteristics: m.p. 95-96 °C; ^{1}H NMR (300 MHz, CDCl$_3$) δ [ppm]: 6.61 (s, 1H, PyH), 6.92 (s, 1H, NH), 7.21–7.27 (m, 1H, ArH), 7.36–7.50 (m, 7H, ArH), 8.37–8.41 (m, 2H, ArH); ^{13}C NMR (75 MHz, CDCl$_3$) δ [ppm]: 164.9, 162.1, 160.9, 137.5, 136.5, 131.1, 129.5, 128.4, 128.3, 125.4, 122.6, 100.5; HRMS (ESI+) m/z: 282.0790 ([M+H]$^+$); found: 282.0793.

2.3. Structural Determination

Colorless single crystals of compounds **6** and **7** were obtained by slowly evaporating a methanol solution containing pure compounds **6** and **7** at room temperature. Single crystal X-ray diffraction data of compounds **6** and **7** were obtained using a SuperNova, Dual, Cu at zero, AtlasS2 diffractometer (Agilent, CA, USA) equipped with MoKα radiation (λ = 1.54184 Å) at 100.00(10) K. The crystal dimensions of compounds **6** and **7** were 0.11 × 0.11 × 0.08 mm^3 and 0.14 × 0.13 × 0.12 mm^3, respectively.

A total of 3608 reflections were collected by employing an ω scan mode for compound **6**, 6797 of which were independent with R_{int} = 0.1240, R_{sigma} = 0.1384. The final R_1 was 0.0697 ($I > 2\sigma(I)$) and wR2 was 0.1869 for compound **6**. A total of 4819 reflections were collected by using ω scan mode for compound **7**, 1795 of which were unique with R_{int} = 0.0317 and R_{sigma} = 0.0245. The final R_1 was 0.0372 ($I > 2\sigma(I)$) and wR$_2$ was 0.0990. The structures of compounds **6** and **7** were solved using the ShelXT structure solution program by Intrinsic Phasing and refined with the ShelXL refinement package via Least Squares minimization, using Olex2 [24–26].

The crystal data and structure refinement details of the compounds **6** and **7** are provided in Table 1. The crystallographic data for compounds **6** and **7** are available from the Cambridge Crystallographic Data Centre (CCDC) (www.ccdc.cam.ac.uk/structures/), with CCDC No. 1878381 and 1870401, respectively.

Table 1. Crystal data and structural refinements of compounds 6 and 7.

Compound	6	7
CCDC No.	1878381	1870401
Empirical formula	$C_{21}H_{17}ClN_2O_4$	$C_{16}H_{12}ClN_3$
Formula weight	396.82	281.74
Temperature/K	100.00(10)	100.00(10)
Crystal system	monoclinic	monoclinic
Space group	P2$_1$/c	Cc
a/Å	8.4842(6)	10.2347(7)
b/Å	24.457(2)	18.3224(10)
c/Å	8.9940(6)	7.2447(4)
α/°	90	90
β/°	96.305(6)	92.266(6)
γ/°	90	90
Volume/Å^3	1855.0(2)	1357.50(14)
Z	4	4
ρcalcg/cm^3	1.421	1.379
μ/mm^{-1}	2.092	2.418
F(000)	824.0	584.0
Crystal size/mm^3	0.11 × 0.11 × 0.08	0.14 × 0.13 × 0.12
Radiation	CuKα (λ = 1.54184)	CuKα (λ = 1.54184)
2Θ range for data collection/°	7.228 to 177.332	9.654 to 148.926
Index ranges	−10 ≤ h ≤ 10, −29 ≤ k ≤ 30, −8 ≤ l ≤ 10	−12 ≤ h ≤ 8, −22 ≤ k ≤ 21, −8 ≤ l ≤ 8
Reflections collected	6427	4819
Independent reflections	3608 [R_{int} = 0.1240, R_{sigma} = 0.1384]	1795 [R_{int} = 0.0317, R_{sigma} = 0.0245]
Data/restraints/parameters	3608/54/255	1795/2/181
Goodness-of-fit on F^2	1.053	1.053
Final R indexes [$I \geq 2\sigma$ (I)]	R_1 = 0.0697, wR$_2$ = 0.1650	R_1 = 0.0372, wR$_2$ = 0.0985
Final R indexes [all data]	R_1 = 0.0835, wR$_2$ = 0.1869	R_1 = 0.0376, wR$_2$ = 0.0990
Largest diff. peak/hole/ e Å^{-3}	1.17/−1.33	0.22/−0.30

2.4. Fungicidal Activity

The in vivo fungicidal activity (EC$_{50}$ values) of compounds **6**, **7**, fenclorim, and pyrimethanil against *P. cubensis* were tested according to methods in the reported literature [27,28]. The fungicidal activities of compounds **6**, **7**, fenclorim and pyrimethanil against *P. cubensis*, *E. cichoracearum*, *B. graminis*,

3. Results and Discussion

3.1. Synthesis and Spectroscopic Properties

The synthetic routes for compounds **6** and **7** are described in Scheme 2; Scheme 3. Intermediate **2** was synthesized through the nucleophilic substitution of the acrylate group of methyl (*E*)-3-methoxyacrylate by *N*-iodosuccinimide. The formation of intermediate **3** from intermediate **2** and arylboronic acid was achieved via the Suzuki–Miyaura cross-coupling reaction. The synthesis of intermediate **4**, the precursor of compound **6**, was achieved via the reduction of intermediate **4** using Pd(PPh$_3$)$_4$ as the catalyst under nitrogen atmosphere. Compound **6** was afforded by the condensation of intermediate **4** and fenclorim **5**. Compound **7** was synthesized by a one-step condensation method, using fenclorim and phenylaline as starting materials.

The chemical structures of compound **6** and **7** were characterized by NMR spectroscopy, HRMS, and X-ray diffraction analysis. For compound **6**, signals corresponding to C–H protons in the phenyl ring and pyrimidine were observed at δ 7.21–8.41 and δ 6.61, respectively; signals corresponding to the C–H proton to N–H proton in imino group were observed δ 6.69. For compound **7**, signals corresponding to C–H protons in methoxyl groups were observed at δ 3.54 and δ 3.67, respectively; signals corresponding to the C–H proton to C–H proton in pyrimidine ring were observed at δ 6.63, and signals corresponding to the C–H proton in the phenyl ring were at δ 7.24–8.32. In the compound **6** ^{13}C-NMR spectra, chemical shifts of carbons that resonated at δ 107.18–170.47 were assigned to carbons in the phenyl ring and pyridine ring. The chemical shifts of carbons that resonated at δ 51.59 and 61.93, respectively, were assigned to the carbons in methoxyl groups. The signal at δ 104.46 can be assigned to carbon (C-7) in the acrylate group. In the ^{13}C-NMR spectra of compound **7**, chemical shifts linked to aromatic rings (phenyl ring and pyrimidine ring) appeared at 100.5–164.94. All HRMS data for compounds **6** and **7** were well-matched with theoretical values calculated from their chemical formula.

3.2. Crystal Structures of Compounds 6 and 7

Compounds **6** and **7** both crystallized in the monoclinic system, with a P2$_1$/c space group and Cc space group, respectively. The molecular structures of compounds **6** and **7** are described in Figure 2a,b, and selected molecular structure parameters, including bond lengths and bond angles for compound **6** and **7**, are listed in Tables 2 and 3, respectively. Packing diagrams of compounds **6** and **7** are shown in Figure 3a,b respectively.

The selected bond lengths and bond angles of the phenyl ring and pyrimidine ring in the crystal structure of compounds **6** and **7** are similar to those of compounds reported in the literature, which are in accordance with normal ranges [29–32]. According to the data in Figure 2a, compound **6** is composed of four molecular moieties (two phenyl rings, a chlorine-substituted pyrimidine ring, and a (*Z*)-methyl 2-iodo-3-methoxyacrylate group). The phenyl ring, formed by C(16)–C(17)–C(18)–C(19)–C(20)–C(21), and the pyrimidine ring, formed by C(15)–N(2)–C(14)–C(13)–C(12)–N(1), are linked by a C(15)–C(16) bridge. The bond length of C(15)–C(16), a single bond, is 1.556(5) Å, and the torsion angle of N(2)–C(15)–C(16) is 119.8(3) Å. The phenyl ring, defined as C(1)–C(2)–C(3)–C(4)–C(5)–C(6), and the pyrimidine ring, are linked by an oxygen atom. The bond angle of C(12)–O(1)–C(1) is 115.3(3) Å. The acrylate moiety assumes an *E* configuration double bond C(7)=C(10) (1.391(6) Å) of the vinyl group. The bond lengths of C(8)–O(3) in the acrylate group are 1.229(6) Å, which is similar to the general length reported for C=O, indicating that it is a double bond [33–35]. The dihedral angles between the mean planes of C(15), N(2), C(14), C(13), C(12), N(1) with C(16), C(17), C(18), C(19), C(20), C(21), C(19) and C(1), C(2), C(3), C(4), C(5), C(6) are 3.368(109)° and 66.294(120)°, respectively.

Compound **7** is composed of a chlorine-substituted pyrimidine ring and two phenyl rings (Figure 2b). The phenyl ring, formed by C(1)–C(2)–C(3)–C(4)–C(5)–C(6), is linked with the pyrimidine ring, formed by C(7)–N(1)–C(8)–C(9)–C(10)–N(2) via a C(1)–C(7) bridge. The bond length of C(1)–C(7) is 1.482(4) Å and the torsion angle of N(2)–C(7)–C(1) is 117.3(2) Å. The pyrimidine ring above and phenyl ring defined as C(11)–C(12)–C(13)–C(14)–C(15)–C(16) are linked by a nitrogen atom, with a torsion angle C(10)–N(3)–C(11) of 126.5(2) Å. The dihedral angles between the mean planes of C(7), N(1), C(8), C(9), C(10), N(2) with C(1), C(2), C(3), C(4), C(5), C(6) and C(11), C(12), C(13), C(14), C(15), C(16) are 8.447(74)° and 45.236(88)°, respectively.

Based on whole structural analysis, molecule **6,** forms C–H⋯N (symmetry code: 1 − x, 1 − y, 1 − z) and C–H⋯O hydrogen bonding interactions (symmetry code: 1 + x, y, z) with the phenyl C atom (Table 4), to from three-dimensional networks. The C⋯N distances between donor (D) and acceptor (A) molecules were 3.341(6) Å for C(5)–H(5)⋯N(2), and 2.8711(16) Å for C(11)–H(11B)⋯O(3), respectively. The distances between hydrogen atom and acceptor atom were 2.53 Å for H(5)⋯N(2), and 2.30 Å for H(11B)⋯O(3), respectively. Both of the bond lengths were shorter than sum of van der Waals radii (2.66 Å for H(5)⋯N(2) and 2.63 Å for H(11B)⋯O(3)) [36]. As shown in Table 5, N(3)–H(3)⋯N(1) hydrogen bonds (N⋯N 3.190(3) Å, N–H⋯N 146°; symmetry code: $\frac{1}{2}$ + x, −1/2 − y, $\frac{1}{2}$ + z) link the neighboring molecules of compound **7** to form a three-dimensional framework. Weak hydrogen bonds C(2)–H(2)⋯N(1), C(6)–H(6)⋯N(2), and C(12)–H(12)⋯N(2) also stabilize the crystal structure.

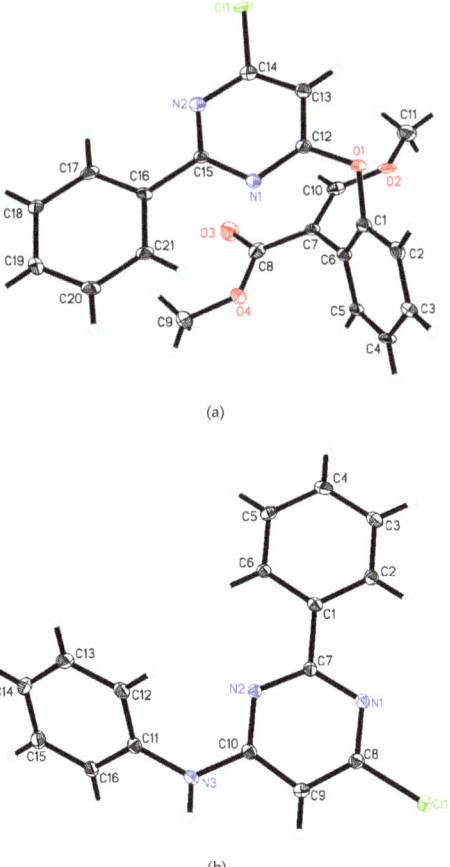

Figure 2. Crystal structure of compound **6** (**2a**) and **7** (**2b**).

Table 2. Selected bond lengths (Å) and bond angles (°) for compound 6.

Bond	Distance (Å)	Bond	Distance (Å)
C(12)–O(1)	1.338(5)	C(1)–O(1)	1.362(5)
C(10)–O(2)	1.386(6)	C(15)–N(1)	1.338(5)
C(11)–O(2)	1.472(6)	C(15)–N(2)	1.308(6)
C(8)–O(4)	1.353(6)	C(14)–N(2)	1.396(6)
C(9)–O(4)	1.537(6)	C(8)–O(3)	1.229(6)
C(12)–N(1)	1.412(5)	C(14)–Cl(1)	1.692(5)
C(15)–C(16)	1.556(5)	C(14)–C(13)	1.367(6)
C(1)–C(6)	1.397(6)	C(5)–C(4)	1.380(6)
C(12)–C(13)	1.362(6)	C(20)–C(19)	1.371(6)
C(15)–C(16)	1.556(5)	C(7)–C(10)	1.391(6)
Angle	(°)	Angle	(°)
C(12)–O(1)–C(1)	115.3(3)	O(1)–C(12)–C13	112.2(4)
C(10)–O(2)–C(11)	116.7(4)	N(1)–C(15)–C16	118.7(4)
C(8)–O(4)–C(9)	118.7(4)	N(2)–C(15)–N1	121.5(4)
C(15)–N(1)–C(12)	117.7(4)	N(2)–C(15)–C16	119.8(3)
C(15)–N(2)–C(14)	118.2(4)	O(1)–C(1)–C2	115.0(4)
O(1)–C(12)–N(1)	122.2(4)	O(1)–C(1)–C(6)	119.9(4)
N(2)–C(14)–C(11)	118.7(3)	C(13)–C(14)–N(2)	126.4(4)
O(4)–C(8)–C(7)	115.5(3)	O(3)–C(8)–O(4)	118.3(4)

Table 3. Selected bond lengths (Å) and bond angles (°) for compound 7.

Bond	Distance (Å)	Bond	Distance (Å)
Cl(1)–C(8)	1.732(3)	C(1)–C(2)	1.399(4)
N(3)–C(11)	1.413(4)	C(1)–C(6)	1.401(4)
N(3)–C(10)	1.356(4)	C(5)–C(6)	1.384(4)
N(1)–C(7)	1.343(4)	C(5)–C(4)	1.389(4)
N(1)–C(8)	1.339(4)	C(9)–C(8)	1.360(4)
N(2)–C(7)	1.337(3)	C(9)–C(10)	1.412(4)
N(2)–C(10)	1.341(4)	C(15)–C(14)	1.390(4)
C(11)–C(16)	1.393(4)	C(2)–C(3)	1.383(4)
C(11)–C(12)	1.395(4)	C(3)–C(4)	1.395(4)
C(1)–C(7)	1.482(4)	C(14)–C(13)	1.383(5)
Angle	(°)	Angle	(°)
C(10)–N(3)–C(11)	126.5(2)	N(2)–C(7)–C(1)	117.3(2)
C(8)–N(1)–C(7)	114.6(2)	N(1)–C(8)–Cl(1)	114.9(2)
C(7)–N(2)–C(10)	117.3(2)	N(1)–C(8)–C(9)	125.2(3)
C(16)–C(11)–N(3)	118.5(2)	C(9)–C(8)–Cl(1)	119.9(2)
C(16)–C(11)–C(12)	119.6(3)	N(3)–C(10)–C(9)	119.5(2)
C(12)–C(11)–N(3)	121.9(2)	N(2)–C(10)–N(3)	119.4(2)
C(15)–C(16)–C(11)	120.3(3)	N(2)–C(10)–C(9)	121.1(2)
C(2)–C(1)–C(7)	120.7(2)	C(3)–C(2)–C(1)	120.7(3)
C(2)–C(1)–C(6)	118.6(3)	C(2)–C(3)–C(4)	120.2(3)
C(6)–C(1)–C(7)	120.7(2)	C(5)–C(6)–C1	120.6(3)

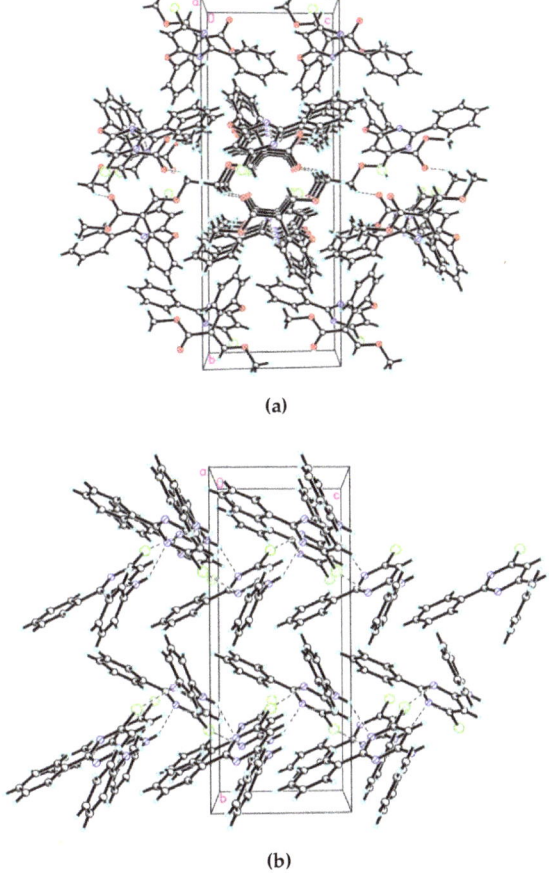

Figure 3. Packing diagram of compound **6** (**3a**) and **7** (**3b**). Dashed lines represent hydrogen bonds.

Table 4. Hydrogen bonding interactions in compound 7.

D–H···A	d(D–H)/(Å)	d(H···A)/(Å)	d(D···A)/(Å)	<(DHA)/(°)
C(5)–H(5)···N(2)	0.93	2.53	3.341(6)	146
C(11)–H(11B)···O(3)	0.96	2.30	3.162(7)	148

Symmetry transformations used to generate the equivalent atoms: #1: 1 − x, 1 − y, 1 − z; #2: 1 + x, y, z.

Table 5. Hydrogen bonding interactions in compound 6.

D–H···A	d(D–H)/(Å)	d(H···A)/(Å)	d(D···A)/(Å)	<(DHA)/(°)
N(3)–H(3)···N(1)	0.86	2.44	3.190(3)	146
C(2)–H(2)···N(1)	0.93	2.48	2.802(4)	100
C(6)–H(6)···N(2)	0.93	2.50	2.817(4)	100
C(12)–H(12)···N(2)	0.93	2.57	2.930(4)	104

Symmetry transformations used to generate the equivalent atoms: $\frac{1}{2}$ + x, −1/2 − y, $\frac{1}{2}$ + z.

3.3. Fungicidal Activities

The in vivo fungicidal activities (EC_{50} values) of compound **6**, compound **7**, positive control fenclorim and pyrimethanil against *B. cinerea* are listed in Table 6. Compound **6** displayed the greatest activity with an EC_{50} value of 20.84 mg/L, which was much greater than that of compound **7** (215.45 mg/L), fenclorim (319.95 mg/L) and pyrimethanil (30.72 mg/L). This result indicates that the combination of the (Z)-methyl-2-iodo-3-methoxyacrylate group substituted phenoxyl group with fenclorim could improve the in vivo fungicidal activity of fenclorim against *Botrytis cinerea*.

Table 6. The in vivo EC_{50} values of compounds **6** and **7** and pyrimethanil against *Botrytis cinerea*.

Comp.	EC_{50} (± SD) (mg/L)	Comp.	EC_{50} (± SD) (mg/L)
6	20.84 ± 4.04	7	215.45 ± 55.43
fenclorim	319.95 ± 30.62	pyrimethanil	30.72 ± 3.78

To further study the fungicidal activity of compounds **6** and **7**, the in vitro inhibitory rate of compounds **6**, **7**, fenclorim, and pyrimethanil against *P. cubensis*, *E. cichoracearum*, *B. graminis*, *R. Solani*, and *P. polysora* were evaluated at different concentrations (Table 7). At 200 mg/L, compound **6** displayed the strongest fungicidal activity against *P. cubensis* (94.00% control) and against *R. Solani* (91.67% control), while compound **7** showed the strongest fungicidal activity against *E. cichoracearum* (91.00% control), *B. graminis* (90.67% control) and *P. polysora* (90.67% control). Furthermore, fenclorim exhibited no activity against the *E. cichoracearum* control and pyrimethanil only displayed good fungicidal activity against *P. cubensis* (89.00% control). As the concentration decreased, most of the fungicidal activity of these compounds brought to gradually. Surprisingly, compound **6** exhibited 80.33% activity of that of the control against *P. cubensis*, when pyrimethanil displayed only 20.67% of that of the control, when at 25 mg/L. These results revealed that the combination of active groups in commercial fungicides with the lead fenclorim could improve the in vitro fungicidal activity of fenclorim significantly.

Table 7. The in vitro fungicidal activities of compounds **6** and **7**.

Compounds	Dose (mg/L)	P. Cubensis	E. Cichoracearum	B. Graminis	R. Solani	P. Polysora
				Inhibitory Rate (%)		
6	200	94.00 ± 1.73	1.67 ± 2.88	40.67 ± 1.15	91.67 ± 2.89	50.00 ± 0
	50	90.00 ± 2.00	0	41.33 ± 1.15	59.33 ± 1.15	8.33 ± 2.89
	12.5	80.33 ± 1.53	0	27.00 ± 1.73	58.33 ± 2.89	0
7	200	93.33 ± 2.89	91.00 ± 3.61	90.67 ± 1.15	70.67 ± 1.15	90.67 ± 2.31
	50	71.67 ± 2.89	89.00 ± 3.61	59.33 ± 1.15	11.67 ± 2.89	58.33 ± 2.89
	12.5	26.67 ± 2.89	31.67 ± 2.89	14.00 ± 1.73	7.67 ± 2.52	0
Fenclorim	200	92.33 ± 2.52	0	23.33 ± 2.89	26.67 ± 2.89	38.33 ± 2.89
	50	85.67 ± 2.08	0	22.33 ± 2.52	28.33 ± 2.89	21.67 ± 1.89
	12.5	22.33 ± 2.52	0	0	6.67 ± 2.89	0
Pyrimethanil	200	89.00 ± 3.61	31.00 ± 3.61	28.33 ± 2.89	10 ± 0	31.33 ± 1.15
	50	80.67 ± 1.15	6.00 ± 1.73	26.00 ± 1.73	9.33 ± 1.15	9.33 ± 1.15
	12.5	20.67 ± 1.15	0	19.33 ± 1.15	0	0

P. cubensis: *Pseudoperonospora cubensis*; *E. cichoracearum*: *Erysiphe cichoracearum*; *B. graminis*: *Blumeria graminis*; *R. solani*: *Rhizoctonia solani*; and *P. polysora*: *Puccinia polysora*.

4. Conclusions

In conclusion, two fenclorim derivatives (compounds **6** and **7**) were synthesized by the linking of active sub-structures method. The chemical structures of the two compounds were confirmed by NMR spectroscopy, HRMS, and X-crystal diffraction, and their fungicidal activity against plant fungi were tested. Compound **6** displayed the greatest activity (EC_{50} value of 20.84 mg/L), which was much greater than that of pyrimethanil (30.72 mg/L) against *B. cinerea* in vivo. Additionally, compound **6** at 25 mg/mL exhibited 80.33% of the control EC_{50} value against *P. cubensis*, when pyrimethanil displayed only 20.67% control EC_{50} value at 25 mg/L in vitro. Moreover, compound **7** exhibited 89% of the control

EC$_{50}$ value against *E. cichoracearum* at 50 mg/L in vitro, while pyrimethanil only exhibited 6% of that of the control. Compounds **6** and **7** could be used further as pyrimidine fungicides in the future.

Author Contributions: Conceptualization, K.-J.X.; methodology, K.X; software, K.-J.X.; validation, K.-J.X.; formal analysis, K.-J.X.; investigation, K.-J.X.; resources, K.-J.X.; data curation, K.-J.X.; writing—original draft preparation, K.-J.X.; writing—review and editing, K.-J.X.; visualization, K.-J.X.; supervision, K.-J.X.; project administration, F.-P.D.; funding acquisition, F.-P.D. All authors have read and agreed to the published version of the manuscript.

Funding: This research and the APC were funded by the National Natural Science Foundation of China (No. 31772182).

Conflicts of Interest: The authors declare no conflict of interest.

References

1. Mardanova, A.; Lutfullin, M.; Hadieva, G.; Akosah, Y.; Pudova, D.; Kabanov, D.; Shagimardanova, E.; Vankov, P.; Vologin, S.; Gogoleva, N.; et al. Structure and variation of root-associated microbiomes of potato grown in alfisol. *World J. Microbiol. Biotechnol.* **2019**, *35*, 1–16. [CrossRef]
2. Liu, H.; Xia, D.G.; Hu, R.; Wang, W.; Cheng, X.; Wang, A.L.; Zhang, Q.; Lv, X.H. A bioactivity-oriented modification strategy for SDH inhibitors with superior activity against fungal strains. *Pestic. Biochem. Physiol.* **2020**, *163*, 271–279. [CrossRef] [PubMed]
3. Sarkar, C.; Saklani, B.K.; Singh, P.K.; Asthana, R.K.; Sharma, T.R. Variation in the LRR region of Pi54 protein alters its interaction with the AvrPi54 protein revealed by in silico analysis. *PLoS ONE* **2019**, *14*, e0224088. [CrossRef] [PubMed]
4. Xavier, W.D.; de Souza Silva, J.V.; Guimaraes, C.M.; Sousa Ferreira, J.L.; Turozi, T.A.; Colodel, S. Use of copper-based pesticides to control fungal diseases of soybean in Northern Brazil. *J. Exp. Agric. Int.* **2019**, *33*, 1–10. [CrossRef]
5. Zhang, X.; Lei, P.; Sun, T.; Jin, X.; Yang, X.; Ling, Y. Design, Synthesis, and fungicidal activity of novel thiosemicarbazide derivatives containing piperidine fragments. *Molecules* **2017**, *22*, 2085. [CrossRef]
6. Da Rocha Neto, A.C.; Luiz, C.; Maraschin, M.; Di Piero, R.M. Efficacy of salicylic acid to reduce *Penicillium expansum* inoculum and preserve apple fruits. *Int. J. Food Microbiol.* **2016**, *221*, 54–60. [CrossRef]
7. Matsuzaki, Y.; Yoshimoto, Y.; Arimori, S.; Kiguchi, S.; Harada, T.; Iwahashi, F. Discovery of metyltetraprole: Identification of tetrazolinone pharmacophore to overcome QoI resistance. *Bioorg. Med. Chem.* **2020**, *28*, 115211. [CrossRef].
8. Odilbekov, F.; Edin, E.; Mostafanezhad, H.; Coolman, H.; Grenville-Briggs, L.J.; Liljeroth, E. Within-season changes in *Alternaria solani* populations in potato in response to fungicide application strategies. *Eur. J. Plant Pathol.* **2019**, *155*, 953–965. [CrossRef]
9. Vaghefi, N.; Hay, F.S.; Kikkert, J.R.; Pethybridge, S.J. Genotypic diversity and resistance to azoxystrobin of *Cercospora beticola* on processing table beet in New York. *Plant Dis.* **2016**, *100*, 1466–1473. [CrossRef]
10. Zhang, H.Y.; Li, M. Transcriptional profiling of ESTs from the biocontrol fungus *Chaetomium cupreum*. *Sci. World J.* **2012**, 1–7.
11. Zhao, J.; Bi, Q.; Wu, J.; Lu, F.; Han, X.; Wang, W. Occurrence and management of fungicide resistance in *Botrytis cinerea* on tomato from greenhouses in Hebei, China. *J. Phytopathol.* **2019**, *167*, 413–421. [CrossRef]
12. Zheng, W.N.; Zhu, Z.Y.; Deng, Y.N.; Wu, Z.C.; Zhou, Y.; Zhou, X.M.; Bai, L.Y.; Deng, X.L. Synthesis, Crystal structure, herbicide safening, and antifungal activity of N-(4,6-dichloropyrimidine-2-yl) benzamide. *Crystals* **2018**, *8*, 75. [CrossRef]
13. Deng, X.L.; Zheng, W.N.; Zhou, X.M.; Bai, L.Y. The effect of salicylic acid and 20 substituted molecules on alleviating metolachlor herbicide injury in rice (*Oryza sativa*). *Agronomy* **2020**, *10*, 317. [CrossRef]
14. Swiecilo, A.; Krzepilko, A.; Michalek, S. Evaluation of azoxystrobin toxicity to saprophytic fungi and radish in the early stages of growth. *Ecol. Chem. Eng. A* **2018**, *25*, 81–92.
15. Berry, E.A.; Huang, L.S. Conformationally linked interaction in the cytochrome bc1 complex between inhibitors of the Qo site and the Rieske iron-sulfur protein. *Biochim. Biophys. Acta-Bioenerg.* **2011**, *1807*, 1349–1363. [CrossRef]

16. Tang, R.; Tang, T.; Tang, G.; Liang, Y.; Wang, W.C.; Yang, J.L.; Niu, J.F.; Tang, J.Y.; Zhou, Z.Y.; Cao, Y.S. Pyrimethanil ionic liquids paired with various natural organic acid anions for reducing its adverse impacts on the environment. *J. Agric. Food Chem.* **2019**, *67*, 11018–11024. [CrossRef]
17. Milling, R.J.; Richardson, C.J. Mode of action of the anilino-pyrimidine fungicide pyrimethanil. 2. Effects on enzyme secretion in *Botrytis cinerea*. *Pestic. Sci.* **1995**, *45*, 43–48. [CrossRef]
18. Miao, H.J.; Zhang, J.W.; Yuan, H.Z.; Li, Y.; Xu, Y.; Li, H.; Yang, X.L.; Ling, Y. Synthesis and fungicidal activities of nucleoside compounds containing substituted benzoyl thiourea. *Chin. J. Org. Chem.* **2012**, *32*, 915–921. [CrossRef]
19. Sun, J.; Zhou, Y. Design, synthesis and insecticidal activity of some novel diacylhydrazine and acylhydrazone derivatives. *Molecules* **2015**, *20*, 5625–5637. [CrossRef]
20. Wang, C.; Song, H.; Liu, W.; Xu, C. Design, synthesis and antifungal activity of novel thioureas containing 1,3,4-thiadiazole and thioether skeleton. *Chem. Res. Chin. Univ.* **2016**, *32*, 615–620. [CrossRef]
21. Liu, Y.G.; Luo, Y.; Lu, Y. A concise synthesis of azoxystrobin using a Suzuki cross-coupling reaction. *J. Chem. Res.* **2015**, *39*, 586–589. [CrossRef]
22. Liu, Y.; Weng, Y.B.; Chen, Z.B.; Wang, Y.L. Synthesis and anticoccidial activities of quinoline carboxylate derivatives with methyl (E)-2-(3-methoxy) acrylate moiety. *Asian. J. Chem.* **2013**, *25*, 8509–8512. [CrossRef]
23. Zhou, Y.L.; Xue, C. Synthesis of pyrimethanil. *Pestic. Sci. Admin.* **2005**, *26*, 24–25.
24. Dolomanov, O.V.; Bourhis, L.J.; Gildea, R.J.; Howard, J.A.K.; Puschmann, H. OLEX2: A complete structure solution, refinement and analysis program. *J. Appl. Crystallogr.* **2009**, *42*, 339–341. [CrossRef]
25. Sheldrick, G.M. Crystal structure refinement with SHELXL. *Acta Crystallogr. Sect. C* **2015**, *71*, 3–8. [CrossRef]
26. Sheldrick, G.M. SHELXT—Integrated space-group and crystal-structure determination. *Acta Crystallogr. Sect. A* **2015**, *71*, 3–8. [CrossRef]
27. Li, H.C.; Guan, A.Y.; Huang, G.; Liu, C.L.; Li, Z.N.; Xie, Y.; Lan, J. Design, synthesis and structure-activity relationship of novel diphenylamine derivatives. *Bioorg. Med. Chem.* **2016**, *24*, 453–461. [CrossRef]
28. Guan, A.; Liu, C.; Chen, W.; Yang, F.; Xie, Y.; Zhang, J.; Li, Z.; Wang, M. Design, synthesis, and structure-activity relationship of new pyrimidinamine derivatives containing an aryloxy pyridine moiety. *J. Agric. Food Chem.* **2017**, *65*, 1272–1280. [CrossRef]
29. Li, Z.Y.; Jia, G.K.; Yuan, L.; Bai, P.F.; He, H.; Zhou, Q. Syntheses, crystal structures and biological activities of three new Schiff bases derived from substituted salicylaldehyde and tris base. *Chin. J. Struct. Chem.* **2017**, *36*, 1797–1802.
30. Mahgoub, M.Y.; Elmaghraby, A.M.; Harb, A.E.A.; Mahgoub, M.Y.; Ferreira, D.S.J.L.; Justino, G.C.; Marques, M.M. Synthesis, crystal structure, and biological evaluation of fused thiazolo [3,2-a] pyrimidines as new acetylcholinesterase inhibitors. *Molecules* **2019**, *24*, 2306. [CrossRef]
31. Deng, X.L.; Zhou, X.M.; Wang, Z.Y.; Rui, C.H.; Yang, X.L. Synthesis, crystal structure and insecticidal activity of N-(pyridin-2-ylmethyl)-1-phenyl-1,4,5,6,7,8-hexahydrocyclohepta[c]pyrazole-3-carbox amide. *Chin. J. Struct. Chem.* **2018**, *37*, 551–556.
32. Shi, J.T.; Gong, Y.L.; Li, J.; Wang, Y.; Chen, Y.; Ding, S.; Liu, J. Synthesis, structure and biological activity of 2-[2-(4-fluorobenzylidene)hydrazinyl]-4-(1-methyl-1H-indol-3-yl)thieno[3,2-d]pyrimidine. *Chin. J. Struct. Chem.* **2019**, *38*, 1530–1536.
33. Tao, Y.; Han, L.; Sun, A.; Sun, K.; Zhang, Q.; Liu, W.; Du, J.; Liu, Z. Crystal structure and computational study on methyl-3-aminothiophene-2-carboxylate. *Crystals* **2020**, *10*, 19. [CrossRef]
34. Manchado, A.; Salgado, M.M.; Vicente, A.; Diez, D.; Sanz, F.; Garrido, N.M. Crystal structure of methyl (4R)-4-(4-meth-oxy-benzo-yl)-4-{(1R)-1-phenyl-eth-ylcarbamo-yl}butanoate. *Acta Crystallogr. Sect. E* **2017**, *73*, 503–506. [CrossRef]
35. Shen, Z.H.; Shi, Y.X.; Yang, M.Y.; Sun, Z.H.; Weng, J.Q.; Tan, C.X.; Liu, X.H.; Li, B.J.; Zhao, W.G. Synthesis, crystal structure, DFT studies and biological activity of a novel schiff base containing triazolo 4,3-a pyridine moiety. *Chin. J. Struct. Chem.* **2016**, *35*, 457–464.
36. Herschlag, D.; Pinney, M.M. Hydrogen bonds: Simple after all? *Biochemistry* **2018**, *57*, 3338–3352. [CrossRef]

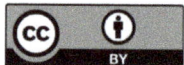

© 2020 by the authors. Licensee MDPI, Basel, Switzerland. This article is an open access article distributed under the terms and conditions of the Creative Commons Attribution (CC BY) license (http://creativecommons.org/licenses/by/4.0/).

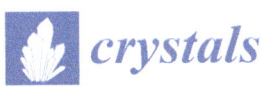

Review

Application of Fundamental Techniques for Physicochemical Characterizations to Understand Post-Formulation Performance of Pharmaceutical Nanocrystalline Materials

Bwalya A. Witika [1,2,*], Marique Aucamp [3], Larry L. Mweetwa [2] and Pedzisai A. Makoni [4,*]

1. ApotheCom | A MEDiSTRAVA Company (Medical Division of Huntsworth), London WC2A 1AN, UK
2. Department of Pharmacy, DDT College of Medicine, Gaborone P.O. Box 70587, Botswana; larrymweetwa1@gmail.com
3. School of Pharmacy, Faculty of Natural Sciences, University of the Western Cape, Private Bag X17, Bellville 7535, South Africa; maucamp@uwc.ac.za
4. Division of Pharmacology, Faculty of Pharmacy, Rhodes University, Makhanda 6140, South Africa
* Correspondence: bwalya.witika@apothecom.com (B.A.W.); p.makoni@ru.ac.za (P.A.M.)

Abstract: Nanocrystalline materials (NCM, i.e., crystalline nanoparticles) have become an important class of materials with great potential for applications ranging from drug delivery and electronics to optics. Drug nanocrystals (NC) and nano co-crystals (NCC) are examples of NCM with fascinating physicochemical properties and have attracted significant attention in drug delivery. NCM are categorized by advantageous properties, such as high drug-loading efficiency, good long-term physical stability, steady and predictable drug release, and long systemic circulation time. These properties make them excellent formulations for the efficient delivery of a variety of active pharmaceutical ingredients (API). In this review, we summarize the recent advances in drug NCM-based therapy options. Currently, there are three main methods to synthesize drug NCM, including top-down, bottom-up, and combination methods. The fundamental characterization methods of drug NCM are elaborated. Furthermore, the applications of these characterizations and their implications on the post-formulation performance of NCM are introduced.

Keywords: nanocrystalline materials; physicochemical characterization; vibrational spectroscopy; X-ray analysis; thermal analysis; critical quality attributes

1. Introduction

There has been an increasing interest in developing drug delivery systems that circumvent the challenges associated with conventional drug delivery [1]. Among those challenges are poor drug solubility and formulation stability, low bioavailability, and undesirable side effect profiles [1]. Solutions to some of these shortcomings have been suggested and have included the use of nanotechnology. Nanotechnology is defined as the engineering and manufacture of materials at an atomic or molecular scale resulting in nanoparticles [2]. The definition of nanoparticles regarding particle size is constantly under deliberation. This has resulted in different disciplines adopting different definitions. As an example, colloid chemistry describes nanoparticles as having particle sizes below 100 nm or and in some instances 20 nm. In the pharmaceutical domain, nanoparticles are identified as having a size ≤ 1000 nm [3]. Therefore, in this review, we define nanocrystalline (NCM) as crystalline materials composed of nanoparticles having dimensions <1000 nm [4,5]. Some of the desirable properties of nanoparticles are that they often maintain crystallinity after their manufacturing process. Crystallinity relates to the extent of structural order in a solid and is characterized by atomic or molecular arrangement being regular and periodic—the production of nanoparticles that exhibit crystallinity results in the formation of NCM. The production of NCM requires a combination of crystal engineering and nanotechnological approaches.

Crystal engineering is the manipulation of non-covalent interactions between molecular or ionic components for the rational design of solid-state structures that may exhibit desirable electrical, magnetic, and optical properties [6]. Intermolecular hydrogen bonds can be used to assemble supramolecular structures that, at the very minimum, control or influence dimensionality [6,7]. Crystal engineering can also be described as the knowledge of intermolecular interactions in the context of crystal packing and the use of such understanding in the design of new solid materials with desirable physicochemical properties [8,9].

Co-crystals are single-phase crystalline solids that are composed of two or more different molecular or ionic compounds, generally in a stoichiometric ratio [10]. Co-crystals can be constructed using several types of molecular interactions such as hydrogen bonds, ionic interactions, π–π stacking, and van der Waal's forces [11–14].

Two general methods are used to manufacture NCM. The first utilizes collision forces to cause particle size reduction to nanometer dimensions and is called the top-down approach [15,16], while the second approach makes use of nucleation and crystal growth. A suitable stabilizer is utilized to prevent crystal growth into the micrometre range and is termed the bottom-up approach [17,18]. In the broadest sense, NCM used in drug delivery can be subdivided into organic and inorganic NCM. In this review, we focus on the characterization of organic NCM for the delivery of active pharmaceutical ingredients (API). More specifically, we highlight the characterization techniques most applicable to NC and NCC as models NCM for the delivery of API.

Drug NC are crystals with a size in the nanometre range. This means that they are nanoparticles that exhibit a high degree of crystallinity [3]. Similarly, drug NCC are crystalline solids existing as a single phase that is composed of different molecules that have nanometric dimensions [19]. In the case of both types of the aforementioned NCM, crystal growth from the nanometer to the micrometre range is inhibited by stabilizers [20–22].

In drug delivery, these NCM have found a broad range of applications in circumventing the shortcomings of conventional drug delivery while exhibiting flexibility regarding the routes of administration.

When applied in transdermal delivery, NCM are expected to pack tightly and form a dense layer that hydrates the skin and improves drug penetration and permeation. Dissolved NCM may be topically retained for a sufficient period and offer sustained API release [23]. As a way of example, a formulation of L-ascorbic acid demonstrated long-term stability as NC dispersed in an oil base. The NC oil dispersion exhibited improved penetration and stability when compared to conventional technologies [24].

Oral administration remains the most preferred route and is generally considered a safe and suitable drug delivery route [25]. Dissolution is often the rate-determining step for absorption, and because NCM generally provide a larger surface area for dissolution, increase saturation solubility, and ultimately increase the dissolution extent, they have been shown to enhance API absorption [26]. Rapamune®, a formulation composed of sirolimus NC blended with additional excipients and directly compressed into tablets, was the first US FDA-approved nanocrystalline drug launched in 2000 by Wyeth Pharmaceuticals (Madison, NJ, USA) for oral use. The oral bioavailability of the API from the nanocrystalline tablets was 21% higher than that of sirolimus delivered in aqueous solution [27]. Similarly, the advantages of nano-drug delivery have been applied to modulate the pharmacokinetic profile of aprepitant (Emend®), which requires delivery at an absorption window in the gastrointestinal tract [28].

Drug delivery to the eye is hindered by pharmacokinetic, physiological, and in some instance's environmental factors. Conventional formulations are rapidly cleared from the site of administration due to rapid eye movement such as blinking and/or lacrimation, resulting in low ocular bioavailability. Consequently, repeated dosing and subsequent reduction in adherence results in poor clinical outcomes. Frequent dosing may also lead to an increase in dose-dependent side effects [29,30]. NCM technologies can play a critical role in drug delivery to the eye by improving the solubility of poorly soluble API. This was explored and showed favourable outcomes when utilized in formulations containing budesonide, dexamethasone, hydrocortisone, prednisolone [31], and fluorometholone [31,32]. A technique based on combining microfluidic and milling technologies resulted in the production of NC of hydrocortisone. The ocular bioavailability of the NC was evaluated in vivo using albino rabbits. Extended duration of action and a significant improvement in the area under the curve (AUC) for hydrocortisone delivered using the NC were observed when compared to coarse hydrocortisone [33].

Parenteral drug delivery ensures a shorter onset of action, higher bioavailability, and use of reduced doses when compared to oral drug delivery. These benefits are ideal target parameters for drug delivery; however, the use of the intravenous route is challenging as only a limited number of solvents and excipients can be used during formulation development. This is due to an increased possibility of adverse outcomes in addition to those caused by the API. NC of ascularine [34], melarsoprol [35], oridonin [36], itraconazole [37], and curcumin [38] have been successfully developed and resulted in increases in their C_{max} and $AUC_{0-\infty}$.

Targeted delivery approaches have been implemented in combination with NC and NCC technology for drugs that exhibit low bioavailability, poor aqueous solubility and stability, and limited in vitro–in vivo correlations (IVIVC) [39,40]. Buparvaquone NC suspended in a mucoadhesive system of Carbopol® 934, 971, 974, 980 or 0.5 % w/w Noveon® AA-1 was used for targeting the gastrointestinal parasite, *Cryptosporidium parvum*, and resulted in better targeting and greater stability than pure buparvaquone [41].

Surface modification of NCM can also be used to reduce the potential toxicity of API to selected cell lines. For instance, surface modification of lamivudine-zidovudine NCC with sodium dodecyl sulphate (SDS) and α-tocopheryl polyethylene glycol succinate 1000 (TPGS 1000) was reported to have reduced cytotoxic effect on HeLa cells [42].

Despite their success in drug delivery, NCM have to undergo rigorous characterization prior to their use in humans. Many of these techniques are centred on developing quality into the product and ensuring that critical process parameters (CPP) do not have a significant impact on the critical quality attributes (CQA) of the product [43]. Consequently, the resultant NC or NCC meets the quality target product profile (QTPP) that could lead to inclusion into suitable dosage forms and subsequent human use.

Formulation and morphology of drug NCM, including fundamental characterizations and their implications on post-formulation performance are described below.

2. Formulation and Morphology of NCM

Two formulation approaches have been shown to produce NC viz., the top-down technique that relies on shear forces for particle size reduction into the nanometre range [15,16] and the bottom-up approach that allows for nucleation and growth of individual monomers, which remain nanosized because of a stabiliser [17,18].

2.1. Top-Down Production Approaches

High-energy mechanical forces are involved in top-down approaches and are provided by media milling (MM) techniques, including NanoCrystals® or high-pressure homogenization (HPH), Insoluble Drug Delivery—Particles (IDD-P™), DissoCubes®, and Nanopure®, to comminute large crystals into crystals of smaller dimensions [16,44]. Top-down processes are commonly used for the preparation of crystalline nanoparticles [45] and are flexible following scale-up production [46]. Consequently, the process has been widely adopted for commercial scale preparation of nanocrystals. With the exception of Triglides produced by IDD-P®, the majority of the other products are commercially produced using NanoCrystals®. However, high-energy input, lengthy operational units, and the potential to introduce contamination from the use of grinding media are drawbacks of this technology. For instance, high pressures of up to 1700 bar with 50–100 cycles of homogenisation are often required to achieve a desired particle size distribution and size [3,47]. Furthermore, the milling time varies from hours to days depending on the properties of the API, milling media, and extent of required particle size reduction [46,48]. Since contamination from grinding media may lead to unexpected side-effects and/or toxicities, the top-down production method is not a suitable option for the preparation of parenterally administered NC [49,50].

2.1.1. HPH (IDD-P®, DissoCubes®, and Nanopure®)

During the process of HPH, API-loaded suspensions are introduced into a high-pressure homogeniser and forced through a narrow orifice in sudden bursts under high pressure. Owing to this, cavitation, high-shear forces, and particle collisions result in fracture of API particles. Generally, the HPH method occurs via the following steps: of (i) crude API powder is dispersed in pure solution or in a solution containing a stabiliser, (ii) a reduction of particle size occurs by high-speed shearing or homogenization under low pressure, (iii) HPH is used to achieve the target particle size and size distribution.

Based on the instrumentation and solutions used, HPH processes can be sub-divided into three patented technologies, including microfluidics for IDD-P® technology, piston gap homogenisation for DissoCubes® in aqueous media, and Nanopure® for non-aqueous media. Nonetheless, attainment of formulation optimization requires an investigation into the effect of various formulation and process parameters.

2.1.2. MM (NanoCrystals®)

In this technique, NC are obtained by subjecting API to a media-milling process. The media mill consists of a milling chamber, milling shaft, and recirculation chamber [16]. The generation of high energy and shear forces as a result of milling media and API collisions provide the requisite energy to disintegrate microparticulate drugs into nano-sized particles. The milling media may be glass, zirconium oxide, or highly cross-linked polystyrene resin. During this process, the milling chamber is initially charged with milling media, water or buffer, API and stabiliser. The system is then rotated at a very high shear rate, and the milling process is performed under controlled temperature conditions in either batch or recirculation mode. When using the batch mode, dispersions with unimodal size distribution profiles and mean diameters <200 nm are produced in approximately 30–60 min. The media milling process can successfully process micronized and un-micronized drug crystals. Following the optimization of formulation and the process parameters, minimal batch-to-batch variability is observed when evaluating the quality of resultant dispersion(s).

However, the generation and introduction of milling media residue into the final product due to media erosion is of major concern. This phenomenon could be problematic during the production of nanosuspensions intended for chronic administration. However, the advent of polystyrene resin-based milling media has led to the reduced occurrence of the aforementioned issue, for which residual polymeric monomers are typically 50 ppb and the residuals generated during the milling process of not more than (NMT) 0.005 % w/w of the final product or resulting solid dosage form [50,51].

MM has been used with considerable success to yield NCC containing furosemide and caffeine, acetamide, urea and nicotinamide as co-formers, carbamazepine, and separately indomethacin with the co-former saccharin [52]. Initially, the manufacture of micronized co-crystals of each was performed using liquid assisted grinding (LAG) with methanol, acetonitrile, or acetone, or using a slurry technique [52]. Subsequently, the resultant co-crystals were dispersed in a solution containing 0.5 % w/v HPMC and 0.02 % w/v sodium dodecyl sulphate (SDS) in distilled water and wet-milled using zirconia beads. Wet-milling was conducted three times at 2000 rpm for 2 min and then 500 rpm for 2 min cycles. The milling chamber was maintained at −10 °C during the process. Lastly, the resulting suspension and zirconia bead mixture was transferred to a centrifuge filter-mesh chamber to separate and collect the suspensions at 400 rpm for 1 min [52].

Itraconazole nanosuspensions have also been manufactured using wet-milling with Tween® 80 dissolved in a 20 mL vial containing 5 mL demineralised water, followed by the dispersion of 250 mg itraconazole in this aqueous phase. Different concentrations of dicarboxylic acid co-formers (maleic, adipic, glutaric, and succinic acid) were dissolved in the suspension. Zirconium oxide milling pearls (30 g) of 0.5 mm diameter were added to the suspension. The vials were placed on a roller-mill and grinding performed at 150 rpm for 60 h after which the nanoparticles were separated from the pearls by sieving [53].

Witika et al. demonstrated the use of (MM) to produce NCC of lamivudine and zidovudine. The initial step involved the use of solution co-crystallisation to produce co-crystals. During the second step, NCC were manufactured using a top-down method, specifically, wet media milling using an in-house modified jigsaw as the milling chamber. A 115 mg aliquot of the harvested or dried co-crystal was placed in a 1.5 mL stainless steel milling chamber. The milling liquid comprised of different % w/v TPGS 1000 and SLS concentrations as defined by experimental design software. Stainless-steel balls were used as milling media with milling times of 10, 20, or 30 min at a constant milling speed of 65 Hz [54].

2.1.3. Bottom-Up Production Approaches

Bottom-up approaches promote the growth of NC from solution via two crucial steps viz., nucleation and crystal growth. Nucleation is crucial in the production of small uniform NC. An increase in nucleation rate results in an increase in the number of nuclei formed from the supersaturated solution, leading to a decrease in supersaturation and thus reduced growth for each nucleus [49]. If a large number of nuclei are produced concurrently during nucleation, a narrow particle size distribution is likely to occur [49]. Therefore, it is essential to promote rapid and homogeneous nucleation when using a bottom-up process. In general, the drug solution and an anti-solventare combined using conventional mixing equipment, e.g., a magnetic stirrer or an agitator blade [55]. Nucleation can be triggered by mixing with an anti-solvent or removal of solvent [18] or introduction of sonic waves to induce sonoprecipitation [55,56]. Sonoprecipitation has been used successfully to develop NCC to produce caffeine-containing co-crystals using a single-solvent approach by separately adding 60 mg caffeine and 48 mg of 2,4-dihydroxybenzoic acid (DHBA) in 7 mL and 242 mL acetone, respectively. The solutions were rapidly injected into 200 mL of hexane at approximately 0 °C and sonicated for 15 s in a cleaning bath. A two-solvent approach using the same procedure with 125 mg of caffeine and 99 mg DHBA dissolved separately in 1 mL chloroform and 600 mL acetone and rapidly injected into 100 mL of hexane at approximately 0 °C was also successful in the production of co-crystals, with Span® 85 as surfactant stabiliser at a concentration of 5 % w/v in hexane [57].

A phenazopyridine-phthalimide nano-cocrystal suspension was produced by dissolving 213 mg phenazopyridine and 147 mg phthalimide in 2 mL of dimethyl sulfoxide (DMSO) separately, after which the individual solutions were rapidly injected into 50 mL 0.4 % w/v SDS aqueous solution at approximately 2 °C using ultrasonic conditions resulting in the formation of a NCC suspension after 15–30 s [58].

Liu et al. [59] produced NCC using top-down and bottom-up approaches. NCC produced using a solution approach were obtained by dissolving 311 mg myricetin and 402 mg nicotinamide separately in 7 mL and 3 mL methanol, respectively [59]. The solutions were rapidly injected together into a conical flask at 0 °C and sonicated for 30 min using an ultrasonic processor set at a frequency of 40 kHz with a power output of 50 W following which the low-temperature control was stopped but ultrasonic agitation maintained. The resultant precipitate was removed after 10, 20, and 30 min, filtered and dried for 24 h at 25 °C [60].

Witika et al. reported the synthesis of lamivudine and zidovudine NCC using a bottom-up technique [19,42]. The NCC were manufactured using a pseudo one solvent cold sonochemical synthesis technique [19,42]. The individual components were dissolved in methanol and water and injected into a precooled conical flask and sonicated.

3. Nucleation and Crystal Growth

Supramolecular synthons are defined as structural units within super-molecules which can be formed and/or assembled by known synthetic operations involving intermolecular interactions. Supramolecular synthons are spatial arrangements of intermolecular interactions. Therefore, the overall goal of crystal engineering is to recognise and design synthons that are robust enough to be interchanged between network structures [9]. The Cambridge Structural Database may be used to identify stable hydrogen bonding motifs with the ambition that the most robust motifs will remain intact across a family of related structures [61,62].

3.1. Supramolecular Processes in Crystal Growth

Nucleation is a molecular assembly process, where a critical number of molecules are needed to achieve a phase change from the liquid melt or solution to form a crystalline solid. The driving force for achieving the critical point of molecular assembly is linked to the free energy of the process [6]. For solution-based crystallisation, which is predominantly used in processing API, the free energy required is linked to the solubility behaviour of the material in a specific solvent. The magnitude of the difference in solubility exhibited by the molecules that are crystallising from a completely solubilised state at a specified composition and temperature drives the process. The larger the differential between solubilised state and the equilibrium state, the greater the supersaturation. The resultant growth of a crystal is dependent on the solubility behaviour and any competing nucleation, which may also be taking place because of the degree of supersaturation achieved. It is, therefore, this phase change process that distinguishes crystallisation from dissolution [63,64].

3.2. Crystal Habit, Morphology, and Growth

Once nucleation has been achieved, crystal growth dominates and is the process, which leads to the evolution of embryonic crystals into a crystal form of defined size and shape. The key drivers with regard to the shape of the growing crystal are related to the crystal lattice of molecular solids and the effects of the choice of solvent and additives on the process of crystal growth. As such, crystal growth is a layer-by-layer process, with the evolution of layers being defined by crystal packing of the unit cell. The unit cell, in turn, describes the critical elements of how a specific molecular species has been assembled in the crystalline state in three-dimension [6,65].

4. Techniques used in the Physicochemical Characterisations of NCM

The characterization approaches for NCM are a combination of techniques used to determine crystallinity, particle size, particle size distribution, as well as intra- and intermolecular interactions. In addition, beneficial characterization of NCM with regard to chemical composition is often required. Broadly, the characterization of NCM, much like any other nanometric drug delivery systems, can be classified into in vitro and in vivo categories [66].

To understand the potential performance of NCM in vivo, physicochemical characterisations need to be carried out, followed by cell-culture studies. The physicochemical characterisations offer an understanding of how the NCM will perform prior to cell testing [67]. These are often conducted "in-glass". Cellular testing is less ethically ambiguous, is easier to control and reproduce, and is less expensive when compared to animal testing [68]. Once a proof of concept for NCM has been demonstrated in vitro, safety and therapeutic efficacy are then tested in animal models. The results of animal studies play a fundamental role in decision-making with regard to progression towards clinical trials. An animal model that reflects the pathophysiology of human disease is invaluable when predicting therapeutic outcomes in humans [66,69].

A collection of recommendations pertaining to nanomaterial characterization reviewed a consensus on a large number of nanomaterial properties [67]. A condensed list of physicochemical parameters for the risk assessment of nanomaterials was compiled based on this collection and we concluded that the nanomaterial properties that are listed in at least half of the 28 sources analysed were [67];

- Specific surface area
- Particle size
- Particle size distribution or polydispersity index
- Crystallinity
- Surface Reactivity
- Solubility
- Agglomeration
- Surface charge
- Elemental/molecular composition
- Surface chemistry

In this review, we will use this list to correlate characterization procedures to the properties on the list.

4.1. Dynamic Light Scattering (DLS)

Dynamic light scattering (DLS) is commonly used for particle size determination and measures the Brownian motion of particles in suspension by relating velocity, known as the translational diffusion coefficient, to the size of particles according to the Stokes–Einstein equation [70,71].

4.1.1. Particles Size (PS)

Particle size (PS) investigations serve as one of the main determining factors of biodistribution and retention of NCM in target tissues. PS is defined as the size of a hypothetical hard sphere that exhibits the same diffusion characteristics as the NCM being measured. The result is reported as mean particle size and homogeneity of size distribution. The latter parameter is expressed as the polydispersity index (PDI), which is a dimensionless parameter calculated from cumulative analysis of the DLS-measured intensity autocorrelation function [71]. A PDI value in the range <0.25 indicates a desirable homogeneity whereas a PDI value >0.5 indicates heterogeneous particle sizes [72]. While DLS provides a simple and rapid estimate of particle size, several studies suggest that DLS exhibits inherent limitations and is relatively poor at analysing multimodal particle size distributions [72,73].

By way of example, when a mixture of 20- and 100-nm nanometre particles are measured, the signal for the small particles may be lost because the signal intensity of a spherical particle of radius r is proportional to r [74]. Therefore, the scattering intensity of small particles tends to be masked by that of larger particles. Microscopy provides an accurate assessment of the size and shape of a NCM but often requires complicated sample preparation steps specific to the microscopic technique used [73], which in turn may change samples and create artefacts such as NCM agglomeration, which is particularly observed during drying prior to electron microscopy [75]. Furthermore, due to the limited throughput capability, it is difficult to obtain an accurate particle size distribution [74], and the underlying principle is that the sample status in each method is not the same.

4.1.2. Surface Charge

Surface charges, expressed as the Zeta Potential (ZP), critically influences the interaction of NCM with the dispersion media [72]. The ZP is commonly measured using Laser Doppler Electrophoresis (LDE), which evaluates the electrophoretic mobility of suspended NCM in a dispersion medium. It is a measure of the energy potential at the boundary of the outer layer. It is generally accepted that NCM that possess a ZP more positive than +30 mV or more negative than −30 mV exhibit colloidal stability that is maintained by repulsion due to electrostatics. Much like with PS measurements, heterogenous samples have misleading ZP measurements due to the ZP of larger particles dominating the scattering signal to the detriment of smaller particles [76]. The measurement of the ZP is, in part, dependent on the ionic strength and valency in an NCM dispersion. High ionic strength and valency ions compress the electric double layer, resulting in a reduced ZP. The pH also has a significant influence on ZP and in alkaline suspensions, the NCM acquire a negative charge and vice versa. Therefore, ZP should be reported with a corresponding pH at which the measurement was taken [70]. Additionally, it is recommended that information of the suspension be precisely described when reporting the ZP, including the ionic strength, composition of the dispersion medium, and pH [77,78]. However, the ZP is of little consequence if the NCM is stored as a solid intended to be redispersed prior to use.

4.2. Thermal Analysis

NCM exhibit many unique properties, which are often superior to those of coarse-grained materials. Consequently, NCM offer significant potential for use in a variety of pharmaceutical applications. Solidification of nanosuspensions of NCM has been identified as a tool to increase patient acceptance/adherence and long-term stability [79].

Due to a high-volume fraction of grain boundaries, NCM have the intrinsic shortcoming of poor thermal stability that significantly limits their use. To aid in understanding this drawback, thermal stability has become a significant aspect in the field of pharmaceutical NCM research [80]. It is therefore of utmost importance to conduct thermal analyses on NCM to determine their suitability in potential secondary or downstream pharmaceutical applications.

4.2.1. Thermal Gravimetric Analysis (TGA)

TGA is one of the oldest thermal analytical procedures and has been used extensively in the study of material science. The technique monitors changes in sample weight, usually nitrogen, as a function of temperature. TGA can be used to facilitate the assessment of processing temperatures of thermally based secondary manufacturing processes such as hot-melt extrusion while also finding utility in determining the presence of residual solvents or moisture. When used as a pre-formulation tool for hot-melt extrusion, TGA is used to determine the thermal stability of the polymers and nanocrystalline API. It allows for the determination of a range of operating temperatures in hot-melt extrusion. This is done in order to avert thermal degradation that may occur during the manufacturing process. TGA can also be used to determine the moisture or residual solvent contents as well as the presence of a solvate in NCM, especially in the instances where a crystallization step was part of the synthetic process of a given NCM.

4.2.2. Differential Scanning Calorimetry (DSC)

DSC is a thermal analytical technique that provides qualitative and quantitative information as a function of time and temperature in respect of thermal changes in materials that involve endothermic or exothermic processes, or changes in heat capacity [81].

DSC is used for the determination of melting point, glass transition temperature, and purity of samples. When applied to NCM products, it is useful in determining changes in crystallinity, glass transition of stabilizing material, and the presence of more than one polymorphic form of the API. This is especially important for API that occurs in different polymorphic forms. Moreover, some top-down techniques like HPH can lead to a batch with an amorphous fraction. This, in turn, could lead to a significant increase in saturation solubility. The DSC of a pure drug, a physical mixture of drug and excipients (stabilizer), and the final formulation, which may be in dried form, is routinely done as pre-formulation and post-formulation quality tests [82].

Kocbek et al. prepared Pluronic® 68 stabilized ibuprofen nanosuspensions. The study results indicated the formation of a eutectic mixture of the drug and Pluronic® 68. In this case, DSC revealed a lower temperature melting peak representing the melting of the eutectic system, and a second peak representing the melting of the excess ibuprofen. Based on the position of the second peak, it was estimated that ibuprofen was in excess after eutectic formation [83].

Similarly, DSC was used to investigate the changes in the crystallinity of itraconazole (ITR) after the nanoprecipitation and drying processes or possible interactions between the API and excipients [84]. The results obtained indicated a small change in melting temperature of ITR, which were attributable to the reduction in PS and were deemed to not have been a consequence of CPP. The results also showed the presence of an amorphous component of ITR and confirmed the presence of both crystalline and amorphous ITR [84].

Although DSC cannot be used to establish the chemical nature of a sample being tested, the results can be useful for determining whether samples exhibit different thermal properties and can therefore distinguish differences relating to material identity, specific solid-state forms, and/or purity [85].

4.3. X-Ray Techniques

X-ray diffraction (XRD) is one of the most widely used techniques for the characterization of NCM. Ideally, crystalline structure, phase behaviour, lattice parameters, and crystallite grain size are derived from XRD [86]. Crystallite grain size is determined using the Scherrer equation [87]. It utilizes the diffractogram of the sample by analysing the broadening of the peaks of the highest intensity. XRD has the advantage of resulting in volume-averaged values while being statistically representative. Despite its applicability, XRD is often replaced in use by single-crystal X-ray diffraction (ScXRD) as the latter is a more definitive technique for determining three-dimensional crystal lattice structures. ScXRD provides an accurate representation of atomic coordinates and thermal parameters. These are obtained by using parameters such as molecular geometry and intermolecular distances [88]. ScXRD does have a major disadvantage in that it requires the accessibility of a single crystal. Unfortunately, in many instances, polycrystallites are formed, especially when using the top-down methods. In such cases, powder X-ray diffraction (PXRD) is the obvious alternative to ScXRD [88].

X-ray photon spectroscopy (XPS) capitalizes on the photoelectric effect [89]. In XPS, following adsorption of incident photons from an X-ray source, core electrons are emitted from a sample and the kinetic energy determined by conservation of energy. As a result of inelastic processes from scattering deep in the bulk, only surface electrons escape without energy loss. Identification of specific elements is accomplished on the basis that each element has a characteristic set of binding energies. The concentration of the element directly correlates to the number of photoelectrons and as such, after background removal, peak areas can be used as a means to quantify specific elements [89].

4.3.1. Powder X-ray Diffraction (PXRD)

PXRD is a non-destructive analytical technique used for the measurement of crystalline and non-crystalline materials. It is utilized to collect structural data at the anatomic level to understand phase transitions, determine the degree of crystallinity, and identify polymorphic and solvatomorphic phases [90,91]. It is an essential tool in pharmaceutical research as it can be applied to polycrystalline materials in both solid and liquid forms. It has application in all stages of drug development, production, and quality control testing of API, excipients, and final products [90,91]. It is an easy-to-use technique, yields reliable and reproducible results and is relatively inexpensive. Moreover, it is highly sensitive and has applications in both qualitative and quantitative analyses [90].

PXRD is more difficult to use to determine the crystal morphology or habit of an API and excipients, and to investigate crystal morphology changes while these substances maintain crystallinity [92]. Peak broadening for particles below 3 nm in size coupled with non-suitability for amorphous materials are the main drawbacks of this technique [86]. In research conducted by Upadhyay et al., the PS of magnetite nanoparticles were determined using X-ray line broadening. The broadening of XRD peaks was mainly caused by particle/crystallite size and lattice strains other than instrumental broadening [93].

Similarly, Li et al. used XRD and noticed that after preparing copper telluride nanostructures with different shapes (i.e., cubes, plates, and rods), the relative intensities between the different XRD peaks varied in relation to the particle shape [94].

The XRD-derived size is often larger than magnetic size. This is due to smaller domains being present in a particle where all moments are aligned in the same direction, even if the particle is a single domain. Consequently, the use of microscopy is often preferred for size determination over XRD [95].

4.3.2. Small Angle X-ray Scattering (SAXS)

For nanomaterials, SAXS is usually the best choice because below a certain particle size, PXRD is not sufficiently sensitive and the X-rays are scattered in an amorphous halo.

SAXS can be used to elucidate the PS, PDI, and morphology [86]. With regards to PS, more statistically reliable results are obtained with SAXS when compared to transmission electron microscopy (TEM). SAXS has been used successfully to study the structural changes of platinum (Pt) nanoparticles (NP) with changes in temperature [96]. The size obtained by XRD was different from the corresponding SAXS value at certain temperatures. This is because XRD is susceptible to the size of the long-range order region while SAXS is susceptible to the size of the fluctuation region of electronic density [86]. In these experiments, it was observed that the PS obtained with SAXS were slightly larger than those obtained using TEM. The reason is that Pt NP were coated with polyvinyl pyrrolidone (PVP) and the scattering intensity due to the PVP coating could not be easily removed [96].

Cipolla et al. used to SAXS to determine the PS, shape, and asymmetry of liposomes loaded with NC [97,98]. As part of the study outcomes, SAXS was identified as a useful and versatile technique to study the solid state of NC loaded in liposomes and dispersions, as well as to study the behaviour of drug NC in dispersion as a variable of temperature and pH [98].

SAXS has also found use in the solid-state characterization of doxorubicin sulphate nanocrystal loaded liposomal dispersions [99,100].

It has to be noted that SAXS is a low-resolution technique and in certain cases, further studies by XRD and/or electron diffraction techniques are indispensable for the characterization of NCM.

4.3.3. X-Ray Photon Spectroscopy (XPS)

Due to its ability to determine surface elemental composition and by virtue of being non-destructive, XPS has become a key characterization technique for NCM [101]. It can be utilized to provide detailed and qualitative information on chemical elements present on the surface of materials. This is particularly useful for NCM stabilized by polymers and/or surfactants. [102]. Recent advances utilizing special sample cells permits the use of liquid samples and consequently broadens the application of XPS [103], specifically for dispersed NCM.

Due to the nature of NCM, XPS has taken on more significance in the advancement of pharmaceutical nanotechnological applications by being capable of detecting the presence and determining the relative concentrations of elements while also determining the average thickness of surface coatings in NCM. As such, it is a useful technique for analysis of potential adulteration or impurities arising during nanomaterial synthesis and/or handling [89].

Through XPS, Qiu et al. conducted an investigation into the difference in reduction behaviour between nanocrystalline and microcrystalline ceria after Ar^+ bombardment or X-ray irradiation. Despite identical experimental conditions, viz. pellets compacted by uniaxial pressure of 10 MPa and XPS data being recorded before and after bombardment experiments, it was observed that the reduction levels of Ce^{4+} to Ce^{3+} were lower in nanocrystalline than microcrystalline ceria [104].

Chow et al. used XPS to ascertain drug encapsulation and demonstrated that most of the drug was entrapped within the cores of NPs, and that the particle composition of the surface was mainly the adsorbed co-stabilizer and polyethylene glycol (PEG) block [105].

Similarly, Dong et al. used XPS to prove the predominant presence of the PEG shell on the surface of paclitaxel loaded methoxy poly(ethylene glycol)-poly(lactide) (mPEG-PLA) NP [106].

In a study to analyze the external surface of a novel controlled release formulation for the anticancer drug paclitaxel (Taxol®) loaded in PLGA nanoparticles and stabilized by α-tocopheryl polyethylene glycol succinate 1000 using XPS, it is determined that the outermost layer was composed by a majority of TPGS 1000 molecules [107].

4.4. Vibrational Spectroscopy

4.4.1. Fourier Transform Infrared (FTIR) Spectroscopy

FTIR spectroscopy is used for the physical and chemical characterization of powder mixtures in the solid state by evaluating functional groups, identifying bond formation, and comparing bond formation [108,109]. It is a fundamental approach for the study of API-excipient interactions since it permits rapid and simple elucidation of chemical and structural attributes of organic materials as it is sensitive to molecular vibrations that are specific for specific functional groups [108]. Molecular vibrations are categorized based on the energy related to the functional groups within molecules over the 650–4000 cm^{-1} wavenumber range [109].

FTIR is mostly used to identify the purity of drug compounds in the crystal, to ascertain the polymorph in the NCM, and some cases are used to determine whether a solvate form of the NCM is present. FTIR can be of specific use in the determination of polymorphic changes during the nanosizing process. For instance, during HPH, piroxicam demonstrated to undergo polymorphic transformation [110]. The piroxicam nanocrystals were stabilized using poloxamer 188. FTIR was used in conjunction with other characterization techniques and confirmed that the crystalline form I of piroxicam made up the majority of the unprocessed piroxicam. A change of colour from white to yellow following HPH indicated a polymorphic conversion from form I to form III and the monohydrate. Confirmation using XRD, FTIR, and DSC confirmed that NC were a mixture of form III and the monohydrate [110].

Lamivudine-zidovudine NCC were synthesized with or without stabilizer [19,111]. The NCC formulation was stabilized with different stabilizers including SDS, TPGS 1000, Tween® 80, and Span® 80. The FTIR spectrum of the NCC was compared to those of the individual drug compounds to verify the absence of chemical interactions. The FTIR spectrum of the NCC revealed the presence of a monohydrate with the presence of a water peak without any peaks corresponding to the API [19,111].

FTIR was used to identify polymorphic changes in wet-milling using an HPH for an experimental anti-cancer compound, SN 30191. The process-induced transformations were studied as a function of time and pressure using infrared spectroscopy, and it was determined that conversion from form II to form I was pressure-dependent [112].

4.4.2. Raman Spectroscopy (RS)

RS is a versatile analytical technique that can be used in drug and formulation development, process control, as well as post-sale analyses [88]. Multivariate data analysis techniques are valuable for opening spectra to interpretation, allowing quantification of compounds, and simplification of large spectral data sets. In the pharmaceutical industry, multivariate techniques, such as partial least squares (PLS) analysis has permitted compounds or properties of compounds to be quantified. API quantification and the ability to determine interactions between API and excipients are examples of this [88].

RS can be used as a tool to identify the phases and phase transitions of various NCM, determine which regions of a nanomaterial are amorphous or crystalline [113–115], whether there are any defects present in the nanomaterial, determine the size (diameter, lateral dimensions, etc.) of various types of nanomaterials [116,117], whether the nanomaterial is homogenous or whether a dispersion of nanoparticles is uniform in size, determine the shape of nanomaterials (rod, spherical, etc.), and differentiate between different allotropes of the same material [118].

Spironolactone NC were synthesized with different stabilizers including poloxamers 407 and 188, hydroxypropyl methylcellulose (HPMC), and sodium deoxycholate. Preformulation and post-formulation experiments using RS to compare the drug nanosuspensions and raw materials were used. Peak shifts were not observed in spironolactone NC stabilised with poloxamer 188, HPMC, and sodium deoxycholate. However, the Raman spectra revealed API peak disappearance with poloxamer 407 stabilized NC, indicating that interactions between drug and stabiliser had occurred in that case [119].

A novel bottom-up process to fabricate fenofibrate NCM termed as "controlled crystallization during freeze-drying" (CCDF) was used to synthesize NC. The size of the NC in this process was influenced by various factors including the freezing rate. To determine the stage at which solute crystallisation occurred, RS monitoring was used. The in-line Raman measurements showed that the first two steps, the freezing step, and the crystallization step are critical steps that determined the final size of the fenofibrate crystals [120].

4.5. Microscopy Techniques

Microscopy imaging is extremely useful when examining the size, shape, and detailed morphology of particles, and for understanding morphology-related properties of substances, formulations, and/or dosage forms [121]. The techniques are frequently used in research and development, especially for solid dosage forms while only a limited number of examples are referenced here. In the evaluation of pharmaceutical raw materials such as API and excipients, microscopy images reveal the size, shape, and morphology of particles, which helps in understanding some processing properties and the pharmaceutical performance of these materials [122,123]. The impact of different preparation procedures, such as precipitation or milling methods, on important properties (shape, size, chemical composition) of the resulting API or excipient particles in NCM can be investigated using microscopy [124–127].

4.5.1. Scanning Electron Microscopy (SEM)

SEM is an analytical technique used for the characterization of surface morphology of API and excipients microscopically, in particular, differences in crystal habits and the shape of the samples [128,129]. SEM does not convey any information in respect of the chemical structure and/or thermal behaviour of compounds, and is used with other thermal and spectroscopic methods such as DSC, TGA, and FTIR to identify incompatibilities between API and excipients [129].

4.5.2. Scanning Electron Microscopy Energy Dispersive X-ray Spectroscopy (SEM-EDX)

Investigation of a sample by SEM does not only produce images but may also provide specific information in respect of the chemical composition of a sample at specific locations in the sample. Energy-dispersive X-ray spectrometry (EDX) is based on the generation of X-rays following the interaction of an electron beam with the atoms in a sample. SEM-EDX has potential applications in NC and NCC use particularly in determining contamination that could arise from milling media. EDX has been successfully used for this application. EDX can also be used to surmise the overall presence of coating agents through determining the presence of coating agent-specific atoms or by observing an increase or reduction in atomic % of pure drug elemental components. EDX was specifically used for both of these applications for the determination of the presence of TPGS 1000 and SDS in NC prepared using the bottom-up method, and the presence of chromium and iron contamination from the steel media milling media during the top-down manufacture of lamivudine-zidovudine NCC [42,111].

4.5.3. Transmission Electron Microscopy (TEM)

Conventional transmission electron microscopes are electron-optical instruments analogous to light microscopes [130]. The main difference being that in TEM, the illumination of the specimen is by an electron beam as opposed to light. An increase in acceleration voltage of the electrons directly results in an increase in resolution. However, a reduction in contrast results from increasing acceleration voltage as a consequence of the scattering of the electrons being decreased at higher velocity [131].

TEM is particularly useful for the study of colloidal and nanostructured drug delivery systems including NCM [88,132]. Much like SEM, TEM is more useful in determining surface morphology, differences in crystal habit, and determining particle shape. TEM is widely the most applied method for evaluation, is used in many characterisation approaches, and is considered the gold standard for PS determination.

4.6. Quantitative Techniques

4.6.1. (Ultra) High-Performance Liquid Chromatography ((U)HPLC)

During different stages of pharmaceutical development, including synthesis and isolation of API, dosage form development, and pharmacological testing, gas or liquid chromatographic methods of analysis are used for quantitative and/or qualitative purposes [133].

High-Performance Liquid Chromatography (HPLC) is based on the principles and theories of gas chromatography and is a rapid and efficient analytical procedure [134,135]. In the broadest sense, chromatographic separations can be classified as normal (NPC) and reversed-phase (RPC), where the stationary phase is more polar than the mobile phase for NPC, whereas the converse is true for RPC [136].

RP-HPLC is the method of choice for in vitro analysis of API due to the stability and reproducibility of stationary phases used for analyses [137]. A large number of aqueous components in the mobile phase, in addition to the ease of reproducing analytical methods in different laboratory settings, make RP-HPLC an ideal analytical method for product development and quality control purposes in the pharmaceutical industry [137].

The use of stationary phases that have a silica-based backbone chemically bonded to a variety of different organic functional groups, form the basis for separations in RP-HPLC [138]. Separation is achieved when the sample to be analysed partitions between an organic modifier used in the mobile phase and the stationary phase or column [139,140]. In general, non-polar compounds are attracted to hydrophobic stationary phases and polar compounds preferentially partition into polar mobile phase components [139]. The specificity and selectivity of an analytical method is the consequence of interaction(s) between analyte(s) and binding sites of the stationary phase and partitioning in the mobile phase [141]. Silica-based columns with C_3, C_4, C_8, or C_{18} alkyl chains bonded to the backbone are the commonly used non-polar stationary phases in RP-HPLC. Silica-based phases are compatible, do not swell in water, and some organic solvents are, therefore, suitable for use with mobile phases comprised of these solvents [139,141,142].

The mobile phase in RP-HPLC is usually water or a buffered solution with an organic modifier such as methanol or acetonitrile added to the composition in order to reduce the polarity of the mobile phase, thereby facilitating the achievement of appropriate retention characteristics for the compounds of interest [138]. Other factors that affect the retention time of analytes include temperature, pH of the buffer and/or mobile phase, stationary phase properties, polarity of the mobile phase, flow rate, and mobile phase composition [139,140].

4.6.2. Ultraviolet-Visible Spectrophotometry (UV-Vis Spec)

Spectroscopy is a branch of science which deals with the study of electromagnetic radiation and its interaction with matter. The UV-visible spectrophotometry specifically is one of the most often used analytical techniques in the pharmaceutical industry [143,144]. The technique is used to evaluate the concentration of a given organic or biological compound [145,146]. This process is achieved using UV or visible radiations which are absorbed by a substance in solution [143–145]. The ratio or function of the ratio of the intensity of two beams of light in the UV-vis region is measured by instruments known as UV spectrophotometers [144]. Absorption of radiation of a specific wavelength, λ, is an indication of the presence of one or more chromophores [147]. A chromophore is a molecular group that has a pi, π, bond which when inserted into a saturated hydrocarbon, produces a compound with absorption between 185 nm and 1000 nm [148]. Temperature and pH may also cause changes in both the intensity and the λ of the absorbance maxima [149,150].

Analysis of compounds using spectroscopy is governed by the Beer–Lambert law [144]. Beer's law states that the intensity of a beam of parallel monochromatic radiation decreases exponentially with the number of absorbing molecules [144,151–153]. Thus, according to Beer, the concentration of a compound is proportional to the absorbance produced [144,150]. Lambert's law states that the intensity of a beam of parallel monochromatic radiation decreases exponentially as it passes through a medium of homogenous thickness [152,154]. As both laws deal with the intensity of monochromatic radiation, a combination of the two laws has been used to yield the Beer–Lambert law [144,151–154].

Different NCM manufacturing methods and conditions have an influence on the solid state form while environmental conditions affect the thermodynamic stability of the polymorphic form [155]. PXRD, DSC, SEM, FTIR, and RS are the most commonly used methods to establish and monitor the solid-state forms of NCM. The use of microscopy techniques is the mainstay of PS, particle shape, and morphology determination. A summary of techniques and their applications is depicted in Table 1.

Table 1. Characterizations associated with NCM (Adapted from [86]).

Entity to Be Characterized	Techniques *
Size and morphology	DLS, SEM, TEM
Surface charge	ZP
Surface chemical analysis	XPS, EDX
Crystal structure	SAXS, PXRD, DSC
Growth kinetics	SAXS, NMR, TEM, cryo-TEM, liquid-TEM
Agglomeration state	ZP, DLS, DCS, UV-Vis, SEM, Cryo-TEM, TEM
Ligand binding/density/mass/surface composition /bulk composition	XPS, FTIR, NMR,
Dispersion of NCM in matrices/supports	TEM, SEM
Dissolution Testing	(U)HPLC, UV

* Physical state of samples: DLS, ZP, TEM, UV-Vis, NMR, and HPLC; liquid state. All other techniques; solid state.

5. Applications of Characterization Techniques on Prediction of NCM Performance

5.1. Prediction of Physical and Chemical Stability of NCM

The success of API delivery to target tissues is largely dependent on the maintenance of stability by the NCM in systemic circulation. The fate of NCM, in vivo, is in part determined by the ability to retain size and payload external to target tissues and to release API to the cells at predetermined rates in appropriate quantities. Ideally, a nanometric drug carrier must remain stable by resisting aggregation or degradation while maintaining API concentrations in the blood until it reaches the target site(s). Altered biodistribution as well as premature drug release can occur as a result of NCM instability, subsequently compromising the performance and efficacy of the delivery system. As such, it is of utmost importance to evaluate NCM with regards to estimating the success of the drug delivery system.

It is important to conduct a series of in vitro tests to investigate the stability of NCM in different biologically relevant media. It is ultimately desirable to conduct investigations into the stability of NCM in vivo since these techniques provide reasonable assessments and prediction of the likely stability of the formulation in physiological environments.

5.1.1. Suspension Stability

The main role of stabilizers in NCM synthesis is to prevent the growth of crystals resulting in micro or macroparticles. However, most stabilizers may offer "stealth" properties, enhance permeation, prevent efflux, enhance cell-targeting, or prevent clearance. By careful formulation, the dissolution and stability can be enhanced while also improving permeation. Consequently performance may be altered by the selection of stabilizers as part of the critical formulation parameters (CFP) [156].

The majority of stabilizing agents are amphiphilic moieties that have the ability to adsorb to the surfaces of newly formed drug particles by utilizing hydrophilic-hydrophobic interactions. This results in an enhancement in the wetting of NC or NCC [155]. In its most classical form, the DLVO theory describes nanoparticle stabilization based on steric and/or electrostatic interactions. Steric stabilization, by use of polymers or non-ionic surfactants, has been more commonly utilized, and has an added facet of being temperature sensitive. Conversely, electrostatic stabilization is achieved with ionic polymers or surfactants. In systems where stabilization is achieved only by electrostatic forces, the ZP should be higher than |30| mV. As previously stated, this value is vulnerable to changes in pH, the presence of ionic species, and changes in hydration (drying) [155].

The physical stability of NCM is usually predicted in the suspension state by the value of the ZP [76]. The use of ZP as a predictor of stability has been shown to be applicable in nano-formulations containing nevirapine [157], efavirenz [158], and curcumin [105]. More specifically, NCM nanosuspensions of miconazole [159], indomethacin [160], and ascorbyl palmitate [161] exhibited ZP-dependent stability.

5.1.2. Phase Behaviour

For crystal cell units, it is important to confirm that the API exists, and in the case of NCC, co-former exist as a co-crystal by non-ionic interaction using appropriate analytical techniques [162]. Furthermore, the extent of polymorphism must be considered when determining the stability of a system and attempting to predict API release from that system.

The most frequently used techniques for investigating the phase behavior of NCM include the use of DSC, TGA, PXRD, and ScXRD. By investigating the thermal behavior and crystallinity of such systems, valuable complementary information can be generated for the characterization and quality control of NCM formulations and technologies [163].

Modulated temperature DSC (MTDSC) is sensitive and has a high separation capacity with overlapping thermal events as quasi-static material properties, and frequency dependency of thermal events are monitored, whereas TGA measures sample mass during the heating process and is convenient for determining the presence of solvates and hydrates [163].

5.1.3. Determination of Critical Aggregation or Micelle Concentration

The critical micelle concentration (CMC) can be used as a measure of the stability of self-assembling NC or NCC systems including polymeric or surfactant stabilized NCM systems. The CMC is defined as the concentration at which self-assembled particles may form. This is a quantitative measure of the physical stability of NCM in solution. A relatively low CMC is indicative of more stable NCM systems than those in which a high CMC is likely. In other words, NCM prepared using stabilizers with a low CMC are more likely to maintain state as a consequence of dilution in the blood [164–168].

5.1.4. Chemical Degradation Analysis

The most standard approach to monitor and/or detect chemical degradation is analysis using (U)HPLC. Impurities or degradation products often present as new peaks; however, recognition of additional products often requires the use of techniques such as liquid chromatography-mass spectrometry (LC-MS). Degradation of molecules can be induced using harsh processing conditions, and exact knowledge of the chemistry of unwanted products is crucial in order to recognize and avoid potentially problematic process steps [163].

Vibrational spectroscopic methods may also be used to determine whether a chemical change has taken place during the process of manufacture and storage. The disappearance of peaks associated with key frequencies of the API could be an indication of degradation. FTIR and RS have been used to ascertain that NCM formulated for the delivery of lamivudine-zidovudine [19,42,111], tadalafil [169], and diclofenac [170] had not undergone chemical degradation or chemically interacted with the stabilizers.

While less commonly used for the purposes of determination chemical degradation, SEM-EDX may offer valuable information regarding the state of the NCM within a bulk. The technique was effectively used to determine whether chemical degradation had occurred by revealing the disappearance of elemental peaks of the appearance of new ones. In addition, the percentage of abundance was equally used as a determinant of chemical degradation for the NCM [42].

5.2. In Vitro Dissolution and Kinetics of Drug Release

When NCM is used for delivery of API, the release of the API is evaluated over time in order to determine the availability of API for absorption and ultimately at target sites thereby influencing therapeutic outcomes [72]. Three possible mechanisms of release from NCM can be envisaged viz., desorption of adsorbed API (A), API diffusion from a polymer/surfactant matrix (B), and/or release following polymer/surfactant erosion (C) as depicted in Figure 1.

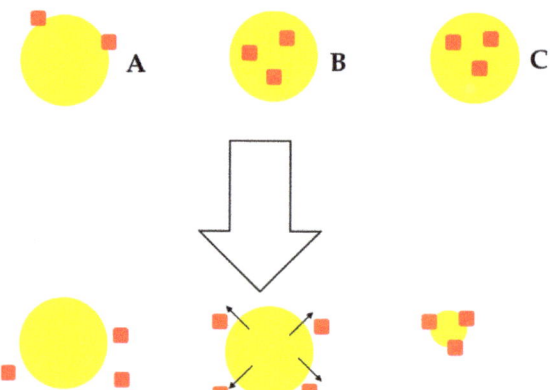

Figure 1. Possible mechanisms of drug release from NCM; desorption-controlled drug release (**A**), diffusion-controlled drug release (**B**) and erosion-controlled drug release (**C**).

In the case of matrix-type polymer/surfactant NCM in which the crystalline API is uniformly distributed or embedded in the matrix, drug release would be predominantly controlled by diffusion through the matrix and/or erosion of the matrix. Depending on the API and matrix physicochemical properties, either one of these mechanisms can be the dominant one. If diffusion occurs more rapidly than matrix/surfactant degradation, diffusion is likely to be the main mechanism of release. In many instances, an initial rapid initial release is noticed and attributable to the crystalline material fraction adsorbed or weakly bound to the surface(s) or that is not entirely embedded in the system (Figure 1A) [171].

API release from NCM is investigated in a number of ways. These are by dialysis membrane diffusion, membrane-less diffusion, sampling and separation, or the use of an in situ analytical technique [172]. When using the sampling and separation technique, API release is determined by separating the released API from the sample by filtration, centrifugation, or centrifugal filtration, and subsequent quantification using an appropriate analytical method such as (U)HPLC or UV spectroscopy.

The NCM are augmented with fresh release medium, preferably simulated bodily fluids and resuspended and incubated further until the next sampling interval. Despite this method having the capability of being performed with a small sample size and simple analytical equipment, several drawbacks exist: the separation methods is slow, tedious, and inefficient, making it inappropriate for studying rapid/immediate release NCM. In addition, the force of centrifugation or shear stress during filtration required for NCM separation tends to increase with a reduction in NCM PS. This can ultimately alter the release kinetics of the API. The main advantage of the dialysis membrane diffusion technique is that he diffusion of the NCM is continuous across the dialysis membrane and not subject to destructive separation processes, making sample acquisition simple and rapid [163,173,174].

The use of dialysis membranes may attenuate API release as it is a diffusion barrier that may behave as an adsorptive surface. Thus, this approach should be conducted with control experiments in which free API is used to assess membrane effects. The dialysis membrane diffusion method typically makes use of large volumes of dissolution media. While large volumes maintain sink conditions for release, API analysis may be hindered due to the low concentrations to be tested. An in situ analytical technique is useful for studying NCM, which are prepared almost exclusively of an API. This technique is used to analyse the properties of NCM in situ to indirectly determine the quantity of API released. Various analytical techniques, including electrochemical analysis, solution calorimetry, or turbidometric and the light scattering techniques have been used for this purpose [172]. These approaches do not need separation of NCM and enable real-time assessment of the release kinetics of API.

While the aforementioned characterizations may be generally applicable, it may not always be applicable to use all of them. The role of PS, PDI, ZP, and polymorphism on NCM performance with regards to processability, content uniformity, and stability of a drug product is recognizable. The possible effect of PS and polymorphism on solubility, dissolution, and bioavailability parameters being strictly related to each other is one of the primary concerns. Definitions of specifications are required particularly when the product performance is affected by PS and polymorphism. We provide an appropriate decision tree in Figure 2, that is closely adapted to that in the ICH Q6A guidelines [175], on what characterization is required and to which performance parameter it relates.

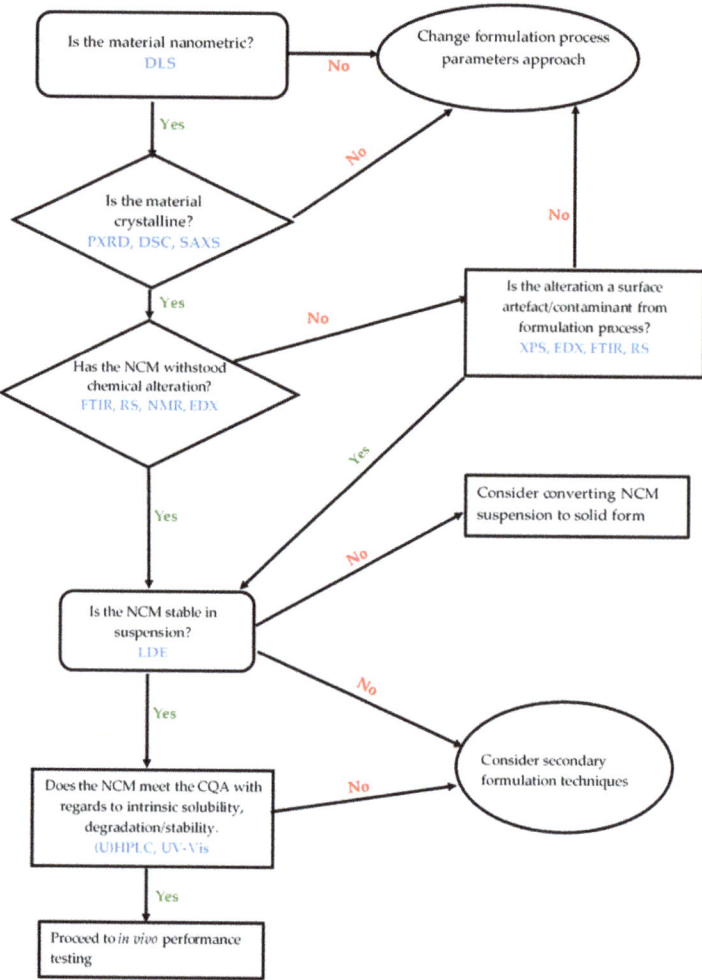

Figure 2. Decision tree relating to NCM characterization.

6. Conclusions

NCM are non-toxic crystalline carriers composed almost entirely of API and very little excipients.

Unlike other nanoparticle technologies such as solid lipid nanoparticles (SLN), nano lipid carriers (NLC), and nanocapsules, NCM are suitable for the delivery of hydrophilic and hydrophobic compounds with very high efficiency. NCM are also relatively easy to prepare and synthesize when compared to other nanoparticle technologies such as liposomes and nanocapsules that require multiple steps and use of organic solvents. NCM have the added advantage of exhibiting better stability than other nanoparticles due to the crystalline state of the particles. In addition, NCM formulations prevent the accumulation of the payload in cells and tissues of healthy organs and often exhibit improved bioavailability for some API. The suitability of the carriers has been proven since they are already on the market (Rapamune® and Emend®). NCM fulfil the key prerequisites for the introduction of the technology to the clinic trial phases and the market, that is, they are in line with regulatory requirements and provide the possibility of qualified industrial large-scale production. Furthermore, NCM exhibit flexibility in terms of the route of administration and have been used for oral, parenteral, ophthalmic, and topical delivery of a variety of compounds.

The characterization of NCM delivery systems is an area that requires the formulation development and production of a products of high quality. Ideally, NCM should be in the nano range with a PDI < 0.500, determined using DLS and Photon Correlation Spectroscopy (PCS) in combination with Laser Diffraction (LD). However, PCS and DLS cannot be used to characterize the shape, surface morphology, and elemental composition of NCM and additional analytical tools are required. Therefore, TEM, SEM, and EDX should be used to assess the shape and surface morphology of NCM in the solid-state and dispersions. The crystalline nature and polymorphic transition of NCM are characterised using DSC, TGA, PXRD, and FTIR/Raman spectroscopy to investigate potential interactions between the API and excipients to be used. Laser Doppler Anemometry (LDA) is used to establish electrophoretic mobility and the ZP of NCM, which should be > +30 mV or < −30 mV in dispersion.

Other characterisations perhaps not considered the most fundamental but worth additional exploration include two-dimensional (2D) nuclear magnetic resonance (NMR) techniques such as correlation spectroscopy (COSY), diffusion-ordered spectroscopy (DOSY), and cross-polarization magic-angle spinning (CPMAS). These are used to generate additional information in terms of the stability of the nanocarriers in solution and solid-state in addition to the presence of hydrogen bonding.

Author Contributions: Conceptualization, B.A.W.; writing—original draft preparation, B.A.W. and M.A.; writing—review and editing, B.A.W., M.A., L.L.M. and P.A.M. All authors have read and agreed to the published version of the manuscript.

Funding: This research was not funded with an external research grant.

Institutional Review Board Statement: Not applicable

Informed Consent Statement: Not applicable

Acknowledgments: The authors acknowledge the Research Committee of Rhodes University (P.A.M.).

Conflicts of Interest: The authors declare no conflict of interest.

References

1. Tiwari, G.; Tiwari, R.; Bannerjee, S.; Bhati, L.; Pandey, S.; Pandey, P.; Sriwastawa, B. Drug delivery systems: An updated review. *Int. J. Pharm. Investig.* **2012**, *2*, 2. [CrossRef] [PubMed]
2. Farokhzad, O.C.; Langer, R. Impact of Nanotechnology on Drug Discovery & Development Pharmanext. *ACS Nano* **2009**, *3*, 16–20. [PubMed]
3. Junghanns, J.U.A.H.; Müller, R.H. Nanocrystal technology, drug delivery and clinical applications. *Int. J. Nanomed.* **2008**, *3*, 295–309. [CrossRef]
4. Müller, R.H. Lipid nanoparticles: Recent advances. *Adv. Drug Deliv. Rev.* **2007**, *59*, 375–376. [CrossRef]
5. Muller, R.H.; Keck, C.M. Challenges and solutions for the delivery of biotech drugs—A review of drug nanocrystal technology and lipid nanoparticles. *J. Biotechnol.* **2004**, *113*, 151–170. [CrossRef]
6. Blagden, N.; de Matas, M.; Gavan, P.T.; York, P. Crystal engineering of active pharmaceutical ingredients to improve solubility and dissolution rates. *Adv. Drug Deliv. Rev.* **2007**, *59*, 617–630. [CrossRef]
7. Subramanian, S.; Zaworotko, M.J. Manifestations of noncovalent bonding in the solid state. 6. [H 4 (cyclam)] 4+ (cyclam = 1,4,8,11-tetraazacyclotetradecane) as a template for crystal engineering of network hydrogen-bonded solids. *Can. J. Chem.* **1995**, *73*, 414–424. [CrossRef]
8. Desiraju, G.R. Crystal Engineering: The design of Organic Solids. *J. Appl. Crystallogr.* **1991**, *24*, 265. [CrossRef]
9. Desiraju, G.R. Supramolecular Synthons in Crystal Engineering. *Angew. Chem. Int. Ed.* **1995**, *34*, 2311–2327. [CrossRef]
10. Aakeroy, C.B.; Aakeroy, A.; Sinha, A.S. *Co-Crystals: Introduction and Scope*; Royal Society of Chemistry: London, UK, 2018; Volume 11.
11. Bolton, O.; Matzger, A.J. Improved stability and smart-material functionality realized in an energetic cocrystal. *Angew. Chem. Int. Ed.* **2011**, *50*, 8960–8963. [CrossRef]
12. Brittain, H.G. Pharmaceutical cocrystals: The coming wave of new drug substances. *J. Pharm. Sci.* **2013**, *102*, 311–317. [CrossRef]
13. Brittain, H.G. Cocrystal Systems of Pharmaceutical Interest: 2010. *Cryst. Growth Des.* **2011**, *36*, 361–381. [CrossRef]
14. Sekhon, B. Pharmaceutical co-crystals—A review. *ARS Pharm.* **2009**, *150*, 99–117.

15. Merisko-Liversidge, E.; Liversidge, G.G. Nanosizing for oral and parenteral drug delivery: A perspective on formulating poorly-water soluble compounds using wet media milling technology. *Adv. Drug Deliv. Rev.* **2011**, *63*, 427–440. [CrossRef] [PubMed]
16. Merisko-Liversidge, E.; Liversidge, G.G.; Cooper, E.R. Nanosizing: A formulation approach for poorly-water-soluble compounds. *Eur. J. Pharm. Sci.* **2003**, *18*, 113–120. [CrossRef]
17. Sinha, B.; Muller, R.H.; Moschwitzer, J.P. Bottom-up approaches for preparing drug nanocrystals: Formulations and factors affecting particle size. *Int. J. Pharm.* **2013**, *8*, 384–392. [CrossRef] [PubMed]
18. De Waard, H.; Frijlink, H.W.; Hinrichs, W.L.J. Bottom-up preparation techniques for nanocrystals of lipophilic drugs. *Pharm. Res.* **2011**, *28*, 1220–1223. [CrossRef]
19. Witika, B.A.; Smith, V.J.; Walker, R.B. A comparative study of the effect of different stabilizers on the critical quality attributes of self-assembling nano co-crystals. *Pharmaceutics* **2020**, *12*, 182. [CrossRef]
20. Choi, J.Y.; Yoo, J.Y.; Kwak, H.S.; Nam, B.U.; Lee, J. Role of polymeric stabilizers for drug nanocrystal dispersions. *Curr. Appl. Phys.* **2005**, *5*, 472–474. [CrossRef]
21. Ghosh, I.; Bose, S.; Vippagunta, R.; Harmon, F. Pharmaceutical Nanotechnology Nanosuspension for improving the bioavailability of a poorly soluble drug and screening of stabilizing agents to inhibit crystal growth. *Int. J. Pharm.* **2011**, *409*, 260–268. [CrossRef]
22. Raghava Srivalli, K.M.; Mishra, B. Drug nanocrystals: A way toward scale-up. *Saudi Pharm. J.* **2016**, *24*, 386–404. [CrossRef]
23. Al Shaal, L.; Müller, R.H.; Keck, C.M. Preserving hesperetin nanosuspensions for dermal application. *Pharmazie* **2010**, *65*, 86–92. [CrossRef] [PubMed]
24. Piao, H.; Kamiya, N.; Cui, F.; Goto, M. Preparation of a solid-in-oil nanosuspension containing l-ascorbic acid as a novel long-term stable topical formulation. *Int. J. Pharm.* **2011**, *420*, 156–160. [CrossRef]
25. Patel, D.A.; Patel, M.R.; Patel, K.R.; Patel, N.M. Buccal mucosa as a route for systemic drug delivery: A review. *Int. J. Drug Dev. Res.* **2012**, *1*, 15–30.
26. Dressman, J.B.; Reppas, C. In vitro–in vivo correlations for lipophilic, poorly water-soluble drugs. *Eur. J. Pharm. Sci.* **2000**, *11*, S73–S80. [CrossRef]
27. Kesisoglou, F.; Panmai, S.; Wu, Y. Nanosizing—Oral formulation development and biopharmaceutical evaluation. *Adv. Drug Deliv. Rev.* **2007**, *59*, 631–644. [CrossRef]
28. Wu, Y.; Loper, A.; Landis, E.; Hettrick, L.; Novak, L.; Lynn, K.; Chen, C.; Thompson, K.; Higgins, R.; Batra, U.; et al. The role of biopharmaceutics in the development of a clinical nanoparticle formulation of MK-0869: A Beagle dog model predicts improved bioavailability and diminished food effect on absorption in human. *Int. J. Pharm.* **2004**, *285*, 135–146. [CrossRef] [PubMed]
29. Edelhauser, H.F.; Rowe-Rendleman, C.L.; Robinson, M.R.; Dawson, D.G.; Chader, G.J.; Grossniklaus, H.E.; Rittenhouse, K.D.; Wilson, C.G.; Weber, D.A.; Kuppermann, B.D.; et al. Ophthalmic drug delivery systems for the treatment of retinal diseases: Basic research to clinical applications. *Investig. Ophthalmol. Vis. Sci.* **2010**, *51*, 5403–5420. [CrossRef]
30. Makoni, P.A.; Khamanga, S.M.; Walker, R.B. Muco-adhesive clarithromycin-loaded nanostructured lipid carriers for ocular delivery: Formulation, characterization, cytotoxicity and stability. *J. Drug Deliv. Sci. Technol.* **2020**, *61*, 102171. [CrossRef]
31. Kassem, M.A.; Abdel Rahman, A.A.; Ghorab, M.M.; Ahmed, M.B.; Khalil, R.M. Nanosuspension as an ophthalmic delivery system for certain glucocorticoid drugs. *Int. J. Pharm.* **2007**, *340*, 126–133. [CrossRef]
32. Baba, K.; Nishida, K. Steroid nanocrystals prepared using the nano spray dryer B-90. *Pharmaceutics* **2013**, *5*, 107–114. [CrossRef]
33. Ali, H.S.M.; York, P.; Ali, A.M.A.; Blagden, N. Hydrocortisone nanosuspensions for ophthalmic delivery: A comparative study between microfluidic nanoprecipitation and wet milling. *J. Control Release* **2011**, *149*, 175–181. [CrossRef]
34. Ganta, S.; Paxton, J.W.; Baguley, B.C.; Garg, S. Formulation and pharmacokinetic evaluation of an asulacrine nanocrystalline suspension for intravenous delivery. *Int. J. Pharm.* **2009**, *367*, 179–186. [CrossRef]
35. Ben Zirar, S.; Astier, A.; Muchow, M.; Gibaud, S. Comparison of nanosuspensions and hydroxypropyl-β-cyclodextrin complex of melarsoprol: Pharmacokinetics and tissue distribution in mice. *Eur. J. Pharm. Biopharm.* **2008**, *70*, 649–656. [CrossRef]
36. Zhang, D.; Chen, M.; Zheng, T.; Wang, S. Preparation and Characterization of an Oridonin Nanosuspension for Solubility and Dissolution Velocity Enhancement AU—Gao, Lei. *Drug Dev. Ind. Pharm.* **2007**, *33*, 1332–1339. [CrossRef]
37. Rabinow, B.; Kipp, J.; Papadopoulos, P.; Wong, J.; Glosson, J.; Gass, J.; Sun, C.S.; Wielgos, T.; White, R.; Cook, C.; et al. Itraconazole IV nanosuspension enhances efficacy through altered pharmacokinetics in the rat. *Int. J. Pharm.* **2007**, *339*, 251–260. [CrossRef] [PubMed]
38. Li, Z.; Sun, M.; Guo, C.; Yu, A.; Xi, Y.; Cui, J.; Lou, H.; Zhai, G. Preparation and characterization of intravenously injectable curcumin nanosuspension AU—Gao, Yan. *Drug Deliv.* **2011**, *18*, 131–142. [CrossRef]
39. Lu, Y.; Wang, Z.H.; Li, T.; McNally, H.; Park, K.; Sturek, M. Development and evaluation of transferrin-stabilized paclitaxel nanocrystal formulation. *J. Control Release* **2014**, *176*, 76–85. [CrossRef] [PubMed]
40. Sarnes, A.; Kovalainen, M.; Häkkinen, M.R.; Laaksonen, T.; Laru, J.; Kiesvaara, J.; Ilkka, J.; Oksala, O.; Rönkkö, S.; Järvinen, K.; et al. Nanocrystal-based per-oral itraconazole delivery: Superior in vitro dissolution enhancement versus Sporanox® is not realized in in vivo drug absorption. *J. Control Release* **2014**, *180*, 109–116. [CrossRef] [PubMed]
41. Müller, R.H.; Jacobs, C. Buparvaquone mucoadhesive nanosuspension: Preparation, optimisation and long-term stability. *Int. J. Pharm.* **2002**, *237*, 151–161. [CrossRef]
42. Witika, B.A.; Smith, V.J.; Walker, R.B. Quality by Design Optimization of Cold Sonochemical Synthesis of Zidovudine-Lamivudine Nanosuspensions. *Pharmaceutics* **2020**, *12*, 367. [CrossRef] [PubMed]

43. Aucamp, M.; Milne, M. The physical stability of drugs linked to quality-by-design (QbD) and in-process technology (PAT) perspectives. *Eur. J. Pharm. Sci.* **2019**, *139*, 105057. [CrossRef]
44. Shegokar, R.; Müller, R.H. Nanocrystals: Industrially feasible multifunctional formulation technology for poorly soluble actives. *Int. J. Pharm.* **2010**, *399*, 129–139. [CrossRef] [PubMed]
45. Rabinow, B.E. Nanosuspensions in drug delivery. *Nat. Rev. Drug Discov.* **2004**, *3*, 785. [CrossRef]
46. Muller, R.H.; Jacobs, C.; Kayser, O. Nanosuspensions as particulate drug formulations in therapy: Rationale for development and what we can expect for the future. *Adv. Drug Deliv. Rev.* **2001**, *47*, 3–19. [CrossRef]
47. Keck, C.M.; Müller, R.H. Drug nanocrystals of poorly soluble drugs produced by high pressure homogenisation. *Eur. J. Pharm. Biopharm.* **2006**, *62*, 3–16. [CrossRef]
48. Li, X.; Zhou, L.; Ma, J.; Gao, L.; Wang, X.; Liu, G. Drug nanocrystals: In vivo performances. *J. Control Release* **2012**, *160*, 418–430. [CrossRef]
49. Lu, Y.; Li, Y.; Wu, W. Injected nanocrystals for targeted drug delivery. *Acta Pharm. Sin. B* **2016**, *6*, 106–113. [CrossRef]
50. Juhnke, M.; Martin, D.; John, E. Generation of wear during the production of drug nanosuspensions by wet media milling. *Eur. J. Pharm. Biopharm.* **2012**, *81*, 214–222. [CrossRef]
51. Van Eerdenbrugh, B.; Van den Mooter, G.; Augustijns, P. Top-down production of drug nanocrystals: Nanosuspension stabilization, miniaturization and transformation into solid products. *Int. J. Pharm.* **2008**, *364*, 64–75. [CrossRef] [PubMed]
52. Karashima, M.; Kimoto, K.; Yamamoto, K.; Kojima, T.; Ikeda, Y. A novel solubilization technique for poorly soluble drugs through the integration of nanocrystal and cocrystal technologies. *Eur. J. Pharm. Biopharm.* **2016**, *107*, 142–150. [CrossRef]
53. De Smet, L.; Saerens, L.; De Beer, T.; Carleer, R.; Adriaensens, P.; Van Bocxlaer, J.; Vervaet, C.; Remon, J.P. Formulation of itraconazole nanocrystals and evaluation of their bioavailability in dogs. *Eur. J. Pharm. Biopharm.* **2014**, *87*, 107–113. [CrossRef]
54. Witika, B.A.; Smith, V.J.; Walker, R.B. Top-Down Synthesis of a Lamivudine-Zidovudine Nano Co-Crystal. *Crystals* **2021**, *11*, 33. [CrossRef]
55. Xia, D.; Cui, Y.G. and F. Application of Precipitation Methods for the Production of Water-insoluble Drug Nanocrystals: Production Techniques and Stability of Nanocrystals. *Curr. Pharm. Des.* **2014**, *20*, 408–435. [CrossRef] [PubMed]
56. Dalvi, S.V.; Yadav, M.D. Effect of ultrasound and stabilizers on nucleation kinetics of curcumin during liquid antisolvent precipitation. *Ultrason. Sonochem.* **2015**, *24*, 114–122. [CrossRef] [PubMed]
57. Sander, J.R.G.; Bučar, D.K.; Henry, R.F.; Zhang, G.G.Z.; MacGillivray, L.R. Pharmaceutical nano-cocrystals: Sonochemical synthesis by solvent selection and use of a surfactant. *Angew. Chem. Int. Ed.* **2010**, *49*, 7284–7288. [CrossRef]
58. Huang, Y.; Li, J.-M.; Lai, Z.-H.; Wu, J.; Lu, T.-B.; Chen, J.-M. Phenazopyridine-phthalimide nano-cocrystal: Release rate and oral bioavailability enhancement. *Eur. J. Pharm. Sci.* **2017**. [CrossRef]
59. Hong, C.; Xie, Y.; Yao, Y.; Li, G.; Yuan, X.; Shen, H. A Novel strategy for pharmaceutical cocrystal generation without knowledge of stoichiometric ratio: Myricetin cocrystals and a ternary phase diagram. *Pharm. Res.* **2015**, *32*, 47–60. [CrossRef] [PubMed]
60. Liu, M.; Hong, C.; Li, G.; Ma, P.; Xie, Y. The generation of myricetin-nicotinamide nanococrystals by top down and bottom up technologies. *Nanotechnology* **2016**, *27*. [CrossRef] [PubMed]
61. Allen, F.H. The Cambridge Structural Database: A quarter of a million crystal structures and rising. *Acta Crystallogr. Sect. B Struct. Sci.* **2002**, *58*, 380–388. [CrossRef] [PubMed]
62. Bruno, I.J.; Cole, J.C.; Edgington, P.R.; Kessler, M.; Macrae, C.F.; McCabe, P.; Pearson, J.; Taylor, R. New software for searching the Cambridge Structural Database and visualizing crystal structures. *Acta Crystallogr. B* **2002**, *58*, 389–397. [CrossRef] [PubMed]
63. Vance, E.J. Growth and Perfection of Crystals. *J. Am. Chem. Soc.* **1959**, *81*, 3489–3490. [CrossRef]
64. Doremus, R.; Roberts, B.; Turnbull, D. Growth and Perfection of Crystals. *J. Polym. Sci.* **1959**, *38*, 2053–2054. [CrossRef]
65. Gagniere, E.; Mangin, D.; Veesler, S.; Puel, F. *Co-Crystallization in Solution and Scale-up Issues*; Royal Society of Chemistry: London, UK, 2012; ISBN 9781849733502.
66. Cho, E.J.; Holback, H.; Liu, K.C.; Abouelmagd, S.A.; Park, J.; Yeo, Y. Nanoparticle characterization: State of the art, challenges, and emerging technologies. *Mol. Pharm.* **2013**, *10*, 2093–2110. [CrossRef]
67. Stefaniak, A.B.; Hackley, V.A.; Roebben, G.; Ehara, K.; Hankin, S.; Postek, M.T.; Lynch, I.; Fu, W.-E.; Linsinger, T.P.J.; Thünemann, A.F. Nanoscale reference materials for environmental, health and safety measurements: Needs, gaps and opportunities. *Nanotoxicology* **2013**, *7*, 1325–1337. [CrossRef]
68. Lewinski, N.; Colvin, V.; Drezek, R. Cytotoxicity of nanopartides. *Small* **2008**, *4*, 26–49. [CrossRef] [PubMed]
69. Almeida, J.P.M.; Chen, A.L.; Foster, A.; Drezek, R. In vivo biodistribution of nanoparticles. *Nanomedicine* **2011**, *6*, 815–835. [CrossRef]
70. Malvern Instruments Ltd. Surfactant micelle characterization using dynamic light scattering. *Malvern Instrum.* **2006**, *MRK809-01*, 1–5.
71. *Malvern Instruments White Paper: Dynamic Light Scattering, Common terms defined*; Malvern Instruments Limited: Worcestershire, UK, 2011; pp. 1–6.
72. Lu, X.-Y.; Wu, D.-C.; Li, Z.-J.; Chen, G.-Q. Polymer nanoparticles. *Prog. Mol. Biol. Transl. Sci.* **2011**, *104*, 299–323. [CrossRef] [PubMed]
73. Hoo, C.M.; Starostin, N.; West, P.; Mecartney, M.L. A comparison of atomic force microscopy (AFM) and dynamic light scattering (DLS) methods to characterize nanoparticle size distributions. *J. Nanopart. Res.* **2008**, *10*, 89–96. [CrossRef]

74. Boyd, R.D.; Pichaimuthu, S.K.; Cuenat, A. New approach to inter-technique comparisons for nanoparticle size measurements; using atomic force microscopy, nanoparticle tracking analysis and dynamic light scattering. *Colloids Surfaces A Physicochem. Eng. Asp.* **2011**, *387*, 35–42. [CrossRef]
75. Mahl, D.; Diendorf, J.; Meyer-Zaika, W.; Epple, M. Possibilities and limitations of different analytical methods for the size determination of a bimodal dispersion of metallic nanoparticles. *Colloids Surfaces A Physicochem. Eng. Asp.* **2011**, *377*, 386–392. [CrossRef]
76. Murdock, R.C.; Braydich-Stolle, L.; Schrand, A.M.; Schlager, J.J.; Hussain, S.M. Characterization of nanomaterial dispersion in solution prior to in vitro exposure using dynamic light scattering technique. *Toxicol. Sci.* **2008**, *101*, 239–253. [CrossRef]
77. Kirby, B.J.; Hasselbrink, E.F. Zeta potential of microfluidic substrates: 2. Data for polymers. *Electrophoresis* **2004**, *25*, 203–213. [CrossRef] [PubMed]
78. Kirby, B.J.; Hasselbrink, E.F. Zeta potential of microfluidic substrates: 1. Theory, experimental techniques, and effects on separations This. *Electrophoresis* **2004**, *25*, 187–202. [CrossRef]
79. Malamatari, M.; Somavarapu, S.; Taylor, K.M.; Buckton, G. Solidification of nanosuspensions for the production of solid oral dosage forms and inhalable dry powders Solidification of nanosuspensions for the production of solid oral dosage forms and inhalable dry powders. *Expert Opin. Drug Deliv.* **2016**. [CrossRef]
80. Peng, H.R.; Gong, M.M.; Chen, Y.Z.; Liu, F. Thermal stability of nanocrystalline materials: Thermodynamics and kinetics. *Int. Mater. Rev.* **2017**, *62*, 303–333. [CrossRef]
81. Verdonck, E.; Schaap, K.; Thomas, L.C. A discussion of the principles and applications of Modulated Temperature DSC (MTDSC). *Int. J. Pharm.* **1999**, *192*, 3–20. [CrossRef]
82. Chogale, M.M.; Ghodake, V.N.; Patravale, V.B. Performance parameters and characterizations of nanocrystals: A brief review. *Pharmaceutics* **2016**, *8*, 26. [CrossRef]
83. Kocbek, P.; Baumgartner, S.; Kristl, J. Preparation and evaluation of nanosuspensions for enhancing the dissolution of poorly soluble drugs. *Int. J. Pharm.* **2006**, *312*, 179–186. [CrossRef] [PubMed]
84. Valo, H.; Kovalainen, M.; Laaksonen, P.; Häkkinen, M.; Auriola, S.; Peltonen, L.; Linder, M.; Järvinen, K.; Hirvonen, J.; Laaksonen, T. Immobilization of protein-coated drug nanoparticles in nanofibrillar cellulose matrices-Enhanced stability and release. *J. Control Release* **2011**, *156*, 390–397. [CrossRef]
85. Clas, S.; Dalton, C.; Hancock, B. Differential scanning calorimetry: Applications in drug development. *Pharm. Sci. Technol. Today* **1999**, *2*, 311–320. [CrossRef]
86. Mourdikoudis, S.; Pallares, R.M.; Thanh, N.T.K. Characterization techniques for nanoparticles: Comparison and complementarity upon studying nanoparticle properties. *Nanoscale* **2018**, *10*, 12871–12934. [CrossRef] [PubMed]
87. Ingham, B.; Toney, M.F. X-Ray Diffraction for Characterizing Metallic Films. In *Metallic Films for Electronic, Optical and Magnetic Applications: Structure, Processing and Properties*; Elsevier Ltd.: Amsterdam, The Netherlands, 2013; pp. 3–38. ISBN 9780857090577.
88. Müllertz, A.; Perrie, Y.; Rades, T. *Advances in Delivery Science and Technology: Analytical Techniques in the Pharmaceutical Sciences*; Rathbone, M.J., Ed.; Springer Science and Business Media LLC: New York, NY, USA, 2016; ISBN 9781493940271.
89. Engelhard, M.H.; Droubay, T.C.; Du, Y. X-ray Photoelectron Spectroscopy Applications. In *Encyclopedia of Spectroscopy and Spectrometry*; Elsevier: Amsterdam, The Netherlands, 2017; pp. 716–724. ISBN 9780128032244.
90. Chauhan, A. Powder XRD Technique and its Applications in Science and Technology. *J. Anal. Bioanal. Tech.* **2014**, *5*. [CrossRef]
91. Kirtansinh, G.; Piyushbhai, P.; Natubhai, P. Application of Analytical Techniques in Preformulation Study: A Review. *Int. J. Pharm. Biol. Arch.* **2011**, *2*, 1319–1326.
92. Hirsch, P.B. *Elements of X-Ray Diffraction*, 2nd ed.; Wesley-Addion Publishing Company: Reading, MA, USA, 1957; Volume 8, ISBN 0201610914.
93. Upadhyay, S.; Parekh, K.; Pandey, B. Influence of crystallite size on the magnetic properties of Fe_3O_4 nanoparticles. *J. Alloys Compd.* **2016**, *678*, 478–485. [CrossRef]
94. Li, W.; Zamani, R.; Rivera Gil, P.; Pelaz, B.; Ibáñez, M.; Cadavid, D.; Shavel, A.; Alvarez-Puebla, R.A.; Parak, W.J.; Arbiol, J.; et al. CuTe nanocrystals: Shape and size control, plasmonic properties, and use as SERS probes and photothermal agents. *J. Am. Chem. Soc.* **2013**, *135*, 7098–7101. [CrossRef]
95. Yan, W.; Mahurin, S.M.; Overbury, S.H.; Dai, S. Nanoengineering catalyst supports via layer-by-layer surface functionalization. *Top. Catal.* **2006**, *39*, 199–212. [CrossRef]
96. Wang, W.; Chen, X.; Cai, Q.; Mo, G.; Jiang, L.S.; Zhang, K.; Chen, Z.J.; Wu, Z.H.; Pan, W. In situ SAXS study on size changes of platinum nanoparticles with temperature. *Eur. Phys. J. B* **2008**, *65*, 57–64. [CrossRef]
97. Cipolla, D.; Wu, H.; Salentinig, S.; Boyd, B.; Rades, T.; Vanhecke, D.; Petri-Fink, A.; Rothin-Rutishauser, B.; Eastman, S.; Redelmeier, T.; et al. Formation of drug nanocrystals under nanoconfinement afforded by liposomes. *RSC Adv.* **2016**, *6*, 6223–6233. [CrossRef]
98. Li, T.; Mudie, S.; Cipolla, D.; Rades, T.; Boyd, B.J. Solid State Characterization of Ciprofloxacin Liposome Nanocrystals. *Mol. Pharm.* **2019**, *16*, 184–194. [CrossRef] [PubMed]
99. Schilt, Y.; Berman, T.; Wei, X.; Barenholz, Y.; Raviv, U. Using solution X-ray scattering to determine the high-resolution structure and morphology of PEGylated liposomal doxorubicin nanodrugs. *Biochim. Biophys. Acta* **2016**, *1860*, 108–119. [CrossRef]
100. Li, X.; Hirsh, D.J.; Cabral-Lilly, D.; Zirkel, A.; Gruner, S.M.; Janoff, A.S.; Perkins, W.R. Doxorubicin physical state in solution and inside liposomes loaded via a pH gradient. *Biochim. Biophys. Acta* **1998**, *1415*, 23–40. [CrossRef]
101. Matthew, J. *Surface Analysis by AUGER and X-Ray Photoelectron Spectroscopy*; Briggs, D., Grant, J.T., Eds.; John Wiley & Sons, Ltd.: Chichester, UK, 2004; Volume 36, ISBN 1-901019-04-7.

102. Ray, S.; Shard, A.G. Quantitative Analysis of Adsorbed Proteins by X-ray Photoelectron Spectroscopy. *Anal. Chem.* **2011**, *83*, 8659–8666. [CrossRef]
103. Beloqui Redondo, A.; Jordan, I.; Ziazadeh, I.; Kleibert, A.; Giorgi, J.B.; Wörner, H.J.; May, S.; Abbas, Z.; Brown, M.A. Nanoparticle-Induced Charge Redistribution of the Air–Water Interface. *J. Phys. Chem. C* **2015**, *119*, 2661–2668. [CrossRef]
104. Qiu, L.; Liu, F.; Zhao, L.; Ma, Y.; Yao, J. Comparative XPS study of surface reduction for nanocrystalline and microcrystalline ceria powder. *Appl. Surf. Sci.* **2006**, *252*, 4931–4935. [CrossRef]
105. Chow, S.F.; Wan, K.Y.; Cheng, K.K.; Wong, K.W.; Sun, C.C.; Baum, L.; Chow, A.H.L. Development of highly stabilized curcumin nanoparticles by flash nanoprecipitation and lyophilization. *Eur. J. Pharm. Biopharm.* **2015**, *94*, 436–449. [CrossRef]
106. Dong, Y.; Feng, S.S. Methoxy poly(ethylene glycol)-poly(lactide) (MPEG-PLA) nanoparticles for controlled delivery of anticancer drugs. *Biomaterials* **2004**, *25*, 2843–2849. [CrossRef]
107. Mu, L.; Feng, S.S. A novel controlled release formulation for the anticancer drug paclitaxel (Taxol®): PLGA nanoparticles containing vitamin E TPGS. *J. Control Release* **2003**, *86*, 33–48. [CrossRef]
108. El-Hagrasy, A.S.; Morris, H.R.; D'Amico, F.; Lodder, R.A.; Drennen, J.K. Near-infrared spectroscopy and imaging for the monitoring of powder blend homogeneity. *J. Pharm. Sci.* **2001**, *90*, 1298–1307. [CrossRef]
109. Robert, M.S.; Webster, F.X.; Kiemle, D.J.; Bryce, D.L. *Spectrometric Identification of Organic Compounds*, 3rd ed.; Wiley: Hoboken, NJ, USA, 1976; Volume 30, ISBN 0471393622.
110. Lai, F.; Pini, E.; Corrias, F.; Perricci, J.; Manconi, M.; Fadda, A.M.; Sinico, C. Formulation strategy and evaluation of nanocrystal piroxicam orally disintegrating tablets manufacturing by freeze-drying. *Int. J. Pharm.* **2014**, *467*, 27–33. [CrossRef] [PubMed]
111. Witika, B.A. Formulation Development, Manufacture and Evaluation of a Lamivudine-Zidovudine Nano Co-Crystal Thermo-Responsive Suspension. Ph.D. Thesis, Rhodes University, Makhanda, South Africa, 2020.
112. Sharma, P.; Zujovic, Z.D.; Bowmaker, G.A.; Denny, W.A.; Garg, S. Evaluation of a crystalline nanosuspension: Polymorphism, process induced transformation and in vivo studies. *Int. J. Pharm.* **2011**, *408*, 138–151. [CrossRef] [PubMed]
113. Loridant, S.; Lucazeau, G.; Le Bihan, T. A high-pressure Raman and X-ray diffraction study of the perovskite $SrCeO_3$. *J. Phys. Chem. Solids* **2002**, *63*, 1983–1992. [CrossRef]
114. Colomban, P. ReviewRaman Studies of Inorganic Gels and of Their Sol-to-Gel, Gel-to-Glass and Glass-to-Ceramics Transformation. *J. Raman Spectrosc.* **1996**, *27*, 747–758. [CrossRef]
115. Durán, P.; Capel, F.; Tartaj, J.; Gutierrez, D.; Moure, C. Heating-rate effect on the $BaTiO_3$ formation by thermal decomposition of metal citrate polymeric precursors. *Solid State Ion.* **2001**, *141–142*, 529–539. [CrossRef]
116. Parayanthal, P.; Pollak, F.H. Raman Scattering in Alloy Semiconductors: "Spatial Correlation" Model. *Phys. Rev. Lett.* **1984**, *52*, 1822–1825. [CrossRef]
117. Ager, J.W.; Veirs, D.K.; Rosenblatt, G.M. Spatially resolved Raman studies of diamond films grown by chemical vapor deposition. *Phys. Rev. B* **1991**, *43*, 6491–6499. [CrossRef]
118. Critchley, L. Is Raman Spectroscopy Useful in Nanomaterial Analysis? Available online: https://www.azonano.com/article.aspx?ArticleID=5273 (accessed on 21 March 2021).
119. Mu, S.; Li, M.; Guo, M.; Yang, W.; Wang, Y.; Li, J.; Fu, Q.; He, Z. Spironolactone nanocrystals for oral administration: Different pharmacokinetic performances induced by stabilizers. *Colloids Surfaces B Biointerfaces* **2016**, *147*, 73–80. [CrossRef]
120. De Waard, H.; De Beer, T.; Hinrichs, W.L.J.; Vervaet, C.; Remon, J.P.; Frijlink, H.W. Controlled crystallization of the lipophilic drug fenofibrate during freeze-drying: Elucidation of the mechanism by in-line raman spectroscopy. *AAPS J.* **2010**, *12*, 569–575. [CrossRef] [PubMed]
121. Swarbick, J. *Encyclopedia of Pharmaceutical Technology*, 3rd ed.; CRC Press: Boca Raton, FL, USA, 2018; ISBN 0824725387.
122. Klienebudde, P. The Crystallite-Gel-Model for microcrystalline Celluslose in Wet Granulation, Extrusion and Spheronization. *Pharm. Res.* **1997**, *14*, 804–809. [CrossRef] [PubMed]
123. Pitchayajittipong, C.; Price, R.; Shur, J.; Kaerger, J.S.; Edge, S. Characterisation and functionality of inhalation anhydrous lactose. *Int. J. Pharm.* **2010**, *390*, 134–141. [CrossRef] [PubMed]
124. Crisp, J.L.; Dann, S.E.; Blatchford, C.G. Antisolvent crystallization of pharmaceutical excipients from aqueous solutions and the use of preferred orientation in phase identification by powder X-ray diffraction. *Eur. J. Pharm. Sci.* **2011**, *42*, 568–577. [CrossRef]
125. Ho, R.; Naderi, M.; Heng, J.Y.Y.; Williams, D.R.; Thielmann, F.; Bouza, P.; Keith, A.R.; Thiele, G.; Burnett, D.J. Effect of milling on particle shape and surface energy heterogeneity of needle-Shaped crystals. *Pharm. Res.* **2012**, *29*, 2806–2816. [CrossRef] [PubMed]
126. Kubavat, H.A.; Shur, J.; Ruecroft, G.; Hipkiss, D.; Price, R. Investigation into the influence of primary crystallization conditions on the mechanical properties and secondary processing behaviour of fluticasone propionate for carrier based dry powder inhaler formulations. *Pharm. Res.* **2012**, *29*, 994–1006. [CrossRef]
127. Otte, A.; Teresa, C. Assessment of Milling-Induced Disorder of Two Pharmaceutical Compounds. *J. Pharm. Sci.* **2012**, *101*, 322–332. [CrossRef]
128. Park, M.H.; Kim, J.H.; Jeon, J.W.; Park, J.K.; Lee, B.J.; Suh, G.H.; Cho, C.W. Preformulation studies of bee venom for the preparation of bee venom-loaded PLGA particles. *Molecules* **2015**, *20*, 15072–15083. [CrossRef]
129. Patel, P.; Ahir, K.; Patel, V.; Manani, L.; Patel, C. Drug-Excipient compatibility studies: First step for dosage form development. *Pharma Innov. J.* **2015**, *4*, 14–20.
130. Ruska, E.; Knoll, M.; Ruska, E. Das Elektronenmikroskop. *Zeitschrift Phys.* **1932**, *78*, 318–339. [CrossRef]

131. Kuntsche, J.; Horst, J.C.; Bunjes, H. Cryogenic transmission electron microscopy (cryo-TEM) for studying the morphology of colloidal drug delivery systems. *Int. J. Pharm.* **2011**, *417*, 120–137. [CrossRef]
132. Klang, V.; Matsko, N.B. Electron microscopy of pharmaceutical systems. *Adv. Imaging Electron. Phys.* **2014**, *181*, 125–208. [CrossRef]
133. Swartz, M.E. Ultra performance liquid chromatography (UPLC): An introduction. *Sep. Sci. Re-Defin.* **2005**, *586*, 8–14.
134. Hamilton, R.J.; Sewell, P.A. *Introduction to High Performance Liquid Chromatography*; Hamilton, R.J., Sewell, P.A., Eds.; Springer: Dordrecht, The Netherlands, 1982; Volume 15, ISBN 978-94-009-5938-5.
135. Davankov, V.A. Separation of enantiomeric compounds using chiral HPLC systems. A brief review of general principles, advances, and development trends. *Chromatographia* **1989**, *27*, 475–482. [CrossRef]
136. Aygün, Ş.F.; Özcimder, M. A comparison of normal(-CN) and reversed (C-18) phase chromatographic behaviour of polycyclic aromatic hydrocarbons. *Turk. J. Chem.* **1996**, *20*, 269–275.
137. de Villiers, A.; Lestremau, F.; Szucs, R.; Gélébart, S.; David, F.; Sandra, P. Evaluation of ultra performance liquid chromatography. Part I. Possibilities and limitations. *J. Chromatogr. A* **2006**, *1127*, 60–69. [CrossRef]
138. Vervoort, R.J.M.; Debets, A.J.J.; Claessens, H.A.; Cramers, C.A.; De Jong, G.J. Optimisation and characterisation of silica-based reversed-phase liquid chromatographic systems for the analysis of basic pharmaceuticals. *J. Chromatogr. A* **2000**, *897*, 1–22. [CrossRef]
139. Snyder, R.J.; Kirkland, J.; Glajch, J.L. *Practical HPLC Method Development*, 2nd ed.; John Wiley and Sons: New York, NY, USA, 1997; Volume 41.
140. Simpson, C. *Practical HPLC*; The Whitefriars Press: London, UK, 1976.
141. Raghavan, R.; Joseph, J. *Chromatographic Methodsof Analysis-High Performance Lquid Chromatography, Enclopedia or Pharmaceutical Technology*; Informa Healthcare USA: New York, NY, USA, 2002.
142. Young, C.S.; Weigand, R.J. An efficient approach to column selection in HPLC method development. *LC-GC N. Am.* **2020**, *20*, 464–473.
143. Ewing, G.W.; Jordan, J. *Instrumental Methods of Chemical Analysis*, 5th ed.; Himalaya Publishing House: New Delhi, India, 1955; Volume 27.
144. Beckett, A.H.; Stenlake, J.B. *Practical Pharmaceutical Chemistry*; John Wiley & Sons, Ltd.: Hoboken, NJ, USA, 1963; Volume 52.
145. Siddiqui, M.R.; AlOthman, Z.A.; Rahman, N. Analytical techniques in pharmaceutical analysis: A review. *Arab. J. Chem.* **2017**, *10*, S1409–S1421. [CrossRef]
146. Butnariu, M.; Coradini, C.Z. Evaluation of Biologically Active Compounds from Calendula officinalis Flowers using Spectrophotometry. *Chem. Cent. J.* **2012**, *6*, 35. [CrossRef] [PubMed]
147. Antosiewicz, J.M.; Shugar, D. UV–Vis spectroscopy of tyrosine side-groups in studies of protein structure. Part 1: Basic principles and properties of tyrosine chromophore. *Biophys. Rev.* **2016**, *8*, 151–161. [CrossRef]
148. Braun, C.S.; Kueltzo, L.A.; Russell Middaugh, C. Ultraviolet absorption and circular dichroism spectroscopy of nonviral gene delivery complexes. *Methods Mol. Med.* **2001**, *65*, 253–284. [CrossRef]
149. Giovannetti, R. The Use of Spectrophotometry UV-Vis for the Study of Porphyrins. In *Macro to Nano Spectroscopy*; IntechOpen: Rijeka, Croatia, 2012.
150. Owen, T. *Fundamentals of UV-Visible Spectroscopy: A Primer*; Agilent Technologies: Waldbronn, Germany, 2000; ISBN 9788578110796.
151. Parnis, J.M.; Oldham, K.B. Beyond the beer-lambert law: The dependence of absorbance on time in photochemistry. *J. Photochem. Photobiol. A Chem.* **2013**, *267*, 6–10. [CrossRef]
152. Allen, H.C.; Brauers, T.; Finlayson-Pitts, B.J. Illustration of Deviations in the Beer-Lambert Law in an Instrumental Analysis Laboratory: Measuring Atmospheric Pollutants by Differential Optical Absorption Spectrometry. *J. Chem. Educ.* **1997**, *74*, 1459. [CrossRef]
153. Ernst, O.; Zor, T. Linearization of the Bradford protein assay. *J. Vis. Exp.* **2010**, 1–6. [CrossRef]
154. Baker, W.B.; Parthasarathy, A.B.; Busch, D.R.; Mesquita, R.C.; Greenberg, J.H.; Yodh, A.G. Modified Beer-Lambert law for blood flow. *Biomed. Opt. Express* **2014**, *5*, 4053. [CrossRef] [PubMed]
155. Peltonen, L.; Strachan, C. Understanding critical quality attributes for nanocrystals from preparation to delivery. *Molecules* **2015**, *20*, 22286–22300. [CrossRef] [PubMed]
156. Chen, Y.; Li, T. Cellular Uptake Mechanism of Paclitaxel Nanocrystals Determined by Confocal Imaging and Kinetic Measurement. *AAPS J.* **2015**, *17*, 1126–1134. [CrossRef]
157. Witika, B.A.; Walker, R.B. Development, manufacture and characterization of niosomes for the delivery for nevirapine. *Pharmazie* **2019**, *74*, 91–96. [CrossRef] [PubMed]
158. Makoni, P.A.; Kasongo, K.W.; Walker, R.B. Short Term Stability Testing of Efavirenz-Loaded Solid Lipid Nanoparticle (SLN) and Nanostructured Lipid Carrier (NLC) Dispersions. *Pharmaceutics* **2019**, *11*, 397. [CrossRef] [PubMed]
159. Cerdeira, A.M.; Mazzotti, M.; Gander, B. Pharmaceutical Nanotechnology Miconazole nanosuspensions: Influence of formulation variables on particle size reduction and physical stability. *Int. J. Pharm.* **2010**, *396*, 210–218. [CrossRef] [PubMed]
160. Verma, S.; Kumar, S.; Gokhale, R.; Burgess, D.J. Physical stability of nanosuspensions: Investigation of the role of stabilizers on Ostwald ripening. *Int. J. Pharm.* **2011**, *406*, 145–152. [CrossRef] [PubMed]
161. Teeranachaideekul, V.; Junyaprasert, V.B.; Souto, E.B.; Müller, R.H. Development of ascorbyl palmitate nanocrystals applying the nanosuspension technology. *Int. J. Pharm.* **2008**, *354*, 227–234. [CrossRef]

162. Center of Drug Evaluation and Research. *Regulatory Classification of Pharmaceutical Co-Crystals, Guidance for Industry*; US Food&Drug Administration: Silver Spring, MD, USA, 2018.
163. Peltonen, L. Practical guidelines for the characterization and quality control of pure drug nanoparticles and nano-cocrystals in the pharmaceutical industry. *Adv. Drug Deliv. Rev.* **2018**, *131*, 101–115. [CrossRef] [PubMed]
164. Accardo, A.; Tesauro, D.; Roscigno, P.; Gianolio, E.; Paduano, L.; D'Errico, G.; Pedone, C.; Morelli, G. Physicochemical properties of mixed micellar aggregates containing CCK peptides and Gd complexes designed as tumor specific contrast agents in MRI. *J. Am. Chem. Soc.* **2004**, *126*, 3097–3107. [CrossRef] [PubMed]
165. Cheng, C.; Wei, H.; Zhang, X.Z.; Cheng, S.X.; Zhuo, R.X. Thermo-triggered and biotinylated biotin-P(NIPAAm-co-HMAAm)-b-PMMA micelles for controlled drug release. *J. Biomed. Mater. Res. Part A* **2009**, *88*, 814–822. [CrossRef] [PubMed]
166. Toncheva, V.; Schacht, E.; Ng, S.Y.; Barr, J.; Heller, J. Use of block copolymers of poly(ortho esters) and poly (ethylene glycol) micellar carriers as potential tumour targeting systems. *J. Drug Target.* **2003**, *11*, 345–353. [CrossRef]
167. Yang, X.; Li, L.; Wang, Y.; Tan, Y. Preparation, pharmacokinetics and tissue distribution of micelles made of reverse thermo-responsive polymers. *Int. J. Pharm.* **2009**, *370*, 210–215. [CrossRef]
168. Tuomela, A.; Hirvonen, J.; Peltonen, L. Stabilizing agents for drug nanocrystals: Effect on bioavailability. *Pharmaceutics* **2016**, *8*, 16. [CrossRef]
169. Rad, R.T.; Mortazavi, S.A.; Vatanara, A.; Dadashzadeh, S. Enhanced dissolution rate of tadalafil nanoparticles prepared by sonoprecipitation technique: Optimization and physicochemical investigation. *Iran. J. Pharm. Res.* **2017**, *16*, 1335–1348. [CrossRef]
170. Pireddu, R.; Caddeo, C.; Valenti, D.; Marongiu, F.; Scano, A.; Ennas, G.; Lai, F.; Fadda, A.M.; Sinico, C. Diclofenac acid nanocrystals as an effective strategy to reduce in vivo skin inflammation by improving dermal drug bioavailability. *Colloids Surfaces B Biointerfaces* **2016**, *143*, 64–70. [CrossRef]
171. Hoffman, A.S. The origins and evolution of "controlled" drug delivery systems. *J. Control Release* **2008**, *132*, 153–163. [CrossRef] [PubMed]
172. Anhalt, K.; Geissler, S.; Harms, M.; Weigandt, M.; Fricker, G. Development of a new method to assess nanocrystal dissolution based on light scattering. *Pharm. Res.* **2012**, *29*, 2887–2901. [CrossRef] [PubMed]
173. Rodrigues, M.; Baptista, B.; Lopes, J.A.; Sarraguça, M.C. Pharmaceutical cocrystallization techniques. Advances and challenges. *Int. J. Pharm.* **2018**, *547*, 404–420. [CrossRef] [PubMed]
174. Agrawal, Y.; Patel, V. Nanosuspension: An approach to enhance solubility of drugs. *J. Adv. Pharm. Technol. Res.* **2011**, *2*, 81. [CrossRef] [PubMed]
175. European Medicines Agency. *ICH Topic Q6A Specifications: Test Procedures and Acceptance Criteria for New Drug Substances and New Drug Products: Chemical Substances Step*; ECA Academy: London, UK, 2000.

MDPI
St. Alban-Anlage 66
4052 Basel
Switzerland
Tel. +41 61 683 77 34
Fax +41 61 302 89 18
www.mdpi.com

Crystals Editorial Office
E-mail: crystals@mdpi.com
www.mdpi.com/journal/crystals

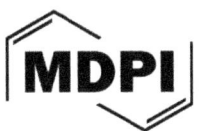

www.ingramcontent.com/pod-product-compliance
Lightning Source LLC
LaVergne TN
LVHW070643100526
838202LV00013B/870